Antiviral Drug Resistance

Antiviral Drug Resistance

Edited by
DOUGLAS D. RICHMAN
University of California, San Diego, USA

JOHN WILEY & SONS
Chichester · New York · Brisbane · Toronto · Singapore

Other Wiley Editorial Offices

John Wiley & Sons. Inc., 605 Third Avenue,
New York, NY 10158-0012, USA

Jacaranda Wiley Ltd, 33 Park Road, Milton,
Queensland 4064, Australia

John Wiley & Sons (Canada) Ltd, 22 Worcester Road,
Rexdale, Ontario M9W 1L1, Canada

John Wiley & Sons (Asia) Pte Ltd, 2 Clementi Loop #02-01,
Jin Xing Distripark, Singapore 0512

Library of Congress Cataloging-in-Publication Data

Antiviral drug resistance/edited by Douglas D. Richman.
    p.   cm.
    Includes bibliographical references and index.
    ISBN 0-471-96120-5 (hbk. : alk. paper)
    1. Drug resistance in microorganisms.   2. Antiviral agents.
  I. Richman, Douglas D.
    [DNLM: 1. Drug Resistance.   2. Viral Diseases—drug therapy.
    3. Antiviral Agents.   WC 501 A633 1996]
    QR177.A59   1996
    616'.0194—dc20
    DNLM/DLC
    for Library of Congress   96-13385
                                                                   CIP

British Library Cataloguing in Publication Data

A catalogue record for this book is available from the British Library

ISBN 0-471-96120-5

Typeset in 10/12 pt Palatino by Mathematical Composition Setters Ltd, Salisbury, Wiltshire.
Printed and bound in Great Britain by Biddles Ltd, Guildford.
This book is printed on acid-free paper responsibly manufactured from sustainable
forestation, for which at least two trees are planted for each one used for paper production.

To
Eva, Sara and Matthew

Contents

Contributors

F. Baldanti PhD
Viral Diagnostic Service, IRCCS Policlinico S Matteo, University of Pavia, Via Taramelli 5, Pavia, Italy

Karen K. Biron PhD
Department of Virology, Glaxo Wellcome, 5 Moore Drive, Research Triangle Park NC 27709, USA

William C. Buhles PhD
Otsuka American Pharmaceutical Inc., 1290 Page Mill Road, Palo Alto CA 94304, USA

Donald M. Coen PhD
Department of Biological Chemistry and Molecular Pharmacology, Harvard Medical School, 250 Longwood Avenue, Boston MA 02115, USA

John M. Coffin PhD
Department of Molecular Biology and Microbiology, Tufts University, 136 Harrison Avenue, Boston MA 02111, USA

Richard T. D'Aquila MD
Massachusetts General Hospital, Infectious Disease Unit, 149 13th Street, Boston MA 02129, USA

W. Lawrence Drew MD, PhD
Mount Zion Medical Center of UCSF, Clinical Laboratory, 1600 Divisadero Street, San Francisco CA 94115, USA

Emilio A. Emini PhD
Department of Antiviral Research, Merck Research Laboratories, Bldg 16, Room 225, West Point PA 19486, USA

Diane Havlir MD
Department of Medicine, University of California, San Diego, CA 92103, USA

Alan J. Hay PhD
Division of Virology, National Institute for Medical Research, The Ridgeway, Mill Hill, London NW7 1AA, UK

Frederick G. Hayden MD
Department of Internal Medicine, Box 473, University of Virginia, Health Sciences Center, Charlottesville VA 229008, USA

David D. Ho MD
The Aaron Diamond AIDS Research Center, Rockefeller University, 455 First Avenue—7th Floor, New York NY 10016, USA

Brendan A. Larder PhD
Clinical Virology Unit, Glaxo Wellcome Medicines Research Centre, Stevenage, Hertfordshire SG1 2NY, UK

Martin Markowitz MD
The Aaron Diamond AIDS Research Center, Rockefeller University, 455 First Avenue—7th Floor, New York NY 10016, USA

Anne G. Mosser PhD
Institute of Molecular Virology, 1525 Linden Drive, University of Wisconsin, Madison WI 53706, USA

Douglas D. Richman MD
Departments of Pathology and Medicine 0679, University of California, San Diego, 9500 Gilman Drive, La Jolla CA 92093-0679, USA

Roland R. Rueckert PhD
Institute of Molecular Virology, 1525 Linden Drive, University of Wisconsin, Madison WI 53706, USA

Sharon Safrin MD
San Francisco General Hospital, Division of AIDS/Infectious Diseases, University of California, San Francisco, 945 Potrero Bldg 80 Ward 84, San Francisco CA 94110, USA

1
Antiviral Drug Resistance: Issues and Challenges

DOUGLAS D. RICHMAN

Drug-resistant mutants were recognized in the 1960s for poxviruses with thiosemicarbazone[1], for poliovirus with guanidine[2], for influenza A virus with amantadine[3,4], and for herpes simplex virus (HSV) with iododeoxyuridine[5,6]. The rate-limiting factors to the identification of drug-resistant virus mutants have been the availability of antiviral drugs and the initiative to search.

The small and efficient genomes of viruses have lent themselves to the intensive investigation of the molecular genetics, structure and replicative cycles of most important human viral pathogens. As a consequence the sites and mechanisms have been characterized for both the activity of and resistance to antiviral drugs more precisely than have those for any other class of drugs[7]. For example, the X-ray crystallographic structures have been reported for four viral proteins that are the targets for antiviral drugs and the binding sites for their inhibitors[8-11]. The characterization of interactions of drugs with drug-resistant mutants has facilitated the design of new and more effective drugs.

The characterization of drug-resistant mutants has also permitted the identification of the existence of previously unrecognized viral proteins. For example, the characterization of the M2 protein of influenza A virus and the UL97 protein of cytomegalovirus (CMV) was an important byproduct of studies of drug resistance. Despite these advances, the challenge remains to identify therapeutic strategies to delay the acquisition of drug resistance and inhibit the replication of resistant virus.

The likelihood that resistant mutants will emerge is a function of at least four factors: the viral mutation frequency; the intrinsic mutability

Antiviral Drug Resistance. Edited by Douglas D. Richman © 1996 John Wiley & Sons Ltd

of the viral target site with respect to a specific antiviral; the selective pressure of the antiviral drug; and the magnitude and rate of virus replication. With regard to the first factor, for single-stranded RNA viruses, whose genomic replication lacks a proofreading mechanism, the mutation frequencies are approximately 3×10^{-5} [12,13]. Thus a single 10 kb genome, such as that of the human immunodeficiency virus (HIV), would be expected to contain on average one mutation for every three progeny viral genomes. The mutation rate of herpesviruses, in contrast, would be expected to be lower because of the fidelity of DNA polymerases and the proofreading mechanisms for double-stranded DNA available in host cells.

The second factor, the intrinsic mutability of the viral target site to a specific antiviral drug, can significantly affect the likelihood of resistant mutants. Zidovudine (AZT) selects for mutations in the reverse transcriptase of HIV more readily *in vitro* and *in vivo* than does the other approved thymidine analog stavudine (d4T). This difference is probably attributable to the presence of the relatively large 3'-azido group on AZT, which differs from the physiologic nucleoside thymidine much more than does d4T. The reverse transcriptase molecule can more readily mutate to interact differently with this unphysiologic sugar moiety on AZT, thus selecting for mutations more easily than against d4T. A similar explanation—a distinctive sugar moiety—probably accounts for the high-level resistance rapidly attainable against lamivudine (3TC) in the reverse transcriptase of HIV, in contrast to zalcitabine (ddC), for example[14-16]. Compared to HIV, resistance of hepatitis B virus to lamivudine occurs relatively slowly, although both virus infections are characterized by high levels of virus replication. The overlapping reading frame for the hepatitis B virus surface antigen with that of the polymerase gene probably constrains mutational options in the polymerase open reading frame, which contains the YMDD amino acid domain that mutates to confer lamivudine resistance.

Resistance to acyclovir occurs in HSV much more readily as a consequence of mutations in thymidine kinase than in DNA polymerase (see Chapters 5 and 6). Similarly, ganciclovir resistance in CMV occurs more readily as a consequence of mutations in UL97 than in DNA polymerase (see Chapters 7 and 8). These observations can probably be explained by the greater dispensability of these kinases, both *in vitro* and *in vivo*, than of DNA polymerase.

One definition of an antiviral drug is a compound that confers sufficient selective pressure on virus replication to select for drug-resistant mutants[17]. Regarding the third factor, with increasing drug exposure the selective pressure on the replicating virus population increases to promote the more rapid emergence of drug-resistant mutants (Figure 1.1). For example, higher doses of AZT tend to select for drug-resistant virus more readily than do lower doses[18]. This increasing selective pressure for resistant mutants increases the likelihood of such mutants as long as significant levels of virus replication are sustained. As antiviral drug activity increases still more, the amount of virus replication diminishes to the point where the likelihood of resistance emerging begins to diminish. This likelihood becomes nil when virus replication is completely inhibited. Thus the ultimate goal of the chemotherapy of viral infection—no different from that for the chemotherapy of tuberculosis or malignancy—is to identify drug regimens that completely inhibit virus replication.

The fourth factor, the magnitude and rate of replication of the virus population, has major consequences on the likelihood of emergence of resistant mutants. This interaction, and its relationship with viral fitness, is well described in Chapter 14. Many virus infections are characterized by high levels of virus replication, with high rates of virus turnover. This is especially true of the chronic infections with HIV, hepatitis B virus and hepatitis C virus. The likelihood of emergence of AZT resistance increases in HIV-infected patients with diminishing CD4 lymphocyte counts[18], which are associated with increasing levels of HIV replication. Acyclovir resistance occurs much more frequently in isolates of herpes

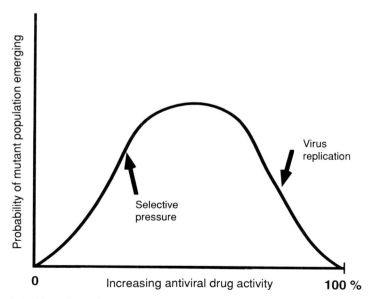

Figure 1.1   *Hypothetical impact of antiviral drug activity upon the probability of the emergence of drug resistance (Reproduced from reference 41 with permission)*

simplex virus from immunosuppressed patients because of the greater levels and duration of viral replication in these patients[19].

Higher levels of virus increase the probability of pre-existing mutants. Luria and Delbrück[20] were probably the first to show that the emergence of a resistant population (in their case the susceptibility of *Escherichia coli* to bacterial virus) results from the survival and selective proliferation of a previously existing subpopulation that randomly emerges in the absence of selective pressure. As mentioned earlier, viruses have a baseline mutation rate. With calculations of approximately 10^{10} new virions being generated daily during HIV infection[21], a mutation rate of 10^{-4}–10^{-5} per nucleotide guarantees the pre-existence of almost any mutation at any time during HIV infection. In fact, drug-resistant mutants have been identified in isolates obtained from patients with no prior drug exposure[22-26]. The pre-existence of drug-resistant picornavirus mutants at a rate of approximately 10^{-5} is also well documented[27,28].

As Coffin elaborates in Chapter 14, the selective pressure of drug treatment permits the outgrowth of these pre-existing mutants. With continuing viral replication in the absence of completely suppressive antiviral drug activity, the cumulative acquisition of multiple mutations can occur over time, as has been described for AZT and protease inhibitors of HIV[29-31].

The emergence of drug-resistant viruses raises the practical question of how to dissect out the component of clinical failure in patients treated with antiviral drugs that is attributable to the acquisition of drug resistance. Ascertaining the contribution of drug resistance to drug failure is difficult because patients who are more likely to develop drug resistance are more likely to have other confounding factors that will predispose to a poor prognosis[32]. Moreover, associations of resistant virus with clinical endpoints is complicated by the fact that patients contain mixtures of viruses with different susceptibilities, and these different populations may be represented differently in different organs of the patients under treatment. For example, is the susceptibility to ganciclovir of CMV that is causing retinitis reflected by the susceptibility of the more accessible isolates in the blood or urine?

The association of drug resistance with loss of activity of antiviral therapy is reviewed in detail in the chapters addressing the clinical implications of drug resistance. How do we, then, contend with the compromise of antiviral efficacy by drug resistance? Complete suppression of virus replication is the obvious answer. Analogous to other chemotherapeutic challenges, such as tuberculosis and malignancy, in which there is a large, chronically replicating biologic population, the combination of highly effective drugs is the most logical solution. As indicated in Figure 1.1, resistant mutants do not emerge if a regimen can prevent the outgrowth of pre-existing mutants and block ongoing replication which permits the emergence of new mutants. A second approach to the emergence of resistant viruses in the face of drug therapy is to switch to an alternative therapy against which the population has no cross-resistance. The limiting factor to both these approaches is the availability of effective antiviral drugs.

With the inevitable emergence of resistance in many viral infections, as with HIV for example, strategies must be designed to optimize treatment in the face of resistant virus populations. Three theoretical mechanisms to sustain antiretroviral drug activity despite the development of drug resistance can be proposed:

1. Plasma drug levels can be generated that exceed the susceptibility of drug-resistant virus. This assumes appropriate pharmacologic characteristics of the drug and constraints on the mutability of the target viral protein. An example of some limited success with this strategy is the non-nucleoside reverse transcriptase inhibitor of HIV, nevirapine (see Chapter 12)[33].
2. Drug resistance mutations, which confer a clear selective advantage in the face of drug pressure, may still impair the replicative capacity of the virus compared to that of the wild-type virus in the absence of treatment. Such attenuated virus may contribute to the activity of lamivudine and perhaps some protease mutants[34-36].
3. For two drugs targeted to the same viral protein (convergent therapy) mutations induced by drug 1 may sensitize the virus to drug 2, or may prevent the emergence of viable mutants to drug 2[37]. The mutation from methionine to valine at residue 184 of reverse transcriptase, which emerges with lamivudine treatment, suppresses the critical mutation at residue 215 that confers resistance to AZT[15,36]. Combinations of protease inhibitors may also exploit this strategy. It seems logical that a potent inhibitor can be designed for the active site of viruses highly resistant to other protease inhibitors, and that the combination of two such protease inhibitors would represent a promising regimen[38].

Strategies to identify effective combination regimens to control virus infections, especially those characterized by chronically high levels of virus replication, must exploit these three approaches to achieve the goal of suppressing virus replication to as great a magnitude as possible for as long as possible.

In addition to new drugs and strategies to confront the challenge of drug resistance, we need to address several very pragmatic methodologic issues. Assays of drug susceptibility that are standardized, affordable, precise and reliable, for both research and clinical applications, are needed. These assays are complicated by the need to isolate, amplify and titer viruses before performing phenotypic analyses. Isolation and propagation are confounded by selection bias and mixtures of virus phenotypes. Titered stocks are necessary to control for the effect of inoculum size upon assay results.

One issue that recurs in discussions of viral susceptibility assays is the drug concentration used to define susceptibility. The 50% inhibitory concentration (IC_{50}) is the most precise value to use for this purpose. The relationship between the inhibition of virus replication and the log of the drug concentration is usually a sigmoid curve. The IC_{50} thus provides the most precise measurement, being in the center of the linear portion of the curve. The use of the IC_{50} disturbs some people because it is unlikely that this concentration will be clinically effective, especially when compared to an IC_{90}, IC_{95}, IC_{99}, etc. These more demanding values may permit the detection of a heterogenous population with mixtures of susceptibilities[39]; nevertheless, their calculation is much less precise and subject to artifactual errors. It should be clear that the IC_{50} determination of susceptibility makes no claim for a therapeutic target concentration, which must be determined independently of drug susceptibility.

Genotypic as well as phenotypic characterization of drug resistance requires affordable, reliable and less cumbersome assays for both research and clinical applications. These phenotypic and genotypic assays must deal with issues of mixtures in clinical specimens. We also must address issues of the focal heterogeneity of virus populations such as CMV in retina and blood.

Dissecting out the contribution of antiviral drug resistance to treatment failure is an important challenge. This contribution may be straightforward, as exemplified by acyclovir resistance of HSV in patients with AIDS, or quite complicated as with zidovudine resistance in HIV infection. In the current era of health care this treatment failure should be measured, not just in terms of morbidity and mortality, but with health outcome measures such as quality of life and economic costs.

With some viruses the impact of drug-resistant mutants upon treatment failure, virulence and response to alternative therapies can be satisfactorily addressed with animal models, for example with picornaviruses, HSV and influenza A virus[40]. Infection with other resistant viruses (human cytomegalovirus, varicella zoster virus and HIV) has not been well elucidated by animal models.

In summary, the study of antiviral drug resistance has provided important insights into the structure of virus enzymes, the functions of certain genes, mechanisms of action of antiviral drugs, the design of new antiviral compounds and the pathogenesis of viral diseases. We have learned that we must expect and monitor for the emergence of resistance at all stages of drug development: during the preclinical evaluation of candidate compounds; during the early clinical evaluation of new drugs; and as part of epidemiologic surveillance for the prevalence of resistance during the use of approved treatments. Accumulating understanding of antiviral drug resistance thus reflects progress in the chemotherapy of viral infection.

REFERENCES

1. Appleyard G, Way HJ. Thiosemicarbazone-resistant rabbitpox virus. *Br J Exp Pathol* 1966;47:144–51.
2. Melnick JL, Drowther D, Barrera-Oro J. Rapid development of drug-resistant mutants of poliovirus. *Science* 1961;134:557.
3. Cochran KW, Maassab HF, Tsunoda A, Berlin BS. Studies on the antiviral activity of amantadine hydrochloride. *Ann N Y Acad Sci* 1965;130:423–39.
4. Oxford JS, Logan IS, Potter CW. *In vivo* selection of an influenza A2 strain resistant to amantadine. *Nature* 1970;226:82–3.
5. Jawetz E, Coleman VR, Dawson CR, Thygeson P. The dynamics of IUDR action in herpetic keratitis and the emergence of IUDR resistance *in vivo*. *Ann N Y Acad Sci* 1970;173:282–91.
6. Sery TW, Nagy RM. A stable mutation of herpes virus resistance to IUDR. *Invest Ophthalmol* 1965;4:947 [Abstract].
7. Richman DD. Drug resistance in viruses. *Trends Microbiol* 1994;2:401–7.
8. Smith TJ, Kremer MJ, Luo M *et al.* The site of attachment in human rhinovirus 14 for antiviral agents that inhibit uncoating. *Science* 1986;233:1286–93.
9. Kohlstaedt LA, Wang J, Friedman JM, Rice PA, Steitz TA. Crystal structure at 3.5 Å resolution of HIV-1 reverse transcriptase complexed with an inhibitor. *Science* 1992;256:1783–90.
10. Navia MA, Fitzgerald PMD, McKeever BM *et al.* Three-dimensional structure of aspartyl protease from human immunodeficiency virus HIV-1. *Nature* 1989;337:615–20.
11. Wild K, Bohner T, Aubry A, Folkers G, Schulz GE. The three-dimensional structure of thymidine kinase from herpes simplex virus type 1. *FEBS Lett* 1995;368:289–92.
12. Holland JJ, De La Torre JC, Steinhauer DA. RNA virus populations as quasispecies. *Curr Topics Microbiol Immunol* 1992;176:1–20.
13. Mansky LM, Temin HM. Lower in vivo mutation rate of human immunodeficiency virus type 1 than that predicted from the fidelity of purified reverse transcriptase. *J Virol* 1995;69:5087–94.
14. Schinazi RF, Lloyd RM Jr, Nguyen M-H *et al.* Characterization of human immunodeficiency viruses resistant to oxathiolane-cytosine nucleosides. *Antimicrob Agents Chemother* 1993;37:875–81.
15. Tisdale M, Kemp SD, Parry NR, Larder BA. Rapid *in vitro* selection of human immunodeficiency virus type 1 resistant to 3'-thiacytidine inhibitors due to a mutation in the YMDD region of reverse transcriptase. *Proc Natl Acad Sci USA* 1993;90:5653–6.

16. Gao Q, Gu Z, Parniak MA, Cameron J *et al*. The same mutation that encodes low-level human immunodeficiency virus type 1 resistance to 2',3'-dideoxy-inosine and 2',3'-dideoxycytidine confers high-level resistance to the (−) enantiomer of 2',3'-dideoxy-3'-thiacytidine. *Antimicrob Agents Chemother* 1993;37:1390−2.

17. Herrmann EC Jr, Herrmann JA. A working hypothesis—virus resistance development as an indicator of specific antiviral activity. *Ann N Y Acad Sci* 1977;284:632−7.

18. Richman DD, Grimes JM, Lagakos SW. Effect of stage of disease and drug dose on zidovudine susceptibilities of isolates of human immunodeficiency virus. *J AIDS* 1990;3:743−6.

19. Englund JA, Zimmerman ME, Swierkosz EM *et al*. Herpes simplex virus resistant to acyclovir. *Ann Intern Med* 1990;112:416−22.

20. Luria SE, Delbrück M. Mutations of bacteria from virus sensitivity to virus resistance. *Genetics* 1943;28:491−511.

21. Ho DD, Neumann AU, Perelson AS *et al*. Rapid turnover of plasma virions and CD4 lymphocytes in HIV-1 infection. *Nature* 1995;373:123−6.

22. Nájera I, Richman DD, Olivares I *et al*. Natural occurrence of drug resistance mutations in the reverse transcriptase of human immunodeficiency virus type 1 isolates. *AIDS Res Hum Retroviruses* 1994;10:1479−88.

23. Nájera I, Holguín A, Quiñones-Mateu ME *et al*. pol gene quasispecies of human immunodeficiency virus: mutations associated with drug resistance in virus from patients undergoing no drug therapy. *J Virol* 1995;69:23−31.

24. Havlir D, Eastman S, Gamst A, Richman DD. Nevirapine resistant virus: kinetics of replication and estimated prevalence in untreated patients. *J Virol* 1996; in press.

25. Kozal MJ, Shah N, Shen N *et al*. Extensive polymorphisms observed in HIV-1 clade B protease gene using high density nucleotide arrays: implications for therapy. *Nature Medicine*, in press.

26. Jacobsen H, Haenggi M, Ott M *et al*. Reduced sensitivity to saquinavir: an update on genotyping from phase I/II trials. Fourth International HIV Drug Resistance Workshop, Sardinia, Italy. 6−9 July 1995; [Abstract].

27. Ahmad ALM, Dowsett AB, Tyrrell DAJ. Studies of rhinovirus resistant to an antiviral chalcone. *Antiviral Res* 1987;8:27−39.

28. Heinz BA, Rueckert RR, Shepard DA *et al*. Genetic and molecular analyses of spontaneous mutants of human rhinovirus 14 that are resistant to an antiviral compound. *J Virol* 1989;63:2476−85.

29. Larder BA, Darby G, Richman DD. HIV with reduced sensitivity to zido-vudine (AZT) isolated during prolonged therapy. *Science* 1989;243:1731−4.

30. Larder BA, Kemp SD. Multiple mutations in HIV-1 reverse trans-criptase confer high-level resistance to zidovudine (AZT). *Science* 1989;246:1155−8.

31. Condra JH, Schleif WA, Blahy OM *et al*. *In vivo* emergence of HIV-1 variants resistant to multiple protease inhibitors. *Nature* 1995;374:569−71.

32. Richman DD. Resistance, drug failure, and disease progression. *AIDS Res Hum Retroviruses* 1994;10:901−5.

33. Havlir DV, Johnson VA, Hall DB *et al*. Factors determining sustained antiviral response to nevirapine. Fourth International HIV Drug Resistance Workshop. Sardinia, Italy. 6−9 July 1995; [Abstract].

34. Schuurman R, Nijhuis M, van Leeuwen R *et al*. Rapid changes in human immunodeficiency virus type 1 RNA load and appearance of drug-resistant

virus populations in persons treated with lamivudine. *J Infect Dis* 1995;171:1431−7.

35. Ho DD, Toyoshima T, Mo H *et al.* Characterization of human immunodeficiency virus type 1 variants with increased resistance to a C_2-symmetric protease inhibitor. *J Virol* 1994;68:2016−20.

36. Larder BA, Kemp SD, Harrigan PR. Potential mechanism for sustained antiretroviral efficacy of AZT-3TC combination therapy. *Science* 1995;269:696−9.

37. Chow Y-K, Hirsch MS, Merrill DP *et al.* Replication incompatible and replication compromising combinations of HIV-1 RT drug resistance mutations. *Nature* 1993;361:650−4.

38. Erickson JW. The not-so-great escape. *Nature Struct Biol* 1995;2:529−9.

39. Richman DD, Guatelli JC, Grimes J, Tsiatis A, Gingeras TR. Detection of mutations associated with zidovudine resistance in human immunodeficiency virus utilizing the polymerase chain reaction. *J Infect Dis* 1991;164:1075−81.

40. Kimberlin DW, Kern ER, Sidwell RW, North TW, Whitley RJ. Models of antiviral resistance. *Antiviral Res* 1995;26:415−22.

41. Richman DD. The implications for drug resistance strategies of combination antiviral therapy. *Antiviral Res* 1996;29:31-3.

PICORNAVIRUSES

2
Capsid-binding Agents

ANNE G. MOSSER AND ROLAND R. RUECKERT

INTRODUCTION

Picornaviruses are a family of small ribosome-sized RNA-containing viruses; among them are poliovirus, human hepatitis A virus and rhinoviruses responsible for the common cold. Some agriculturally important agents are also picornaviruses, for example foot-and-mouth disease virus, encephalomyocarditis virus and Theiler's virus. Human picornaviruses are divided into three major genera: rhinoviruses, enteroviruses and hepatitis A virus (Table 2.1). There are some 67 distinct serotypes of human enteroviruses and over 100 of rhinoviruses; a person could thus be infected with several per year and still not experience all the known serotypes in a lifetime. Vaccines, despite their exceptional success in controlling poliomyelitis and hepatitis A, are generally dismissed as impractical for controlling the other picornaviruses because of the large number of antigenically distinct serotypes. Likewise, the large number of serotypes demands that an antipicornaviral agent must have an exceptionally broad spectrum of activity.

Human rhinoviruses are responsible for about one-third of all common colds[5,6]. Adults are estimated to average some three colds per year; the frequency in children is perhaps twice that[5]. In the United States alone this works out to some one billion colds per year, or about 300 million attributable to rhinoviruses. Couch estimates a figure about one-tenth of this[7]. Nonetheless, the market potential for a successful antipicornaviral agent is substantial. Enteroviruses are also responsible for a spectrum of discomforts, ranging from common colds to myalgias, fever, myocarditis, meningitis and fatal infections[2]. The number of enteroviral infections in the United States is estimated to be of the order of 10 million cases per year[8].

Antiviral Drug Resistance. Edited by Douglas D. Richman © 1996 John Wiley & Sons Ltd

Table 2.1   *Classification of human picornaviruses*

	Number of serotypes
Human rhinoviruses	102
Major (ICAM-1) group	91[a]
Minor (LDLR) group	10
HRV87	1
Human enteroviruses	67
Poliovirus	3
Coxsackie virus A	23[b]
Coxsackie virus B	6
Echovirus	31[c]
Numbered enteroviruses	4
Human hepatitis A virus	1[d]

[a] Includes all serotypes of human rhinoviruses except type 87 and the 10 members of the minor receptor group (types 1A, 1B, 2, 29, 30, 31, 44, 47, 49, 62)[1].
[b] Coxsackie virus A1–22, 24. A23 has been reclassified as echovirus 9[2].
[c] Echovirus 1–9, 11–27, 29–33. Echoviruses 10 and 28 have been reclassified as reovirus 1 and human rhinovirus 1A, respectively[3]. A case has been made for reclassification of echoviruses 22 and 23[4].
[d] Human hepatitis A, formerly classified enterovirus 72, is insensitive to capsid-binding drugs.

Picornaviruses were the first animal viruses whose structures were solved to atomic resolution. This, together with their importance as human pathogens, has made them the target of major drug development efforts. Among the most promising antivirals are the capsid-binding agents, which prevent thermal inactivation and receptor-mediated uncoating. Crystallographic studies reveal that capsid-binding agents insert into a hydrophobic pocket in each of the 60 protomers which make up the protein shell. This pocket is normally occupied by still unidentified natural molecules (pocket factor), which may modulate uncoating of virus by its receptors. Resistance to capsid-binding drugs occurs by single amino acid substitutions. Mapping the location of such resistance mutations calls attention to segments of protein likely to be involved in the transduction pathway, by which receptors trigger the release of internal proteins and delivery of the RNA genome into the cell. This information may eventually aid in designing more potent antivirals. Studies on drug-dependent mutants suggest that capsid-binding drugs are analogs of pocket factor with roles in assembly, stability and uncoating of the viruses (see below). The natural function of the drug-binding pocket is not known, but it probably provides the space needed for internal rearrangements which occur during the eclipse step.

This chapter provides a brief account of the discovery and development of antipicornaviral capsid-binding compounds, their mode of action and mechanisms of resistance. It highlights insights on uncoating functions provided by biochemical, genetic and crystallographic studies of resistant mutants, and summarizes the current status of capsid-binding drugs in clinical testing.

Identification of capsid-binding agents

The earliest research on picornaviral capsid-binding inhibitors can be traced to Eggers and co-workers who, in 1970, showed that rhodanine acted at an early step in the infection cycle of echovirus 12[9,10]. By 1977 they had recognized the capsid-binding activity of rhodanine through its ability to protect the infectivity of virions against inactivation by heat[11] and alkaline pH[12]; in addition, they had also pinpointed its locus of action specifically to the uncoating step[11], and showed that rhodanine had little, if any, effect on the viral attachment or penetration steps[12].

The antiviral activity of rhodanine appeared to be highly specific for echovirus 12, with little activity against a variety of other enteroviruses tested. The spark that ignited commercial interest in capsid-binding inhibitors was probably struck with the discovery that arildone inhibited poliovirus. Arildone had been identified as an antiviral in routine pharmaceutical screening at the Sterling Winthrop Institute; it was reported in 1977 as a new chemical class of antiviral (aryl-alkyl-diketones) with *in vitro* activity against equine rhinovirus as well as a number of other RNA and DNA viruses[13]. However, its capsid-binding similarity to rhodanine became apparent only later, when in 1979 it was reported that arildone stabilized poliovirus against inactivation on by heat and alkaline pH[14] and specifically blocked the uncoating step[15].

The high activity of arildone against poliovirus (submicromolar concentrations[15]), and the demonstration that it could prevent poliovirus-induced death in mice[16], underscored the potential of uncoating blockers in the systemic treatment of viral diseases, and fueled the programs of several pharmaceutical research groups toward the development of more effective antipicornavirals. Some of the most extensively studied are shown in Figure 2.1. They include dichloroflavan or 'DCF'[17,18], Ro 09-0410 or 'chalcone'[19,20], R61837[21], Disoxaril[22-25], Pirodavir[26], WIN 54954[27] and WIN 63843[28]. Although structurally diverse, all are elongated hydrophobic molecules which, by binding to the virus particle, neutralize its ability to infect a normally susceptible host cell.

Most human enteroviruses and rhinoviruses are susceptible to capsid-binding drugs; hepatitis A virus is a notable exception. Also unsusceptible

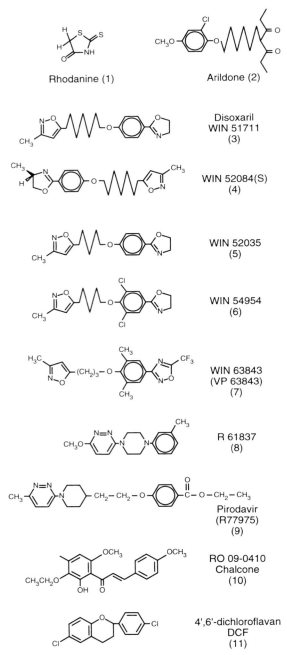

Figure 2.1 *Representative capsid binding-agents with neutralizing activity against human picornaviruses*

are a number of picornaviruses afflicting livestock: foot-and-mouth disease viruses, Theiler's viruses and encephalomyocarditis viruses (not shown in Table 2.1). Crystallographic studies of these viruses show that the entrance to the drug-binding site is blocked[29,30]; thus design of antivirals against picornaviruses of livestock will proceed differently from that of human rhinoviruses and enteroviruses.

With modern diagnostic methods, particularly the polymerase chain reaction, it is now possible to identify a picornavirus in a clinical specimen within a matter of hours[31]. The large number of picornavirus serotypes requires the identification of broad-spectrum antipicornaviral agents. Prospects that such an agent could be found seemed slight until the development of disoxaril[27], which was found to have broad activity against many enterovirus serotypes. Unfortunately, disoxaril eventually had to be rejected for toxicologic reasons (crystals developing in the kidney).

Identification of two antiviral groups, A and B

The continuing search for broad-spectrum compounds revealed two groups of human rhinoviruses, dubbed the 'A' and 'B' antiviral groups

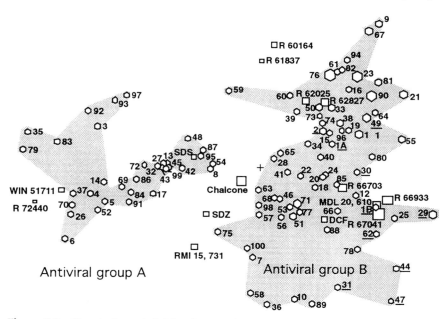

Figure 2.2   *'Spectral map' dividing human rhinoviruses into two antiviral groups, 'A' and 'B'. This is not a conventional X vs Y plot: it was generated by multivariate analysis, incorporating the activity of 15 antiviral compounds against all serotypes. (Reproduced from reference 33 with permission.) The different symbol sizes reflect virus sensitivities (hexagons) or drug potencies (squares). Viruses with low sensitivity to any of the compounds fall near the center of the map (cross-hair)*

(Figure 2.2). Group A viruses (33 serotypes) display above average susceptibility to 'long' capsid-binding compounds, such as disoxaril, whereas group B viruses (67 serotypes) are sensitive to shorter ones, such as dichloroflavan (DCF)[32]. Polioviruses (not shown) and human rhinovirus 14 fall into Group A, but HRV16 is in Group B. This initially suggested that effective treatment of common cold viruses might require the development of two compounds, one specific for each group, but discovery of pirodavir[26] showed that it was possible to find compounds with high activity against both groups.

MECHANISMS OF ACTION

Before discussing the mechanism of action of picornaviral capsid-binding compounds, it is useful to review viral structure and the process of infection. Picornaviruses have a single-stranded, positive-sense RNA surrounded by an icosahedral protein shell composed of 60 copies of each of four capsid proteins, VP1, VP2, VP3 and VP4 (Figure 2.3, A–C). The three larger proteins, VP1, VP2 and VP3, make up the bulk of the capsid and share a common core structure, the eight-stranded antiparallel β barrel[34,35]. VP4 is smaller and is confined to the inner surface of the capsid, in contact with the viral RNA and with the amino termini of VP1 and VP3. The VP1 proteins are contiguous around the fivefold axes of symmetry; loops connecting the β strands, especially the B–C loops, build star-shaped plateaux around the fivefold axes. Surrounding these plateaux are 15Å (1.5 nm)-deep canyons of enteroviruses and rhinoviruses that are acceptors for cellular receptors[36,37].

Discovery of pocket factor, a natural analog of capsid-binding antivirals

Each VP1 harbors a hydrophobic drug-binding pocket[43] accessible to the surface through a 'pore' at the base of the canyon (Figure 2.3D, E). The term 'pocket factor' refers to chemically uncharacterized cellular molecules (natural ligands) residing in this pocket. These were first detected by crystallographic studies in poliovirus[34,44]. Crystallography does not reveal the chemical identity of pocket factor because resolution is insufficient to differentiate the diameter of its atoms (e.g. carbon, nitrogen and oxygen); hence the ambiguous name 'pocket factor'. Moreover, studies with a number of picornaviruses suggests that each virus species may contain a different pocket factor. In the three serotypes of poliovirus, and in Coxsackie virus B3, pocket factor can be modeled as sphingosine or palmitate[44,45]. In human rhinoviruses

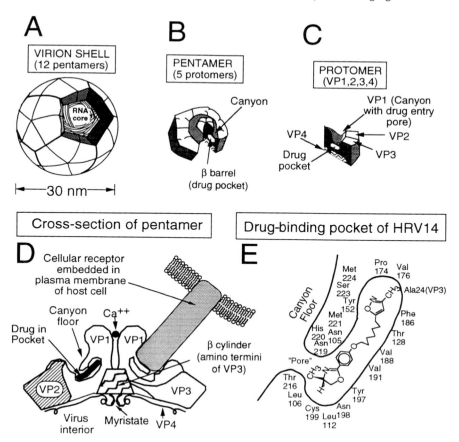

Figure 2.3 *Key features in the structure of human rhinovirus 14. (A) The protein shell
is composed of 60 protein subunits called protomers[38] organized as 12 pentamers[39].
One of the pentamers has been removed to show the tightly packed single-stranded
RNA genome inside. (B) Pentamer with one wedge-shaped protomer removed; filled
ring shows the approximate location of the 'canyon'. Each virion has 12 such canyons
(not shown in panel A). (C) Each protomer is composed of four segments (VP1,2,3
and 4) which are derived by three cleavages of a precursor protein, P1. (D) Cross-
section of a pentamer showing relationships between the drug-binding pocket, the
canyon floor and the cellular receptor. An ion, located at each pentamer center in
HRV 1A, 14 and 16, is tentatively identified as calcium[40], which is necessary for
attachment of some rhinoviruses[41]. (E) Detail showing orientation of WIN 52084 and
identity of amino acid residues lining the canyon floor and drug-binding pocket in a
single protomer. In HRV14 the drug prevents attachment of virus to its receptor,
intercellular adhesion molecule-1 (ICAM-1). WIN 52084 differs from disoxaril by
addition of a methyl group (the one nearest the 'pore'), rendering its carbon ligand in
the oxazoline ring asymmetric. The (S) isomer (methyl group pointing down through
the plane of the page) is 10 times more inhibitory against HRV14 than the (R) isomer,
possibly because of its greater surface complementary with the viral pocket residues[42]*

1A and 16 however, pocket factor is tentatively identified as a fatty acid eight or more carbon atoms long[40,46]. HRV14 differs from the other picornaviruses in that its drug-binding pocket is empty; this does not preclude the possibility that the pocket factor was lost during purification or crystallization[43]. It is also clear from crystallographic studies that pocket factors are displaced from the pocket by WIN drugs.

Steps in entry and uncoating

Infection begins with attachment of the virus to specific receptors in the plasma membrane of susceptible cells. Figure 2.4 provides a current view of the steps by which these receptors mediate transfer of the viral genome from the virion through the lipid bilayer and into the cytoplasm of the cell.

When attached to a single receptor unit (step 1), virus binding is reversible. As receptors are recruited from the fluid membrane reversibility decreases (virus is harder to remove by washing virus–cell complexes) and penetration begins, with invagination of the plasma membrane (step 2). 'Penetration' of the virus (measured, for example, by loss of sensitivity to neutralizing antibody) occurs by normal trafficking of the endosomal pathway (step 3). At some point the virus particle 'uncoats' (step 4). The uncoating process can be separated into two steps: (4a) a major rearrangement of the capsid protein, resulting in ejection of an internal protein, VP4, leaving a non-infective A particle; and (4b) release of RNA from A particles to form empty shells.

Infectosome, the infective uncoating unit

For infection to be successful the RNA must be transferred across the membrane and into the cytoplasm (infectosome). It has not so far been possible to study infectosomes biochemically, probably because fewer than 1% of the attached particles are infectious (produce plaques). This low infective efficiency is attributable at least in part to extracellular 'elution' of non-infective A particles; typically 80% of the attached virus suffers this fate[12,49,50].

A common way of measuring uncoating of the biologically successful particles is to infect cells with virus made photosensitive with neutral red or acridine orange[51], and to measure the rate at which the infectivity of cell-associated virus becomes insensitive to white light[52,53]. This was the method used to demonstrate that capsid-binding drugs block uncoating of a number of viruses including echovirus 12[10], poliovirus

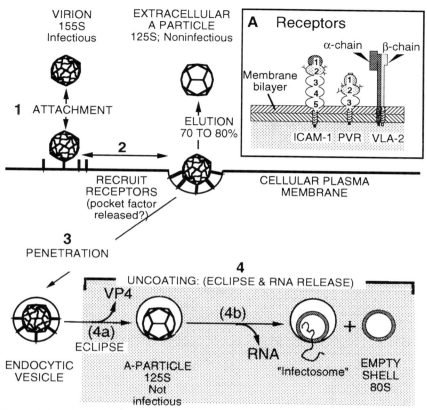

Figure 2.4 *Model illustrating steps in infection (entry) of cells by picornaviruses. The three best-understood picornavirus receptors are illustrated in the inset; all are cellular molecules which the virus has mobilized for its own ends. About 90% of all rhinoviruses use intercellular adhesion molecule-1 (ICAM-1) as a receptor (see 'Major receptor group', Table 2.1). The polioviruses use a second type of receptor (PVR) and echoviruses, a third (VLA-2). For reviews of these receptors and their roles in uncoating see[47,48]. Uncoating (step 4, shaded) consists of two transitions: (4a) loss of VP4 and (4b) release of RNA. Step 4a may be considered a 'melting transition'; under standard conditions it occurs at a temperature characteristic of the virion and decreases as the number of bound receptors increases. Step 4a (melting) is triggered when the temperature of the virion, or receptor–virion complex, reaches a critical temperature. Under a given set of conditions the eclipse temperature is affected by occupancy (natural pocket factor or an analog) of the subcanyon pocket. Treatment of poliovirus by heat, acid or alkaline pH triggers a similar two-stage process*

types 1 and 2, and human rhinovirus 2[24]. The photosensitivity method did not make clear whether the block is at the 'eclipse' transition (ejection of VP4) or at the RNA release step, but biochemical studies indicate that the block is at the eclipse step[50,54].

Single-cycle growth curves

Single-cycle growth experiments in suspension culture provide an instructive tool for illustrating the action of attachment or uncoating inhibitors. In the panels shown in Figure 2.5 the virus was attached to suspended cells at room temperature, and unattached virus was removed by sedimenting and washing virus–cell complexes. To initiate uncoating the virus–cell complexes are simply diluted tenfold in warm growth medium (zero time). Samples are removed at intervals, and virus is released from the cells, then titered for infectivity by plaque assay. Controls, i.e. virus attached and propagated in the absence of drug (bold lines), initially show a marked (100- to 1000-fold) decline of infectivity (eclipse phase) during which the virus is uncoating. This is followed by a rise period which plateaus, indicating that assembly is complete within six hours (polio) to eight hours (HRV14).

The dashed lines show the effects of capsid-binding drugs which prevent the uncoating of poliovirus (left), but prevent attachment of

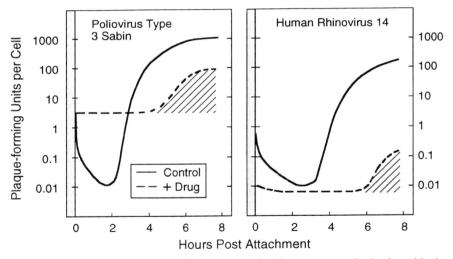

Figure 2.5 *Single-cycle curves showing growth of viruses in which drug blocks specifically at the uncoating step (left) or at the attachment step (right). Where drug was used it was also present during the virus attachment step (Y-axis, left of 0). Virus–cell complexes were sedimented to remove unattached virus, then diluted into warm medium (zero time). At intervals thereafter samples were removed, virus was released from cells by freezing and thawing, then greatly diluted to reduce drug concentration to subinhibitory levels. After a period long enough for dissociation of the drug from virions (1 h at room temperature in this case) infectivity was measured by plaque titration. For details on poliovirus see[54]; for HRV14[50]. Virus produced in the presence of drug (hatched) is enriched in drug-resistant mutants*

HRV14 (right). As seen in the left panel, poliovirus attaches normally in the presence of drug; its infectivity titer at zero time is the same as for untreated virus; however, the eclipse phase is now absent. In the presence of drug, for both PV3 and HRV14, some progeny eventually appear. To some extent this represents leakage of wild-type virus through the drug block; it also represents the presence of resistant mutants in the wild-type population, because this progeny virus is enriched with drug-resistant mutants[54].

Most picornaviral capsid-binding drugs block the virus uncoating step[10,24,25,45,54], but for some virus–drug combinations it is the attachment step, rather than the uncoating step, that is inhibited by capsid-binding compounds[33,50,55–58]. Whether the inhibitory effect of the compounds is on uncoating or on attachment seems to be determined much more by the virus than by the drug. For example, disoxaril specifically inhibits uncoating of polioviruses and rhinoviruses 1A and 2, but inhibits attachment of HRV14. As a rough generalization the attachment–inhibitory activity of capsid-binding drugs is confined to rhinoviruses belonging to the major (ICAM-1) receptor group[27], but there are exceptions. For example, chalcone is reported to inhibit attachment of two minor group rhinoviruses (2 and 29); WIN 51711, on the other hand, did not[59]. Attachment of HRV29 was also partially inhibited by R 61837, whereas that of HRV2 was not. These exceptions probably reflect the dual target effects of capsid-binding compounds in some viruses. It has been shown, for example, that WIN 52035 inhibits uncoating as well as attachment of HRV14, a member of the major receptor group[50].

MECHANISMS OF DRUG RESISTANCE

Selection of resistant variants

When virus-infected cells are cultured in the presence of drug at a concentration sufficient to neutralize the parental virus, resistant virus usually appears within a single growth cycle, illustrating the ease with which mutations arise in picornaviruses[60]. Drug-resistant mutants have been isolated with frequencies of 5×10^{-4} to 10^{-5} [61,62], which is consistent with the model that resistance arises by the selection of pre-existing mutants with single amino acid substitutions. In the laboratory, drug-resistant mutants have been selected either by picking plaques from monolayers infected with diluted virus stocks and incubated under agar in the presence of drug (Figure 2.6A)[54,61], or by one or more passages in the presence of drug, sometimes in increasing concentrations[62,63]. Resistant virus has also been isolated in clinical studies from nasal washings from experimentally infected drug-treated volunteers[64].

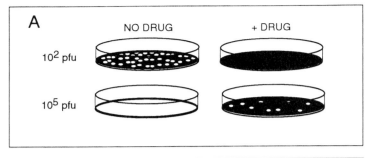

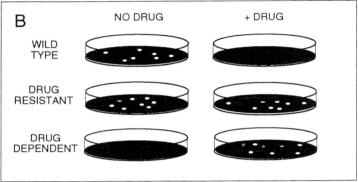

Figure 2.6 *Plaque method for selecting drug-resistant mutants from a plaque-purified virus stock. (**A**) (Top) Using about 100 plaque-forming units (pfu) of virus (left) select a drug concentration (right) which prevents plaque formation. (Bottom) Plating 1000-fold more virus obliterates the cell monolayer in the absence of drug (left) but selects for plaques of drug-resistant mutants (right); in plaque purified stocks of parental (wild-type) virus the mutant frequency is typically of the order of 10*$^{-4}$*[61]. (**B**) Phenotype of wild-type, drug-resistant and drug-dependent mutants. Resistant mutants (technically non-dependent mutants) plate with roughly equal efficiency in the presence or absence of drug. Dependent mutants require drug to form plaques; revertants (able to grow in the absence of drug) can be selected by plating larger amounts of dependent mutants*[54]

Frequently the drug-resistant viruses grow less vigorously in tissue culture than the parental wild-type virus[54,62].

When resistant mutants were titered by plaque assay in the presence and absence of drug, two general classes of mutants were found (Figure 2.6B), those that grew equally well in the presence or absence of drug, and drug-dependent mutants that formed plaques only in the presence of drug. The spectrum of resistance phenotypes varies markedly with the virus serotype. For example, Heinz *et al.*[61] found that none of over 100 mutants of HRV14 resistant to WIN 52084 or 52035 were drug dependent. In contrast, about 10% of the mutants of HRV16 resistant to WIN

52035 (W. Wang, personal communication), two-thirds of PV3S mutants resistant to WIN 51711[54], and all of HRV1A mutants resistant to WIN 56291 (D. Pevear, personal communication) were drug dependent.

Studies on HRV14

The WIN drug-resistant mutants of HRV14 were selected either under high drug concentrations (capable of reducing the number of virus plaques by 10 000-fold) or under somewhat lower concentrations (virus plaques reduced by 100- or 1000-fold). Although none of these mutants was drug dependent they had achieved resistance in two different ways. Some of them (including all of the mutants selected under high drug concentrations) were no longer able to bind enough drug to stabilize the virus against loss of infectivity by heating. These were termed 'drug-exclusion' mutants. Drug-exclusion mutants that are no longer protected by drug against thermal[62,63], acid[62] and alkaline[65] inactivation have been isolated frequently in studies with other virus–drug combinations.

Some of the HRV14 WIN drug-resistant mutants studied by Heinz et al.[61] were stabilized by drug against thermal inactivation. These were called 'compensation' mutants, as they had not lost the ability to bind drug at normally inhibitory concentrations (as measured by ability of added drug to thermostabilize the mutant), and yet they were now able to carry out viral functions normally blocked by drug, in this case cell attachment. Genetic studies with the HRV14 mutants showed that drug-exclusion mutants had amino acid substitutions in the wall of the drug-binding pocket, whereas drug-compensation mutants frequently had amino acid substitutions in other functional parts of the viral capsid (see below).

Studies with poliovirus

All of the WIN drug-resistant mutants of poliovirus type 3[54] appeared to be compensation mutants, since all were thermostabilized by drug. About two-thirds of these were dependent on the presence of drug for plaque formation[54]. In single-cycle growth curve experiments, however, all of these mutants grew as well in the absence of drug as in its presence. This paradoxical behavior was traced to extreme thermolability in the absence of drug at 37 °C, the growth temperature (Figure 2.7A). Thermolability was exhibited only after virus was released from the cell, implying the presence of a cell-associated protective factor. Thus in the absence of thermostabilizing drug, dependent mutants decayed too rapidly after release to permit spread in the plaque assay (Figure 2.7B).

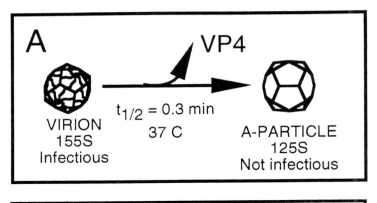

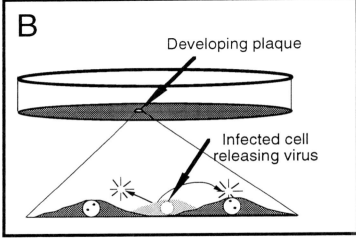

Figure 2.7 Mechanism of drug dependence in poliovirus type 3. (**A**) Unless drug is present the mutant is hyperlabile, decaying to form A particles with a half-life of 0.3 minutes at growth temperature (37 °C). (**B**) The dependent mutant is able to grow at 37 °C because it is stable so long as it remains inside the cell; the virion becomes hyperlabile only after release from the cell. The protective cellular material remains to be identified. Drug protects the released mutant, assuring it a survival time sufficient to spread and form a plaque

The thermodecay product was shown to consist of 125S A particles lacking VP4. Thus these mutants underwent the first (eclipse) step in uncoating (Figure 2.4, step 4a) inappropriately in the absence of receptor. Although not tested in the same ways, the arildone-dependent mutants of poliovirus type 2 studied by Schrom et al.[66] may be similar to these poliovirus type 3 mutants, in that they are extremely thermolabile and are still thermostabilized by the drug.

Studies with other rhinoviruses

Ahmad *et al.*[62] isolated a chalcone-dependent mutant of HRV9 after repeated passages in increasing concentrations of drug. This mutant required drug for the formation of infectious virus in a single-cycle growth curve experiment, but drug did not have to be added until five hours after attachment. Coupled with the fact that viral proteins were synthesized in normal amounts in the absence of drug, this implied that drug was required for assembly of this drug-dependent mutant. Drug-dependent mutants which require drug for assembly have also been isolated for WIN drug-dependent HRV1A (D. Pevear, personal communication) and HRV16 (W. Wang, personal communication).

GENETICS OF DRUG RESISTANCE

Human rhinovirus 14: genetics of attachment inhibition

Most cases of drug resistance studied in *in vitro* systems have been traced to single amino acid substitutions in the coat protein. Heinz *et al.*[61] found that mutations that conferred drug resistance on HRV14 were of two types. One set was called drug-exclusion mutants because they were no longer thermostabilized by drug; they had greatly reduced drug-binding affinity. Sequencing of portions of the genome encoding the capsid proteins of these mutants revealed that all 56 drug-exclusion mutants had single amino acid substitutions at one of two positions: VP1 residues 188 (normally valine) and 199 (normally cysteine) (Figure 2.8). These relatively small residues project towards the cavity of the drug-binding pocket. In drug-exclusion mutants they were replaced with amino acids with bulkier side chains, thus physically preventing the binding of large WIN drugs. This has been verified by X-ray crystallographic studies[61,67,68].

A second set, called compensation mutants, had amino acid replacements in those portions of the polypeptide chains that move when the drug is inserted into the binding pocket. These chains form both the 'roof' of the drug-binding pocket and the floor of the canyon, thought to accept the cellular receptor. Recent X-ray crystallographic studies have shown that some of these residues point into the canyon, where they appear to influence the binding of virus to the cellular receptor, ICAM-1[50,56]. Other residues form part of the pocket lining. They generally reduce the bulk of the side chain within the pocket, and may decrease the binding affinity of drug for virus[69]. Thus both the compensation mutations that line the canyon and those that line the

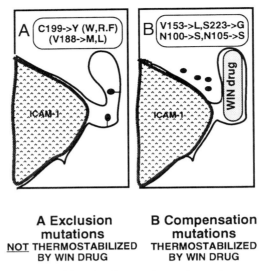

Figure 2.8 *Cross-section of drug-binding pocket at base of receptor-binding canyon, showing the position of single amino acid mutations which give rise to exclusion or compensation resistance to WIN drugs in human rhinovirus 14. Thermostabilization by drug provides a convenient screen for distinguishing mutants which retain the ability to bind drug from those which do not. The right panel suggests how deformation of the canyon floor might prevent the receptor from binding into the bottom of the canyon*

drug-binding pocket may favor the conformational changes necessary for binding to cells and initiating uncoating.

The mechanism by which compensation mutants function is not yet clear. Two different mechanisms might be imagined: full pocket compensation, in which a mutation in the viral shell enables the receptor to attach despite the presence of drug in the pocket; and empty pocket compensation, in which the receptor is able to attach only if the pocket is empty, but by decreasing affinity for drug or increasing affinity for receptor the mutation increases the probability that receptor can bind and trigger uncoating.

Poliovirus type 3: genetics of uncoating inhibition

All of the drug-resistant mutants of PV3S were protected from thermal inactivation by drug, so they are by definition compensation mutants. The non-drug-dependent drug-resistant mutants of poliovirus type 3 had single amino acid replacements defining regions of the viral capsid important in initiating uncoating[70]. Amino acid substitutions were identified in three distinct loci (Figure 2.9, bottom panel): at VP1 residue

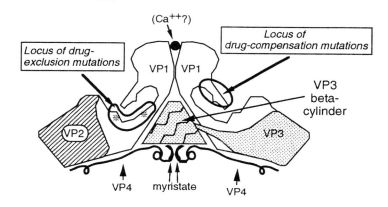

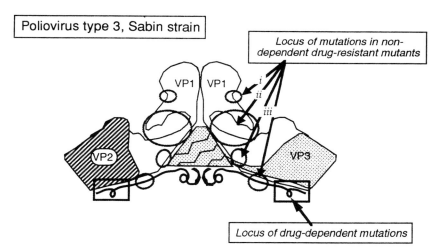

Figure 2.9 *Loci of drug resistance mutations in human rhinovirus 14 and type 3 poliovirus. Schematic side views of a pentamer with sections removed to reveal the anatomy of two drug-binding sites*

105 on the edge of the canyon and potentially involved in receptor binding or action; at VP1 residues 192, 194 and 260 in the lining of the drug-binding pocket; and on or near the inner capsid surface, at VP4 residue 46 or VP1 residue 129. These appear to trace a pathway from the surface, where the virus interacts with its receptor on the cell to trigger the conformational changes that lead eventually to uncoating, through the drug-binding pocket where mutations may influence either the

affinity for drug or the ability of the VP1 β barrel to undergo conformational changes, to the inside of the virus capsid at the locus of structures such as VP4 molecules and the amino termini of VP1, which are expelled from the virion in the formation of the A particle.

Genetics of drug dependence

Attempts to isolate drug-dependent mutants from HRV14 failed, but about two-thirds of the drug-resistant mutants of PV3S were dependent on drug for plaque formation. The drug-dependent mutants of poliovirus type 3[70] had single amino acid substitutions on all four viral capsid proteins. These altered amino acids were clustered in a small volume on the inner capsid surface near the three fold axis of symmetry (rectangular box in Figure 2.9, bottom panel). Because these changes conferred extreme thermolability on the drug-dependent mutants, this area appears to represent a sort of thermostat for the first stage of viral uncoating[70].

CRYSTALLOGRAPHIC STUDIES

Capsid-binding agents neutralize picornaviruses by blocking the eclipse step of uncoating; interference with attachment to receptors is a secondary effect observed only with certain rhinoviruses[55,57]. In HRV14, for example, WIN compounds inhibit not only the attachment step, but also the uncoating step[50]. The reason why capsid inhibitors block attachment in some viruses but not in others is not yet fully understood. However, structural studies on HRV14 and HRV16, both of which are attachment inhibited and use the same receptor (ICAM-1), have revealed two different mechanisms at play. One of these has provided important insights into the interaction of the virus with its receptor.

Two mechanisms for inhibition of receptor attachment

The pioneer study of Smith *et al.*[43], which identified the picornaviral drug-binding site as a hydrophobic pocket in the β barrel of VP1, was carried out with HRV14; this work showed that two different agents, WIN 51711 and WIN 52084, both of which prevent attachment of the virus, deformed the roof of the drug-binding pocket some 0.45 nm outward into the base of the canyon (see Figure 2.3). This same deformation was subsequently observed with a variety of other HRV14-neutralizing compounds[61,71,72]. This work established that in HRV14 the capsid is deformable in the pocket region and can assume an empty ('closed') or full ('open') state (compare left and right pockets in Figure 2.3D). It also suggested that one mechanism of attachment inhibition was 'steric interference', i.e. receptor docking was blocked when drug braced the pocket roof (canyon floor) in the open state.

Realization that there must be a second mechanism of attachment inhibition emerged from crystallographic studies on HRV16. With this virus the canyon as receptor attachment site had been directly visualized by cryoelectron microscopy and image reconstruction[37]. Analysis of virus–drug complexes revealed no significant deformation of the canyon by any of four different compounds that prevent its attachment[40]. This result implied that receptor binding induces inward deformation of the HRV16 canyon. In this case drug probably stiffens the region over the pocket, preventing the deformation required for proper docking of the receptor. One implication of this model is that each bound receptor molecule induces small, probably destabilizing, changes in the configuration of its conjugate protomer. Such small receptor-induced changes provide a physical basis for the destabilizing effect that accompanies receptor recruiting (see Figure 2.5).

The reason why capsid-binding drugs inhibit uncoating of some viruses but attachment in others is not clear. One intriguing possibility is related to the propensity of picornaviruses to equilibrate between two isoelectric forms[73]:

$$B \longleftrightarrow A$$
$$\sim 5 \quad pI \quad \sim 7$$

Arildone reportedly stabilized HRV14 in the A form[43], but stabilized wild-type type 2 poliovirus in the B form[65]. The sample is too small to draw any conclusions and calls for a more thorough search for correlations between the ability of capsid-binding drug to inhibit attachment and to stabilize virus in the isoelectric A form.

Mechanism of uncoating inhibition

As shown in Figure 2.4, uncoating consists of two steps, eclipse and RNA release. Available evidence[50,54] indicates that antiviral compounds prevent step 4a, the eclipse transition in which the virion is transformed to a non-infectious A particle. This transition involves major structural changes: ejection of VP4 and extrusion of the amino terminus of VP1, enabling the A particle to attach to liposomes[74]. It has been suggested[43] that the function of the pocket is to provide the space needed to accommodate the movement of proteins during these major conformational changes, and that the effect of the antiviral is to 'stiffen' VP1 and thereby block the movement necessary for eclipse. This hypothesis imposes no requirement that the antiviral cause any conformational changes when it fills the pocket, and indeed none are observed in poliovirus[75] or in HRV1A[46], where drug blocks uncoating but not attachment.

In several rhinoviruses an ion, tentatively identified as calcium on the basis of its presence in the crystallization liquor and its coordination geometry, is located at each of the 12 pentamer centers. In each case the ion is coordinated by side chains in the VP1 DE loops; the side chains involved are Asp137 in HRV1A[46], carbonyls of Gln141 in HRV14[43], and imidazoles of His134 in HRV16[40]. In the case of HRV14 calcium binding increased with binding of WIN compounds[40] and decreased with decreasing pH[76]. The role of such ions in modulating the effects of WIN drugs does not appear to have been experimentally examined.

Design of antivirals

The goal of drug design is to produce an inhibitory molecule with a target specificity and binding affinity high enough to eliminate drug toxicity. The hydrophobic drug-binding pocket in rhinoviruses and enteroviruses seemed to provide an almost ideal target because it is possible to actually see, through computer imaging, how the drug binds within the intact virus particle. Moreover, pocket residues lie in a highly conserved region of the coat protein[77]. This excited high hopes that it would be possible, through crystallographic analysis of virus–drug complexes, to identify key binding interactions between drug and pocket and then, through medicinal chemistry, to synthesize compounds with the maximum possible binding affinities. Now, despite a decade of experience[67,68,71,72,75,78,79], it must be admitted that the most effective compounds so far achieved, pirodavir and WIN 54954, have been discovered through the tried and trusted empirical screening and medicinal chemical methods[26,80]. This is due in part to the large number of rhinovirus and enterovirus serotypes, the hydrophobic nature of the bonding interactions and the variety of pocket shapes involved. Resolution achieved by X-ray crystallography—possibly as good as a few Angstroms, given the additional resolving power of symmetry and molecular modeling in solving the virus structures—is still generally insufficient to predict binding affinities which, in the case of van der Waal binding, requires knowledge of distances of the order of tenths of an Angstrom. However, demonstration that it is indeed possible to generate broad-spectrum antipicornavirals is a major achievement and spurs optimism that, particularly with continued advances in computational chemistry[81,82], the goal of computing high-affinity drug binding will eventually succeed.

AGENTS OF CLINICAL INTEREST

To be a viable candidate for clinical testing a capsid-binding drug must meet three criteria in cell culture-based assays: it must be potent, it must be active against a wide range of viruses, and it must lack cytotoxicity at effective antiviral concentrations. This has been accomplished. WIN drugs have also been shown to be efficacious in mice even when tissues have high titers of virus[83-86]. A number of experimental capsid-binding compounds have reached the stage of clinical trials using common cold viruses with human volunteers: chalcones[87], R61837[88], pirodavir[89], and WIN 54954[90]. Of these, the two most promising have been pirodavir and WIN 54954.

Pirodavir

At concentrations equal to or less than 0.07 μg/ml pirodavir inhibits 80% (EC80) of 100 rhinovirus serotypes tested; 1.3 μg/ml was required to inhibit 80% of 16 commonly isolated enteroviruses. These values are well below the cytotoxic concentration of 7 μg/ml[58]. In clinical trials intranasal pirodavir significantly decreased cold symptoms and nasal secretion if administered before infection and with frequent doses (six times daily using 2 mg per dose). The lack of protection observed with three times daily dosing is likely to be related to inadequate antiviral activity owing to the rapid mucociliary clearance of the drug[89]. Intranasal pirodavir given six times daily also proved ineffective in treating natural rhinovirus colds, although resistance emergence was not observed[91].

Similar results were obtained with a less potent and narrower-spectrum derivative, R61837[87,88]. Administration of intranasal R61837 six times daily, beginning before viral challenge, reduced the frequency of colds induced with HRV9 by 71%. However, this agent was also associated with the emergence of resistant variants *in vivo*[64]. Approximately 30% of drug-exposed infected volunteers shed resistant virus. Although most isolates showed low-level resistance (four- to eight-fold increases in inhibitory concentrations), one volunteer shed highly resistant virus which had a 100-fold decrease in sensitivity to the drug. In retrospect sequestration by the solubilizing vehicle (hydroxypropyl-β-cyclodextrin) or metabolic destruction of the drug may also have been problems[26].

WIN 54954

As illustrated in the above study intranasal administration is an inconvenient mode of medication and bioavailability of the drug may be compromised by ciliary flushing. Thus the oral route of medication is preferable, but the insolubility of capsid-binding drugs results in slower dissolution rates and potentially lower oral absorption. Encouraging results suggesting that the oral route may be feasible have, however, been obtained with WIN 54954. This compound, though slightly less active against rhinoviruses (EC80 0.28 μg/ml for 52 rhinoviruses tested), is more active than pirodavir against enteroviruses (EC80 0.06 μg/ml for 15 commonly isolated enteroviruses); these concentrations fall well below its cytotoxic level, which is about 4 μg/ml[86]. Given prophylactically (three oral doses per day at 600 mg per dose, starting one day before infection), WIN 54954 was shown to be effective in colds experimentally induced with Coxsackie virus A21[92]. It reduced the number of colds, virus shedding and symptoms, but proved ineffective against HRV16, 39 or 23, apparently because of inadequate distribution of the drug into respiratory secretions, even though plasma levels were high[90].

VP 63843

One likely explanation for the poor showing in clinical tests of capsid-binding drugs with high *in vitro* potency is that they are rapidly metabolized to inactive products. Diana and co-workers have recently reported on WIN 63843 (Figure 2.1), a derivative of WIN 54954 modified by replacing its two chloro groups on the phenyl ring with methyl groups and replacing its acid-labile oxazoline ring with a trifluoromethylated oxadiazole ring. WIN 63843 (now called VP 63843) is reportedly as active as 54954 but with a much longer half-life in the bloodstream[93]. A monkey liver microsomal assay, developed to examine the metabolic activity of capsid-binding drugs, revealed an increased *in vitro* half-life of at least fivefold in a P450 system. This low rate of metabolism should not only help maintain effective blood concentrations but reduce the toxicity encountered with earlier compounds.

The feasibility of developing compounds with the kind of potency and broad action spectrum necessary to deal with human picornaviruses has now been demonstrated, most notably by the research groups at Sterling Winthrop in Rensselear, New York, and at Janssen Research Corporation in Beerse, Belgium[26,27]. The disappointing efficacy of current compounds in clinical tests indicates that a marketable product has still to be developed. However, demonstration that capsid-binding compounds can be active by the oral route is an important advance, and break-throughs in reducing metabolic breakdown have created a climate of optimism for the future.

The magnitude of the resistance problem cannot be assessed until clinically effective antipicornavirals actually become available. There is reason to hope that drug resistance will be a smaller problem with picornaviruses than with viruses producing chronic infections. This is because picornavirus infections are typically short in duration, measured in days. Thus antivirals which suppress infection, even for a day or less, can win precious time needed for the body to mount adequate immune defences.

Limited experience suggests that mutants resistant to capsid drugs are often less vigorous than wild-type parents[54,64,94]. For example, one clinical trial assessed the human pathogenicity of rhinovirus selected for phenotypic resistance to a capsid-binding agent. HRV2 was passaged *in vitro* in the presence of the chalcone RO 09-0410; one variant selected *in vitro* displayed a 16-fold decrease in sensitivity to the drug. Following intranasal inoculation of susceptible volunteers, this variant was found to be over three times less likely to produce infection than the wild-type virus[95]. Among infected volunteers the frequency and severity of colds were comparable to those observed with wild-type virus.

Acknowledgment

We are indebted to Fred Hayden and Mark McKinlay for critical reading of the manuscript. This work was supported by grants from the National Institute of Health (AI31960) and the Lucille P. Markey Charitable Trust.

REFERENCES

1. Uncapher CR, DeWitt CM, Colonno RJ. The major and minor group receptor families contain all but one human rhinovirus serotype. *Virology* 1991;180:814–17.
2. Melnick JL. Enteroviruses. In: Evans AS, ed. *Viral Infections of Humans: Epidemiology and Control*, 3rd edn. New York: Plenum Press, 1989;191–263.
3. Melnick JL. Portraits of viruses: the picornaviruses. *Intervirology* 1983;20:61–100.
4. Hyypia T, Horsnell C, Maaronen M *et al*. A distinct picornavirus group identified by sequence analysis. *Proc Natl Acad Sci USA* 1992;89:8847–51.
5. Gwaltney JM Jr. Rhinoviruses. In: Evans AS, ed. *Viral Infections of Humans: Epidemiology and Control*, 3rd edn. New York: Plenum Press, 1989;593–615.
6. Dick EC, Inhorn SL. Rhinoviruses. In: Feigin RD, Cherry JD, eds. *Textbook of Pediatric Infectious Diseases*, 3rd edn. Philadelphia: WB Saunders, 1992:1507–32.
7. Couch RB. Rhinoviruses. In: Fields BN, Knipe DM, Chanock RM *et al*., eds. *Virology*, 2nd edn. New York: Raven Press, 1990:607–29.
8. Kogon A, Spigland I, Frothingham TE *et al*. Observations on viral excretion, seroimmunity, intrafamilial spread, and illness association in Coxsackie and echovirus infections. *Am J Epidemiol* 1969;89:51–61.
9. Eggers HJ, Koch MA, Furst A *et al*. Rhodanine: a selective inhibitor of the multiplication of echovirus 12. *Science* 1970;167:294–7.

10. Eggers HJ. Inhibition of early stages of virus–cell interactions. *Ann N Y Acad Sci* 1970;173:417–19.
11. Eggers HJ. Selective inhibition of uncoating of echovirus 12 by rhodanine. *Virology* 1977;78:241–52.
12. Rosenwirth B, Eggers HJ. Early processes of echovirus 12-infection: elution, penetration, and uncoating under the influence of rhodanine. *Virology* 1979;97:241–55.
13. Diana GD, Salvador UJ, Zalay ES *et al.* Antiviral activity of some diketones. 2. Aryloxy alkyl diketones. *In vitro* activity against both RNA and DNA viruses. *J Med Chem* 1977;20:757–61.
14. Caliguiri LA, McSharry JJ, Lawrence GW. Effect of arildone on modifications of poliovirus *in vitro*. *Virology* 1980;105:86–93.
15. McSharry JJ, Caliguiri LA, Eggers HJ. Inhibition of uncoating of poliovirus by arildone, a new antiviral drug. *Virology* 1979;97:307–15.
16. McKinlay MA, Miralles JV, Brisson CJ, Pancic F. Prevention of human poliovirus-induced paralysis and death in mice by the novel agent arildone. *Antimicrob Agents Chemother* 1982;22:1022–5.
17. Bauer DJ, Selway JWT, Batchelor JF *et al.* 4',6-dichloroflavan (BW683C), a new antirhinovirus compound. *Nature* 1981;292:369–70.
18. Tisdale M, Selway JWT. Effect of dichloroflavan (BW683c) on the stability and uncoating of rhinovirus type 1B. *J Antimicrob Chemother* 1984;14(Suppl.A):97–105.
19. Ishitsuka H, Ninomiya YT, Obsawa C, Fujiu M. Direct and specific inactivation of rhinovirus by chalcone Ro 09-0410. *Antimicrob Agents Chemother* 1982;22:617–21.
20. Ninomiya Y, Ohsawa C, Aoyama M *et al.* Antivirus agent, Ro 09-0410, binds to rhinovirus specifically and stabilizes the virus conformation. *Virology* 1984;134:269–76.
21. Al-Nakib W, Tyrrell DAJ. A 'new' generation of more potent synthetic antirhinovirus compounds: comparison of their MICs and their synergistic interactions. *Antiviral Res* 1987;8:179–88.
22. Otto MJ, Fox MP, Fancher MJ *et al.* *In vitro* activity of WIN 51711: a new broad-spectrum antipicornavirus drug. *Antimicrob Agents Chemother* 1985;27:883–6.
23. McKinlay M. WIN 51711: a new systemically active broad-spectrum antipicornavirus agent. *J Antimicrob Chemother* 1985;16:284–6.
24. Fox MP, Otto MJ, McKinlay MA. The prevention of rhinovirus and poliovirus uncoating by WIN 51711: a new antiviral drug. *Antimicrob Agents Chemother* 1986;30:110–16.
25. Zeichhardt H, Otto MJ, McKinlay MA, Willingmann P, Habermehl K-O. Inhibition of poliovirus uncoating by disoxaril. *Virology* 1987;160:281–5.
26. Andries K. Discovery of pirodavir, a broad-spectrum inhibitor of rhinoviruses. In: Adams J, Merluzzi V, eds. *The Search for Antiviral Drugs.* Boston: Birkhauser Publishers, 1993:179–209.
27. McKinlay MA, Dutko FJ, Pevear DC *et al.* Rational design of antipicornavirus agents. In: Brinton MA, Heinz FX, eds. *New Aspects of Positive Strand RNA Viruses.* Washington, DC: American Society for Microbiology, 1990:366–72.
28. Diana GD, Rudewicz DC, Pevear DC *et al.* WIN 63843, a metabolically stable broad spectrum antipicornaviral compound. *Antiviral Res* 1995;26:345.
29. Luo M, Vriend G, Kamer G *et al.* The structure of mengovirus at atomic resolution. *Science* 1987;235:182–91.

30. Acharya R, Fry E, Stuart D *et al*. The three-dimensional structure of foot-and-mouth disease virus at 2.9 Å resolution. *Nature* 1989;337:709–15.
31. Rotbart HA, Romero JR. Laboratory diagnosis of enteroviral infections. In: Rotbart HA, ed. *Human Enterovirus Infections*. Washington DC: ASM Press, 1995:401–18.
32. Andries K, Dewindt B, Snoeks J *et al*. Two groups of rhinoviruses revealed by a panel of antiviral compounds present sequence divergence and differential pathogenicity. *J Virol* 1990;64:1117–23.
33. Andries K, Dewindt B, Snoeks J *et al*. A comparative test of fifteen compounds against all known human rhinovirus serotypes as a basis for a more rational screening program. *Antiviral Res* 1991;16:213–25.
34. Hogle JM, Chow M, Filman DJ. Three-dimensional structure of poliovirus at 2.9 Å resolution. *Science* 1985;229:1358–65.
35. Rossmann MG, Arnold E, Erickson JW *et al*. The structure of a human common cold virus (rhinovirus 14) and its functional relations to other picornaviruses. *Nature* 1985;317:145–53.
36. Colonno RJ, Condra JH, Mizutani S *et al*. Evidence for the direct involvement of the rhinovirus canyon in receptor binding. *Proc Natl Acad Sci USA* 1988;85:5449–53.
37. Olson NH, Kolatkar PR, Oliveira MA *et al*. Structure of a human rhinovirus complexed with its receptor molecule. *Proc Natl Acad Sci USA* 1993;90:507–11.
38. Dunker AK, Rueckert RR. Fragments generated by pH dissociation of ME virus and their relation to the structure of the virion. *J Mol Biol* 1971;58:217–35.
39. Rueckert RR. Picornaviral architecture. In: Maramorosch K, Kurstak E, eds. *Comparative Virology*. New York: Academic Press, 1971:255–306.
40. Oliveira MA, Zhao R, Lee W-M *et al*. The structure of human rhinovirus 16. *Structure* 1993;1:51–68.
41. Lonberg-Holm K. Attachment of animal virus to cells, an introduction. In: Lonberg-Holm K, Philipson L, eds. *Receptors and Recognition*. Series B, Vol. 8: *Virus Receptors*. Part 2, *Animal Viruses*. London: Chapman & Hall, 1980:1–20.
42. Zhang A, Nanni RG, Oren DA, Rozhon EJ, Arnold E. Three-dimensional structure–activity relationships for antiviral agents that interact with picornavirus capsids. *Semin Virol* 1992;3:453–72.
43. Smith TJ, Kremer MJ, Luo M *et al*. The site of attachment in human rhinovirus 14 for antiviral agents that inhibit uncoating. *Science* 1986;233:1286–93.
44. Filman DJ, Syed R, Chow M *et al*. Structural factors that control conformational transitions and serotype specificity in type 3 poliovirus. *EMBO J* 1989;8:1567–79.
45. Muckelbauer JK, Kremer M, Minor I *et al*. The structure of Coxsackievirus B3 at 3.5 Å resolution. *Structure* 1995;3:653–67.
46. Kim KH, Willingmann P, Gong ZX *et al*. A comparison of the anti-rhinoviral drug binding pocket in HRV14 and HRV1A. *J Mol Biol* 1993;230:206–27.
47. Rueckert RR. Picornavirus structure and multiplication. In: Fields BN, Knipe DM, Howley PM *et al*., eds. *Virology*, 3rd edn. New York: Raven Press, 1996:609–54.
48. Crowell RL, Tomko RP. Receptors for picornaviruses. In: Wimmer E, ed. *Cellular Receptors of Animal Viruses*. New York: Cold Spring Harbor Laboratory Press, 1994:75–99.

49. Joklik WK, Darnell JE. The adsorption and early fate of purified poliovirus in HeLa cells. *Virology* 1961;13:439–47.
50. Shepard DA, Heinz BA, Rueckert RR. WIN 52035–2 inhibits both attachment and eclipse of human rhinovirus 14. *J Virol* 1993;67:2245–54.
51. Crowther D, Melnick JL. Studies of the inhibitory action of guanidine on poliovirus multiplication in cell culture. *Virology* 1961;15:65–74.
52. Wilson JN, Cooper PD. Aspects of the growth of poliovirus as revealed by the photodynamic effects of neutral red and acridine orange. *Virology* 1963;21:135–45.
53. Wilson JN, Cooper PD. The effect of light on poliovirus grown in neutral red. *Virology* 1965;26:1–9.
54. Mosser AG, Rueckert RR. WIN 51711-dependent mutants of poliovirus type 3: evidence that virions decay after release from cells unless drug is present. *J Virol* 1993;67:1246–54.
55. Pevear DC, Fancher MJ, Felock PJ *et al*. Conformational change in the floor of the human rhinovirus canyon blocks adsorption to HeLa cell receptors. *J Virol* 1989;63:2002–7.
56. Heinz BA, Shepard DA, Rueckert RR. Neutralizing rhinoviruses with antiviral agents that inhibit attachment and uncoating. In: Laver WG, Air GM, eds. *Use of X-ray Crystallography in the Design of Antiviral Agents*. New York: Academic Press, 1990:183–6.
57. Moeremans M, De Raeymaeker M, Daneels G *et al*. Study of the parameters of binding of R61837 to human rhinovirus 9 and immunobiochemical evidence of capsid-stabilizing activity of the compound. *Antimicrob Agents Chemother* 1992;36:417–24.
58. Andries K, Dewindt B, Snoeks J *et al*. In vitro activity of pirodavir (R77975), a substituted phenoxypyridazinamine with broad-spectrum antipicornaviral activity. *Antimicrob Agents Chemother* 1992;36:100–7.
59. Dewindt B, van Eemeren K, Andries K. Antiviral capsid-binding compounds can inhibit the adsorption of minor receptor rhinoviruses. *Antiviral Res* 1994;25:67–72.
60 Holland J, Spindler K, Horodyski F *et al*. Rapid evolution of RNA genomes. *Science* 1982;215:1577–85.
61. Heinz BA, Rueckert RR, Shepard DA *et al*. Genetic and molecular analyses of spontaneous mutants of human rhinovirus 14 that are resistant to an antiviral compound. *J Virol* 1989;63:2476–85.
62. Ahmad ALM, Dowsett AB, Tyrrell DAJ. Studies of rhinovirus resistant to an antiviral chalcone. *Antiviral Res* 1987;8:27–39.
63. Yasin SR, Al-Nakib W, Tyrrell DAJ. Isolation and preliminary characterization of chalcone Ro 09-0410-resistant human rhinovirus type 2. *Antiviral Chem Chemother* 1990;1:149–54.
64. Dearden C, Al-Nakib W, Andries K, Woestenborghs R, Tyrrell DAJ. Drug resistant rhinoviruses from the nose of experimentally treated volunteers. *Arch Virol* 1989;109:71–81.
65. Eggers HJ, Rosenwirth B. Isolation and characterization of an arildone-resistant poliovirus 2 mutant with an altered capsid protein VP1. *Antiviral Res* 1988;9:23–35.
66. Schrom M, Laffin JA, Evans B, McSharry JJ, Caliguiri LA. Isolation of poliovirus variants resistant to and dependent on arildone. *Virology* 1982;122:492–7.
67. Badger J, Minor I, Kremer MJ *et al*. Structural analysis of a series of antiviral agents complexed with human rhinovirus 14. *Proc Natl Acad Sci USA* 1988;85:3304–8.

68. Badger J, Krishnaswamy S, Kremer MJ *et al*. Three-dimensional structures of drug-resistant mutants of human rhinovirus 14. *J Mol Biol* 1989;207:163–74.
69. Hadfield AT, Oliveira MA, Kim KH *et al*. Structural studies on human rhinovirus 14 drug resistant compensation mutants. *J Mol Biol* 1995;253:61–73.
70. Mosser AG, Sgro J-Y, Rueckert RR. Distribution of drug resistance mutations in type 3 poliovirus identifies three regions involved in uncoating functions. *J Virol* 1994;68:8193–201.
71. Chapman MS, Minor I, Rossmann MG. Human rhinovirus 14 complexed with antiviral compound R 61837. *J Mol Biol* 1991;217:455–63.
72. Zhang A, Nanni RG, Oren DA, Rozhon EJ, Arnold E. Three-dimensional structure–activity relationships for antiviral agents that interact with picornavirus capsids. *Semin Virol* 1992;3:453–71.
73. Rueckert RR. Picornaviridae and their replication. In: Fields BN, Knipe DM, Chanock RM *et al*, eds. *Virology*, 2nd edn. New York: Raven Press, 1990:507–48.
74. Flore O, Fricks CE, Filman DJ, Hogle JM. Conformational changes in poliovirus assembly and cell entry. *Semin Virol* 1990;1:429–38.
75. Grant RA, Hiremath CN, Filman DJ *et al*. Structures of poliovirus complexes with anti-viral drugs: implications for viral stability and drug design. *Curr Biol* 1994;4:784–97.
76. Giranda VL, Heinz BA, Oliveira MA *et al*. Acid-induced structural changes in human rhinovirus 14: possible role in uncoating. *Proc Natl Acad Sci USA* 1992;89:10213–17.
77. Palmenberg AC. Sequence alignments of picornaviral capsid proteins. In: Semler B, Ehrenfeld E, eds. *Molecular Aspects of Picornavirus Infection and Detection*. Washington DC: ASM Publications, 1988:211–41.
78. Bibler-Muckelbauer JK, Kremer MJ, Rossmann MG *et al*. Human rhinovirus 14 complexed with fragments of active antiviral compounds. *Virology* 1994;202:360–9.
79. Zhang A, Nanni RG, Li T *et al*. Structure determination of antiviral compound SCH 38057 complexed with human rhinovirus 14. *J Mol Biol* 1993;238:857–67.
80. Andries K. Anti-picornaviral agents. In: Jeffries DJ, DeClercq E, eds. *Antiviral Chemotherapy*. Chichester: John Wiley & Sons, 1995:287–319.
81. McCammon JA. Computer-aided molecular design. *Science* 1987;238:486–91.
82. Harrison SC. Common cold virus and its receptor. *Proc Natl Acad Sci USA* 1993;90:783.
83. McKinlay MA, Steinberg BA. Oral efficacy of WIN 51711 in mice infected with human poliovirus. *Antimicrob Agents Chemother* 1986;29:30–2.
84. See D, Tilles J. WIN 54954 treatment of mice infected with a diabetogenic strain of group B Coxsackievirus. *Antimicrob Agents Chemother* 1993;37:1593–8.
85. See D, Tilles J. Treatment of Coxsackievirus A9 myocarditis in mice with WIN 54954. *Antimicrob Agents Chemother* 1992;36:425–8.
86. Woods MG, Diana GD, Rogge MC *et al*. *In vitro* and *in vivo* activities of WIN 54954, a new broad-spectrum antipicornavirus drug. *Antimicrob Agents Chemother* 1989;33:2069–74.
87. Al-Nakib W, Higgins PG, Barrow GI *et al*. Suppression of colds in human volunteers challenged with rhinovirus by a new synthetic drug (R61837). *Antimicrob Agents Chemother* 1989;33:522–5.
88. Barrow GI, Higgins PG, Tyrrell DAJ, Andries K. An appraisal of the efficacy of the antiviral R 61837 in rhinovirus infections in human volunteers. *Antiviral Chem Chemother* 1990;1:279–83.

89. Hayden FG, Andries K, Janssen PAJ. Safety and efficacy of intranasal pirodavir (R77975) in experimental rhinovirus infection. *Antimicrob Agents Chemother* 1992;36:727–32.

90. Turner RB, Dutko FJ, Goldstein NH, Lockwood G, Hayden FG. Efficacy of oral WIN 54954 for prophylaxis of experimental rhinovirus infection. *Antimicrob Agents Chemother* 1993;37:297–300.

91. Hayden FG, Hipskind GJ, Woerner DH *et al*. Intranasal pirodavir (R77975) treatment of rhinovirus colds. *Antimicrob Agents Chemother* 1995;39:290–4.

92. Schiff GM, Sherwood JR, Young EC, Maxon LJ. Prophylactic efficacy of WIN 54954 in prevention of experimental human Coxsackievirus A21 infection and illness. *Antiviral Res* 1992;17(Suppl): Abstract 92.

93. Diana GD, Rudewicz P, Pevear DC *et al*. Picornavirus inhibitors: trifluoromethyl substitution provides a global protective effect against hepatic metabolism. *J Med Chem* 1995;38:1355–71.

94. Groarke JM, McKinlay MA, Dutko FJ, Pevear DC. Coxsackievirus B3 mutants resistant to WIN 63843 are attenuated for virulence in mice: molecular analysis of the drug resistant phenotype. *Antiviral Res* 1995;26:300.

95. Yasin SR, Al-Nakib W, Tyrrell DA. Pathogenesis for humans of human rhinovirus type 2 mutants resistant to or dependent on chalcone Ro 09-0410. *Antimicrob Agents Chemother* 1990;34:963–6.

INFLUENZA A VIRUSES

3
Amantadine and Rimantadine—Mechanisms

ALAN J. HAY

INTRODUCTION

The target of antiviral drug action is in many instances known or is fairly obvious, whether the drug was 'designed' and developed against a particular target or discovered empirically as, for example, substrate analogues of an enzyme. The closely related anti-influenza drugs amantadine and rimantadine[1] provide an example where this was not so, and where the study of drug resistance not only identified the target but was also instrumental in elucidating its novel function. Thus, although the anti-influenza A activity of these agents was discovered in the early 1960s[2] and amantadine was licensed for clinical use in 1966, more than two decades elapsed before there was any knowledge as to the identity of the target protein, the M2 protein[3], or its functional activity[4].

As well as highlighting the importance and value of investigating the basis of drug resistance, studies of amantadine and rimantadine have also illustrated some potential pitfalls associated with interpreting the results of such investigations. First, in cell culture they possess two different concentration-dependent inhibitory actions directed against distinct targets, only one of which (at micromolar concentrations) is selectively antiviral and specific for influenza A viruses[3,5]. Whether the two actions are synergistic or antagonistic depends on both the drug concentration and the virus strain. In the past this has complicated interpretation of the inhibitory effects of intermediate drug concentrations and of the clinically relevant mode of action. Secondly, the specific

Antiviral Drug Resistance. Edited by Douglas D. Richman © 1996 John Wiley & Sons Ltd

anti-influenza A action of micromolar concentrations of amantadine, directed against the virus M2 protein, can inhibit two different stages in virus infection[3], the relative drug susceptibility of which depends on the particular virus strain. Thirdly, loss of drug susceptibility of recombinant (reassortant) or mutant viruses may be due to changes in another, functionally related, virus protein and reflect a loss of requirement for the function of the target protein rather than its acquisition of resistance to drug action. These features are discussed in the ensuing brief discussion of the molecular bases of susceptibility and resistance of influenza A viruses to the actions of amantadine and rimantadine.

GENETIC BASIS OF DRUG RESISTANCE

Mutants resistant to amantadine and rimantadine have been isolated from 'susceptible' virus stocks and are readily selected following *in vitro* passage of virus in the presence of drug[6], or after treatment of humans, animals or birds with either drug[7-11] (see Chapter 4). Resistant viruses consistently exhibit cross-resistance to amantadine and rimantadine and to other compounds, e.g. cyclo-octylamine, which act in a similar manner against the same target[3,8]. Thus susceptibility and resistance to amantadine and rimantadine are in many contexts considered indistinguishable, and are treated as such in the following discussion.

It is now well established by data from a variety of studies that the principal determinant of susceptibility/resistance to amantadine is the M2 protein, and that this is the target of drug action. Analyses of reassortants between a resistant mutant, selected *in vitro* or *in vivo*, and a susceptible virus showed that the M gene is the major determinant of susceptibility of human influenza subtypes[7,13,14]. Similar studies involving avian virus strains also implicated the haemagglutinin (HA) gene[5,15,16]. However, we can account for the influence of the virus HA on drug susceptibility in terms of an altered requirement for M2 function in the transport of different HAs to the cell surface rather than a direct effect of the drug on HA (see below).

Without exception, resistant viruses selected following passage in cell culture in the presence of amantadine or rimantadine possess mutations in their M genes which cause single amino acid substitutions in the M2 protein, at residues 27, 30, 31 or 34[3,7,11,17] (Table 3.1). These mutations occur downstream of the termination site for translation of the M1, or matrix, protein from the colinear transcript, and therefore only alter the sequence encoding the 97 amino acid M2 protein (Figure 3.1B), which is translated from the spliced mRNA[18]. Similar analyses of viruses isolated following *in vivo* infection have shown a consistent correlation between

Table 3.1 *Amino acid substitutions in the M2 proteins of amantadine- and rimantadine-resistant influenza A viruses selected in vivo or in vitro*

Virus	26†	27	30	31	34
In vivo					
A/New York/83 (H3N2)[7]		Val→Ala (1)*	Ala→Val (2)	Ser→Asn (10)	
A/Virginia/88 (H3N2)[8]		Val→Ala (1)	Ala→Val (1) →Thr (1)	Ser→Asn (14)	
A/Shanghai/87 (H3N2)[9]		Val→Ala (3)	Ala→Val (1) →Thr (1)	Ser→Asn (1)	
A/USA/90 (H3N2)[10]	Leu→Phe (2)			Ser→Asn (2)	
Ck/Pennsylvania/83 (H5N2)[11]		Ile→Ser (1) →Thr (3)	Ala→Ser (1) →Thr (1)	Ser→Asn (1)	
In vitro					
A/Singapore/57 (H2N2)[3]		Val→Ala (7)	Ala→Thr (6)	Ser→Asn (12)	
Ck/Germany/27 (H7N7)[3] (Weybridge)		Val→Ala (3) →Gly (2) →Asp (1)	Ala→Thr (7) →Pro (2)	Ser→Asn (4)	Gly→Glu (29)
Ck/Germany/34 (H7N1)[3] (Rostock)		Ile→Ser (17) →Thr (8) →Ala (1)			
Ck/Germany/34 (H7N1)[12+] (Rostock)	Leu→Hist (1)	Ile→Thr (6) →Ser (2) →Asn (1)	Ala→Thr (4) →Ser (1)	Ser→Asn (4)	Gly→Glu (3)
Rostock (HA, K58I)[12]		Ile→Thr (1)	Ala→Thr (5)	Ser→Asn (12)	

†Amino acid residue
•Number of isolates
+Viruses isolated by plaque selection in presence of amantadine without prior passage in presence of drug

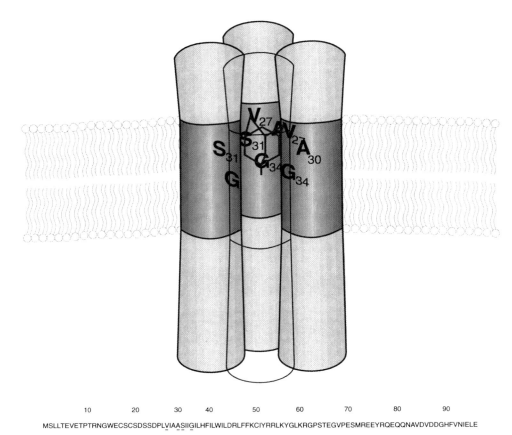

MSLLTEVETPTRNGWECSCSDSSDPLVIAASIIGILHFILWILDRLFFKCIYRRLKYGLKRGPSTEGVPESMREEYRQEQQNAVDVDDGHFVNIELE

External/luminal domain   Transmembrane domain   Internal/cytoplasmic domain

Figure 3.1   (**A**) *Diagrammatic representation of the M2 homotetramer indicating the possible interaction of amantadine with the channel. Amino acids altered in the M2 proteins of amantadine-resistant mutants of A/Chicken/Germany/27 (H7N7, Weybridge strain) are indicated with respect to a putative α-helical transmembrane domain[45]. (**B**) Amino acid sequence of the M2 protein of A/Chicken/Germany/27 indicating its orientation in the membrane. The locations of single amino acid substitutions in proteins of amantadine-resistant mutants are underlined*

resistance to amantadine or rimantadine (as determined by ELISA) and the presence of a resistance-determining amino acid at position 26, 27, 30 or 31 of the transmembrane domain of the M2 protein[7-11] (Table 3.1). Thus, although changes in the virus haemagglutinin have been shown to alter the drug susceptibility of certain avian influenza viruses, the resistance determinant in the M2 protein is dominant since it essentially abolishes drug susceptibility. This lack of susceptibility provides a definitive criterion for identifying the drug-resistant phenotype and is the basis of a simple ELISA test[7,19]. As resistance to amantadine and rimantadine selected *in vivo* and *in vitro* is due to the same amino acid substitutions, it is evident that the activity of M2 inhibited *in vitro* accounts for the clinical efficacy of the drugs.

FUNCTIONS OF THE M2 PROTEIN INHIBITED BY AMANTADINE

On the basis of inhibition by amantadine two roles have been identified for the M2 protein in virus replication: one in the uncoating or disassembly of the virion during endocytosis, and the other in regulating the pH of the *trans* Golgi, both of which appear to be dependent on the ion channel activity of the protein. Although M2 may perform other as yet unidentified roles, in, for example, virion assembly, they are not blocked by amantadine and therefore would not involve its ion channel activity.

Virus uncoating

Early studies showed that amantadine did not irreversibly inactivate virus infectivity, nor prevent the attachment of virus to or penetration of virus into cells[20]. It specifically prevents the initiation of primary transcription as a consequence of inhibiting the dissociation of M1 from the ribonucleoprotein (RNP) and hence blocking the entry of RNP into the nucleus and subsequent activation of the RNA transcriptase[5,17,21-23].

The fact that mutant viruses are resistant to the action of amantadine by virtue of amino acid changes in M2 demonstrated that the M2 protein in the virion is the target. The common basis for resistance of M2 to inhibition by amantadine, the ability of M2 to modulate intravesicular pH, and the selective proton channel activity of M2 have implicated the latter activity in the uncoating process. Thus it was postulated that during endocytosis M2 mediates the passage of protons from the acidic medium of the endosome into the virion to induce low pH disassembly of the RNP/M1 core structure, and that this is required in addition to HA-mediated fusion between the virus membrane and the endosome membrane[24] to effect complete uncoating of the RNP[4,21,23,25]. Other observations consistent with this idea include the reversible dissociation of M1 at reduced pH[26], and the specific reduction by amantadine of the rate of membrane fusion *in vitro* between virus and liposomes, and its enhancement by the Na^+/H^+ ionophore monensin[25,27]. The specific inhibition of M2 involved in this process is quite distinct from the non-specific effect of higher concentrations of amantadine (>100 μM) which, by causing an elevation in the pH of endosomes, indirectly inhibits the low pH-induced changes, particularly in HA, which are necessary for virus infection[3,16,24].

Modification of *trans* Golgi pH

The first clue that the M2 protein had an ion channel activity with the ability to modulate pH came from the observation that, during infection of cells by certain avian influenza A viruses of the H7 subtype, inhibition of M2 by amantadine resulted in expression of the low-pH form of HA on the cell surface[28]. As a consequence the release of infectious virus was prevented and virus replication was inhibited[29]. The HAs of these viruses have a polybasic intervening sequence which renders them susceptible to cleavage into HA1/HA2 by furin-like enzymes during passage through the *trans* Golgi[30], where they become susceptible to an irreversible low pH-induced conformational change[24,28]. That M2 is required to counteract such potential changes in HA by maintaining an appropriate pH within the *trans* Golgi was indicated by a number of observations. The amantandine-induced change in HA was reversed by agents which increase vesicular pH, such as the Na^+/H^+ ionophore monensin, and was abrogated by mutations in M2 alone[28]. Inhibition of M2 by amantadine caused an increase in acidity of the *trans* Golgi, as shown directly using the cytochemical pH probe DAMP (3-(2,4-dinitro-anilino)-3'-amino-N-methyldipropylamine)[31]. Furthermore, coexpression of M2 was shown to be required for the transport of native H7 HA to the surface of transfected cells[32,33].

Susceptibility to this action of amantadine thus depends on both the pH stability of the cleaved HA1/HA2 and the pH of the *trans* Golgi[32,34]. On the one hand, virus infection of chick embryo fibroblasts was more susceptible to amantadine than infection of MDCK cells by the same virus, apparently owing to the lower pH within the *trans* Golgi of the former. On the other hand, mutant viruses with acid-labile HAs were more susceptible than wild type[34]. Furthermore, the amantadine resistance of a mutant, which was selected without prior passage in the presence of drug, was shown to be due to an amino acid change in the HA which increased its pH stability, and not to a mutation in M2[35]. In this case, therefore, resistance was due to a reduced requirement for M2 function and not drug resistance of M2 *per se*. Only following subsequent passage in the presence of amantadine did the virus acquire a second mutation in M2 which removed the residual drug susceptibility[12].

Modification of cytoplasmic pH

A more direct assay of the ability of M2 to modify pH utilized the dual-wavelength fluorescent probe SNARF-1 to monitor changes in cytoplasmic pH. Under conditions where the pH of the cytoplasm of control cells was some 0.3–0.4 pH units higher than that of the extracellular medium, expression of M2, either in virus-infected MDCK cells or M2-expressing mouse erythroleukaemia (MEL) cells, caused a reduction in pH to a level equivalent to the external pH[36,37]. These changes were specifically prevented or reversed by amantadine inhibition unless they were due to an amantadine-resistant M2. An antibody against the N terminus of the protein could block the effects of both susceptible and amantadine-resistant M2 proteins.

In vitro modification of pH in artificial vessels

Another dual-wavelength fluorescent pH indicator, pyranine, was used in an *in vitro* assay to demonstrate that purified M2 incorporated into artificial membrane vesicles can, on its own, mediate changes in vesicular pH[38]. The apparent transfer of protons into the vesicles was once again specifically inhibited by rimantadine.

ION CHANNEL ACTIVITY

Electrophysiological studies of ion permeability associated with the M2 protein expressed in *Xenopus oocytes*[39–41] and mammalian cells[42,43], as well as purified M2 incorporated into lipid bilayers[44], have provided clear evidence that the protein forms an ion channel. Results obtained from different experimental systems have, however, led to different conclusions regarding the characteristics of the channel, in particular its ion selectivity. Studies using all three systems have been reported to show that M2 forms a pH-regulated cation channel. It was concluded from studies of M2 expressed in *X. oocytes*[39,40] and in CV-1 cells[42] that the protein has a high permeability for Na^+ and that the increase in current which occurred on reducing pH from 7 to 6 was due to activation of the channel at lower pH. Purified M2 incorporated into asolectin bilayers formed cation channels which were moderately selective among monovalent cations[44]. Although no direct measurements of H^+ permeability were reported for these systems, it was presumed that the M2 channel would also be permeable to H^+.

The results of direct measurements of H^+ permeability of M2 expressed in another mammalian cell, mouse erythroleukaemia (MEL) cells, showed that the M2 channel expressed in these cells is selective for protons and has a low relative permeability for other physiological ions, including Na^+, K^+ and Cl^- [43]. In this case the increase in ionic current on increasing H^+ concentration at lower pH is simply a concentration-dependent increase in ion flux, which approaches saturation at pH below 5. Activation (i.e. transition from closed to open state) by external pH appeared to occur at somewhat higher pH, between 8 and 7, although there are examples of M2 channels which are active at external pH above 9. How the apparent differences in activation relate to the physiological activity of M2 is unclear.

In spite of the different results reported, certain common characteristics, including pH dependence of the ionic current and specific inhibition by amantadine or rimantadine, do suggest that they are derived from studies of a similar channel activity. Proton permeability readily accounts for the physiological activities of M2 in modifying pH within the *trans* Golgi and cytoplasm of virus-infected and M2-transfected cells, as well as its postulated role in acidification of the virion interior during endocytosis. Its responsiveness to changes in 'external' pH, particularly in the range 6.5–5, and the orientation of M2 in the membrane are also consistent with its functional roles. The dependence of channel conductance on external pH and the higher permeability of M2 to inward current are properties which reflect the function of M2 in promoting proton flow in an N to C terminal direction down the electrochemical proton gradient which exists across the membrane under physiological conditions [43].

MECHANISM OF DRUG ACTION

The correlation between the ability of amantadine and rimantadine to block ion permeation and to prevent M2-mediated changes in pH and inhibit virus replication shows that this is the basis of their antiviral activity. Single amino acid substitutions in M2 which render virus replication resistant to the drugs also largely abolish the block of ion channel activity. Furthermore, the time dependence of inhibition of proton permeation through M2 expressed in MEL cells was similar to that of the reversal by amantadine or rimantadine of M2-mediated changes in cytoplasmic pH in these cells [37,43]. Both inward and outward ion flux were similarly affected. When added intracellularly rimantadine had no effect on M2 current in MEL cells, indicating that interaction with M2 is accessible only from the external N-terminal region of the molecule [43].

The mechanism of M2 block is less clear. Although time and concentration dependence of inhibition indicates binding of one molecule of drug per channel complex, the irreversibility of inhibition has hampered more definitive analyses of the characteristics of the interaction of drug with M2[41,43]. There is no conclusive evidence as to where the molecule binds, or whether it physically blocks the channel or induces a structural change that closes the channel. The original suggestion that the drug interacted with the transmembrane region of a pore formed by the homotetramer[45,46] (Figure 3.1A) was based on the locations of resistance-determining amino acid substitutions. Structure–activity studies of cyclic alkylamines which demonstrated the importance of the size of the aliphatic ring are consistent with this model. In cell culture cyclo-octylamine possesses an activity similar to amantadine, whereas cyclopentylamine is ineffective and cycloheptylamine and cyclohex-ylamine demonstrate intermediate activity[3].

Studies by neutron diffraction of the interaction of amantadine with the membrane-spanning domain of a peptide, corresponding to residues 22–46 of M2, inserted into a lipid bilayer showed that the drug inter-acted specifically with the region between valine 27 and serine 31[47]. Interaction with a mutant peptide in which alanine replaced valine 27 was altered, suggesting that the resistance of proton permeability[48] to block by amantadine may result directly from an alteration in the interaction of drug with this pore region. Similar studies using the intact protein have not been done, so we cannot be sure that these data provide a true picture of the interaction of amantadine with M2.

Characteristics of the inhibition of M2 channel activity were inconsist-ent with a mechanism involving simple non-competitive block of the open channel[41,43,44]. In particular, the pH dependence of the apparent binding constants for interaction of amantadine with three different M2 proteins was interpreted as indicating that the drug had a higher affinity for the closed state of the channel[41]. It therefore appears that inhibition involves an allosteric mechanism whereby interaction of drug, possibly with a site distant from the pore-forming region, induces an irreversible change to an inactive state[41,44].

MECHANISM OF DRUG RESISTANCE

In the absence of a clearer understanding of the mechanism whereby amantadine blocks ion flux, the structure of the channel or the site of interaction of amantadine with M2, it is not possible to explain how the various single amino acid substitutions render the channel conductance refractory to drug action. To date, the amino acids shown to be responsible have all been located in one of five positions: 26, 27, 30, 31 or 34, within a short segment of the transmembrane domain of the molecule (Table 3.1 and Figure 3.1). Whether the initial simplistic explanation that these changes might directly affect the interaction of amantadine with the protein, or whether they affect the consequences of that interaction, has yet to be demonstrated convincingly. Support for the former comes from neutron diffraction studies, which showed that substitution (V27A) of alanine in place of valine 27 interfered with interaction of amantadine with the transmembrane peptide (amino acids 22–46) inserted into lipid bilayers[47]. The same change (V27A) is responsible for abrogating amantadine inhibition of the M2 proteins of both human (H2 and H3 subtypes) and avian (H7 subtype) influenza A viruses.

The variety of resistance-determining amino acid substitutions which occur frequently is fairly restricted (Table 3.1). Valine or isoleucine at position 27 are replaced with a smaller non-polar residue alanine, or an uncharged polar serine or threonine. Alanine at position 30 is replaced by a larger non-polar residue, valine, or a polar serine or threonine. The only change at position 31 is replacement of the serine by asparagine (S31N). The change at position 34 of several amantadine-resistant avian viruses also is exclusively glycine to glutamic acid (G34E). It is not difficult to envisage that the consequences of these various changes may simply be to disturb or destabilize the interaction of the drug, and this has also been considered in terms of computer modelling of the interaction of amantadine with the M2 channel[49]. That some of these amino acid changes reduce the channel activity of certain M2 proteins indicates that they do not simply counteract a reduction in ion flux by the inhibitor.

CONSEQUENCES OF DRUG RESISTANCE

In Chapter 4 Hayden discusses the consequences of resistance mutations on the biological characteristics of amantadine/rimantadine-resistant influenza A viruses. Information presently available indicates that drug-resistance mutations selected *in vivo* appear neither deleterious nor advantageous to the virus. Studies of amantadine-resistant avian viruses showed that they did not differ from the susceptible parent in replication capacity, transmissibility or pathogenicity[11,50]. Rimantadine-resistant human isolates were observed to be similar to the corresponding drug-susceptible viruses in their virulence in ferrets[51] and their ability to cause illness[8,9]. Whether they differ in their ability to cause epidemics is not known. No significant spread of resistant strains within the human population has been observed. Furthermore, relatively few natural isolates and, with the possible exception of early H1N1 viruses, no type

A viruses causing epidemics have been observed to be resistant to amantadine or rimantadine. Whether this is simply coincidental or whether there are structural/functional consequences of the resistance mutations which reduce the epidemic potential of the variants is not known. It is clear, however, that drug-resistance amino acid changes selected *in vitro* can alter M2 function, and may either enhance or impair activity and consequently influence virus replication.

The frequency with which different amino acid substitutions are selected depends on the subtype and strain of virus (Table 3.1). This implies that the amino acid changes do affect M2 function and virus replication, and that their effects depend on the properties of the particular M2 protein. This is evident when comparing human and avian amantadine-resistant viruses, and is also apparent in comparisons of closely related avian strains and of different human virus subtypes. For example, amantadine-resistant mutants of the human H2N2 virus A/Singapore/1/57 with changes V27A, A30T or S31N in M2 were selected with a frequency of 1:1:2. Several studies of the emergence of amantadine- and rimantadine-resistant human strains *in vivo* and *in vitro* have indicated the strong tendency to select for the S31N resistance determinant. In contrast, resistance of 60% of the mutants of A/Chicken/Germany/27 (Weybridge strain) selected *in vitro* was due to substitution of glycine 34 by glutamic acid. On the other hand, resistance of mutants of the closely related strain A/Chicken/Germany/34 (Rostock), selected following passage in the presence of amantadine, was due exclusively to a change in isoleucine 27. The predominance of these mutations in the M2s of the drug-resistant avian viruses can be explained by their enhancing effects on the activity of M2 in increasing *trans* Golgi pH. Mutations which impaired this function were not tolerated. Amino acid changes such as L26H, A30T, S31N and G34E in the M2s of Rostock amantadine-resistant mutants, isolated without prior passage in drug (Table 3.1), were shown to reduce the activity of M2 in this assay and to impair virus growth in cell culture[12]. During subsequent passage in the absence or presence of amantadine these mutants either reverted to a wild-type drug-susceptible phenotype or acquired a second mutation in M2 or HA which suppressed or compensated for the attenuating effect of the first mutation[12]. In particular, the amino acid change I27T, which on its own enhanced M2 activity, suppressed the negative effects of the A30T or S31N changes in the double mutants. A mutation in HA which increased its pH stability complemented the reduced activity of the G34E M2 mutant and the consequent lower pH encountered in the *trans* Golgi during transport to the surface of mutant virus-infected cells.

The differential effects of amino acid changes on the properties of M2 proteins was shown clearly by their effects on the proteins of the closely related avian H7 strains Rostock and Weybridge, which differ in six amino acids. The substitution G34E exerted opposite effects, increasing the activity of the Weybridge protein in contrast to its attenuating effect on the Rostock protein. The effects of amino acid substitutions A30T and S31N on the Weybridge M2 protein were neutral. Such differences in the effects of amino acid substitutions on M2 activity can thus in part account for differences observed in the frequency of selection of particular drug-resistance mutations (Table 3.1).

The influence of pH stability of the HA of these viruses on the selection of M2 mutants was clearly illustrated by the effect of a mutation K58I in the HA2 of Rostock which increased its stability by 0.7 pH units[35]. Although partially resistant to amantadine, passage in the presence of drug selected mutations in M2 which conferred complete resistance. In contrast to viruses with wild-type HA, in which mutations in M2 exclusively affected residue 27, the majority of the double mutants contained amino acid substitutions S31N (67%) or A30T (28%) in their M2s (Table 3.1). As the combined effects of the mutation in HA and threonine 30 in M2 was still suboptimal for HA expression, it is apparent that selection of the M2 mutants depended on some other aspect of M2 function, possibly its role in virus uncoating. However, at present we do not know how the properties of M2 relate to the pH of membrane fusion by HA during endocytosis.

The effects of certain mutations on the ion channel activity of the M2 protein of the human virus A/Udorn/72 (H3N2) have been studied directly in X. oocytes[40]. As observed in the 'HA assay' for the Weybridge M2, substitution of serine 31 by asparagine (S3IN) had little effect on the activity of the Udorn M2. This is consistent with the prominence of this resistance determinant in the M2s of drug-resistant mutants of all three human subtypes. Other substitutions, including valine 27 by alanine, serine or threonine, and glycine 34 by glutamic acid, caused some increase in activity, whereas substitution of alanine 30 by threonine caused substantial attenuation of the Udorn M2 protein. Although the latter amino acid substitution has been shown to be responsible for the *in vivo* rimantadine resistance of more recent 1987 and 1988 H3N2 viruses, and the *in vitro* amantadine resistance of the earlier H2N2 Singapore virus (Table 3.1), there are no reports to indicate whether this resistance determinant would be selected in the case of A/Udorn/72. Substitution of threonine for valine 27 in this M2 did not affect its susceptibility to inhibition by amantadine[40], in contrast to the effect of threonine 27 on certain avian virus M2 proteins (Table 3.1).

Thus, from the limited studies to date it is evident that differences between the M2 proteins of different viruses influence the effects of amino acid substitutions on M2 activity, and on its susceptibility to inhibition by amantadine or rimantadine. Other features of the viruses, in particular the HA, can also influence the selection of particular resistance determinants. In this respect the *in vivo* selection of an 'uncommon' substitution, leucine 26 by phenylalanine, in the M2s of certain amantadine-resistant variants of recent human H3N2 viruses[10] would appear to result from some as yet unidentified change during antigenic drift of these viruses. Whether such influences will have an impact on the persistence of the drug-resistance phenotype among different epidemic variants of human viruses should become apparent from future monitoring of the properties of these viruses.

CONCLUSIONS

Amantadine and rimantadine suppress the replication of influenza A viruses by blocking the proton channel activity of the M2 protein. Single amino acid substitutions within the N-terminal half of the transmembrane pore appear to interfere with the interaction of drug with this region of the channel to abrogate an irreversible allosteric block. The effects of these amino acid changes on the ion-conductance and pH-modulating activity of M2, as well as its susceptibility to drug, depend on the primary structure of the protein. More extensive structure–activity investigations should provide a clearer understanding of the mechanism of proton transfer and regulation of ion permeation, and the mechanisms of inhibition of M2 by and resistance to amantadine and rimantadine. This may also prove helpful in developing alternative inhibitors of M2 and potential drugs against other virus ion channels.

REFERENCES

1. Douglas RG Prophylaxis and treatment of influenza. *New Engl J Med* 1990;322:443–50.
2. Davies WL, Grunert RR, Haff RF *et al*. Antiviral activity of 1-adamantanamine (amantadine). *Science* 1964;144:862–3.
3. Hay AJ, Wolstenholme AJ, Skehel JJ, Smith MH. The molecular basis of the specific anti-influenza action of amantadine. *EMBO J* 1985;4:3021–4.
4. Hay AJ. The mechanism of action of amantadine and rimantadine against influenza viruses. In: Notkins AL, Oldstone MBA, eds, *Concepts in Viral Pathogenesis* Vol. III. New York: Springer Verlag, 1989:361–7.
5. Hay AJ, Zambon MC. Multiple actions of amantadine against influenza viruses. In: Becker Y, ed. *Antiviral Drugs and Interferon: the Molecular Basis of their Activity*. Boston: Martinus Nijhoff, 1984:301–15.
6. Appleyard G. Amantadine resistance as a genetic marker for influenza viruses. *J Gen Virol* 1977;36:249–55.

7. Belshe RB, Hall Smith M, Hall CB, Betts R, Hay AJ. Genetic basis of resistance to rimantadine emerging during treatment of influenza virus infection. *J Virol* 1988;62:1508–12.

8. Hayden FG, Belshe RB, Clover RD *et al*. Emergence and apparent transmission of rimantadine-resistant influenza A virus in families. *New Engl J Med* 1989;321:1696–1702.

9. Mast EE, Harmon MW, Gravenstein S *et al*. Emergence and possible transmission of amantadine-resistant viruses during nursing home outbreaks of influenza A (H3N2). *Am J Epidemiol* 1991;134:988–97.

10. Roumillat F, Rocha E, Regnery H, Wells D, Cox N. Emergence of amantadine-resistant influenza A viruses in nursing homes during the 1989–1990 influenza season (abstract p. 34–42). In: *Abstracts of the VIIIth International Congress of Virology, Berlin,* 1990;p.321.

11. Bean WJ, Threlkeld SC, Webster RG. Biologic potential of amantadine-resistant influenza A virus in an avian model. *J Infect Dis* 1989;159:1050–6.

12. Grambas S, Bennett MS, Hay AJ. Influence of amantadine-resistance mutations on the pH regulatory function of the M2 protein of influenza A viruses. *Virology* 1992;191:541–9.

13. Lubeck MD, Schulman JL, Palese P. Susceptibility of influenza A viruses to amantadine is influenced by the gene coding for M protein. *J Virol* 1978;28:710–6.

14. Hay AJ, Kennedy NTC, Skehel JJ, Appleyard G. The matrix protein gene determines amantadine sensitivity of influenza viruses. *J Gen Virol* 1979;42:189–91.

15. Scholtissek C, Faulkner GP. Amantadine-resistant and -sensitive influenza A strains and recombinants. *J Gen Virol* 1979;44:807–15.

16. Hay AJ, Zambon MC, Wolstenholme AJ, Skehel JJ, Smith MH. Molecular basis of resistance of influenza A viruses to amantadine. *J Antimicrob Chemother* 1986;18(Suppl B):19–29.

17. Kendal AP, Klenk HD. Amantadine inhibits an early, M2 protein-dependent event in the replication cycle of avian influenza (H7) viruses. *Arch Virol* 1991;119:265–73.

18. Lamb RA, Lai C-J, Choppin PW. Sequences of mRNAs derived from genome RNA segment 7 of influenza virus: colinear and interrupted mRNAs code for overlapping proteins. *Proc Natl Acad Sci USA* 1981;78:4170–4.

19. Kendal AP. Reference viruses for use in amantadine sensitivity testing of human influenza A viruses. *Antivir Chem Chemother* 1991;2:115–18.

20. Kato N, Eggers HJ. Inhibition of uncoating of fowl plague virus by 1-adamantanamine hydrochloride. *Virology* 1969;37:632–41.

21. Bukrinskaya AG, Vorkunova NK, Kornilayeva GV, Narmanbetova RA, Vorkunova GK. Influenza virus uncoating in infected cells and effect of rimantadine. *J Gen Virol* 1982;60:49–59.

22. Bukrinskaya AG, Vorkunova NK, Pushkarskaya NL. Uncoating of a rimantadine-resistant variant of influenza virus in the presence of rimantadine. *J Gen Virol* 1982;60:61–6.

23. Martin K, Helenius A. Nuclear transport of influenza virus ribonucleoproteins: the viral matrix protein (M1) promotes export and inhibits import. *Cell* 1991;67:117–30.

24. Wiley DC, Skehel JJ. The structure and function of the haemagglutinin membrane glycoprotein of influenza virus. *Annu Rev Biochem* 1987;56:365–94.

25. Wharton SA, Belshe RB, Skehel JJ, Hay AJ. Role of virion M2 protein in influenza virus uncoating: specific reduction in the rate of membrane fusion between virus and liposomes by amantadine. *J Gen Virol* 1994;75:945–8.
26. Zhirnov OP. Solubilization of matrix protein M1/M from virions occurs at different pH for orthomyxo- and paramyxoviruses. *Virology* 1990;176:274–9.
27. Bron R, Kendal AP, Klenk HD, Wilschut J. Role of the M2 protein in influenza virus membrane fusion: effects of amantadine and monensin on fusion kinetics. *Virology* 1993;195:808–11.
28. Sugrue RJ, Bahadur G, Zambon MC *et al*. Specific structural alteration of the influenza haemagglutinin by amantadine. *EMBO J* 1990;9:3469–76.
29. Ruigrok RWH, Hirst EMA, Hay AJ. The specific inhibition of influenza A virus maturation by amantadine: an electron microscopic examination. *J Gen Virol* 1991;72:191–4.
30. Stieneke-Grober A, Vey M, Angliker H *et al*. Influenza virus haemagglutinin with multibasic cleavage site is activated by furin, a subtilisin-like endoprotease. *EMBO J* 1992;11:2407–14.
31. Ciampor F, Bayley PM, Nermut MV *et al*. Evidence that the amantadine-induced, M2-mediated conversion of influenza virus hemagglutinin to the low pH conformation occurs in an acidic *trans* Golgi compartment. *Virology* 1992;188:14–24.
32. Ohuchi M, Cramer A, Vey M *et al*. Rescue of vector-expressed fowl plague virus hemagglutinin in biologically active form by acidotropic agents and coexpressed M2 protein. *J Virol* 1994;68:920–6.
33. Takeuchi K, Lamb RA. Influenza virus M_2 protein ion channel activity stabilizes the native form of fowl plague virus hemagglutinin during intracellular transport. *J Virol* 1994;68:911–19.
34. Grambas S, Hay AJ. Maturation of influenza A virus hemagglutinin— estimates of the pH encountered during transport and its regulation by the M2 protein. *Virology* 1992;190:11–18.
35. Steinhauer DA, Wharton SA, Skehel JJ, Wiley DC, Hay AJ. Amantadine selection of a mutant influenza virus containing an acid-stable hemagglutinin glycoprotein: evidence for virus-specific regulation of the pH of glycoprotein transport vesicles. *Proc Natl Acad Sci USA* 1991;88:11525–9.
36. Ciampor F, Thompson CA, Grambas S, Hay AJ. Regulation of pH by the M2 protein of influenza A viruses. *Virus Res* 1992;22:247–58.
37. Hay AJ, Thompson CA, Geraghty FM *et al*. The role of the M2 protein in influenza A virus infection. In: Hannoun C, Kendal AP, Klenk HD, Ruben FL, eds. *Options for Control of Influenza II*. Amsterdam: Excepta Medica, 1993:281–8.
38. Schroeder C, Ford CM, Wharton SA, Hay AJ. Functional reconstitution in lipid vesicles of influenza virus M2 protein expressed by baculovirus: evidence for proton transfer activity. *J Gen Virol* 1994;75:3477–84.
39. Pinto LH, Holsinger LJ, Lamb RA. Influenza virus M2 protein has ion channel activity. *Cell* 1992;69:517–28.
40. Holsinger LJ, Nichani D, Pinto LH, Lamb RA. Influenza A virus M_2 ion channel protein: a structure–function analysis. *J Virol* 1994;68:1551–63.
41. Wang C, Takeuchi K, Pinto LH, Lamb RA. Ion channel activity of influenza A virus M_2 protein: characterization of the amantadine block. *J Virol* 1993;67:5585–94.
42. Wang C, Lamb RA, Pinto LH. Direct measurement of the influenza A virus M_2 protein ion channel activity in mammalian cells. *Virology* 1994;205:133–40.

43. Chizhmakov IV, Geraghty FM, Ogden DC *et al*. Selective proton permeability and pH regulation of the influenza virus M2 channel expressed in mouse erythroleukaemia cells. 1996. *J Physiol*, in press.
44. Tosteson MT, Pinto LH, Holsinger LJ, Lamb RA. Reconstitution of the influenza virus M_2 ion channel in lipid bilayers. *J Membrane Biol* 1994;142:117–26.
45. Sugrue RJ, Hay AJ. Structural characteristics of the M2 protein of influenza A viruses: evidence that it forms a tetrameric channel. *Virology* 1991;180:617–24.
46. Holsinger LJ, Lamb RA. Influenza virus M_2 integral membrane protein is a homotetramer stabilized by formation of disulfide bonds. *Virology* 1991;183:32–43.
47. Duff KC, Gilchrist PJ, Saxena AM, Bradshaw JP. Neutron diffraction reveals the site of amantadine blockade in the influenza A M2 ion channel. *Virology* 1994;202:287–93.
48. Duff KC, Ashley RH. The transmembrane domain of influenza A M2 protein forms amantadine-sensitive proton channels in planar lipid bilayers. *Virology* 1992;190:485–9.
49. Sansom MSP, Kerr ID. Influenza virus M2 protein: a molecular modelling study of the ion channel. *Protein Eng* 1993;6:65–74.
50. Beard CW, Brugh M, Webster RG. Emergence of amantadine-resistant H5N2 avian influenza virus during a simulated layer flock treatment program. *Avian Dis* 1987;31:533–7.
51. Sweet C, Hayden FG, Jakeman KJ, Grambas S, Hay AJ. Virulence of rimantadine-resistant human influenza A (H3N2) viruses in ferrets. *J Infect Dis* 1991;164:969–72.

4
Amantadine and Rimantadine—Clinical Aspects

FREDERICK G. HAYDEN

INTRODUCTION

Shortly after the recognition of the anti-influenza activity of amantadine in 1963, studies by Neumayer et al.[1], Grunert et al.[2] and Schild et al.[3] found that influenza A viruses manifested a wide range of susceptibilities to amantadine, both in cell culture and in experimentally infected mice. Certain laboratory-passaged strains (e.g. A/PR8, A/NWS) appeared to be much less susceptible. Development of resistance to the antiviral action of these drugs was demonstrated in 1965, when Cochran et al.[4] reported that an influenza A/Japan/305 (H2N2) strain became insensitive to amantadine following one multiple-cycle passage in the presence of the drug *in vitro*. In contrast, Oxford et al.[5] reported that *in vitro* growth of several influenza A viruses did not lead to the emergence of resistance during three to five passages in the presence of high concentrations of amantadine (50 μg/ml). However, passage of an influenza A/Singapore/1/57 virus in amantadine-treated mice led to selection of a resistant variant with approximately 50-fold reduction of susceptibility *in vitro*. These workers[5] commented that it would be 'of particular interest to determine whether such increased drug resistance occurs in field trials of amantadine in man'.

In 1977 Appleyard[6] demonstrated that coinfection of eggs, cell cultures or mice with sensitive and resistant viruses resulted in the transfer of resistance between strains. This occurred in an all-or-nothing manner independent of the surface antigens of the viruses. Drug-resistant variants were estimated to occur with a frequency of approximately one to four

Antiviral Drug Resistance. Edited by Douglas D. Richman © 1996 John Wiley & Sons Ltd

per 10^{-4} in cell culture-grown virus populations[6,7]. Subsequent work determined that resistance was transferable by genetic reassortment of RNA gene segment 7 (M gene) between sensitive and resistant strains[7,8]. The M2 protein was established as the target of the specific anti-influenza A actions of these drugs[9,10]. As reviewed by Hay (Chapter 3), resistance to amantadine and rimantadine results from point mutations leading to single amino acid substitutions in the membrane-spanning portion of the M2 protein. The anti-influenza action of these agents in blocking the ion channel function of M2 is lost in resistant variants.

Over the past decade recovery of drug-resistant human viruses has been documented in certain patients receiving rimantadine or amantadine[11-14], their contacts[14-17], and less often in non-treated persons[18-20]. As discussed by Bean et al.[21], relevant variables regarding the importance of drug resistance include the frequency and rapidity of resistance emergence; the genetic stability, transmissibility and pathogenicity of resistant variants; and their ability to compete epidemiologically with wild-type viruses in the absence of selective drug pressure. Based on previous reviews of this topic[22-25], this chapter describes methods for assay of virus susceptibility and reviews information available from animal models and human studies that address the biologic characteristics of resistant viruses and the correlations of these factors with particular resistance mutations.

IN VITRO ASSAYS OF DRUG SUSCEPTIBILITY

Phenotypic assays

Most resistant variants of influenza A virus are totally insensitive to the selective action of low concentrations of these drugs ($\leqslant 1$ μg/ml), although their replication may be inhibited by the non-specific action of higher drug concentrations ($\geqslant 10$ μg/ml) in cell culture[10,14]. The threshold concentration of 1 μg/ml also corresponds with the maximal concentrations achievable in blood and respiratory secretions during clinical use at tolerable doses[26]. Interestingly, viruses exhibit cross-susceptibility or cross-resistance to amantadine, rimantadine and related drugs such as cyclo-octylamine[27,28].

Various *in vitro* assays have been used to assess drug susceptibility (Table 4.1). These range considerably in their labor-intensiveness and the time required for completion. Some require prior titration of virus pools to standardize virus inocula, whereas others have been adapted to incorporate a broad range of inoculum sizes. Certain older assays, such as the egg-bit method described by Pemberton et al.[19], or the hemadsorption reduction test used by Heider et al.[20], gave poor drug concentration–

Table 4.1 Representative in vitro susceptibility assays for influenza A viruses to amantadine and rimantadine

Assay type	Cell culture	Multiplicity of infection	Endpoint	Approximate time (days)
Endpoint infectivity[3]	Monkey kidney Chick embryo	Variable	Titer reduction by fixed drug concentration	6–10
Virus yield[7]	MDCK	Low (0.005)	HA titer	1–2
Plaque inhibition[6,27,27a]	Chick embryo	Low ($<10^{-3}$)	Plaque count	3–5
Plaque inhibition[7,29,30]	MDCK	Low ($<10^{-3}$)	Plaque count	2–4
Quantitative[19,28] hemadsorption	BSC-1	High (~10)	OD of hemolyzed GP RBC	1
Hemadsorption[20] reduction test	Ehrlich ascites tumor	0.05	Counting of hemadsorbed GP RBC	2
ELISA-strain specific[12,31,32]	MDCK	Low (variable)	OD	2
ELISA-type specific[33]	Chick embryo	High (variable)	OD	1
ELISA-type specific[15,17,18]	MDCK	Low (variable)	OD	2

GP, guinea pig; MDCK, Madin Darby canine kidney; OD, optical density

response effects and hence potentially ambiguous results. A plaque inhibition assay in chick embryo fibroblasts gave poor correlations with inhibition observed in eggs and *in vivo*[27a]. In contrast, enzyme-linked immunoassays (ELISA), which measure the expression of viral hemagglutinin[12,14,31,32] or the type-specific ribonucleoprotein or matrix protein[15,17,18], provide sensitive assays for amantadine and rimantadine susceptibility. In general, these assays utilize overnight growth of varying viral inocula in the presence of fixed drug concentrations. Their results have been correlated with the presence of specific M2 mutations by RNA sequence analysis of resistant variants. However, the endpoints in this type of assay are significantly influenced by the input virus titer and the type of host cell. For example, Valette *et al.*[32] found that inhibitory concentrations for recent H3N2 subtype viruses averaged approximately 100-fold higher in Vero than in MDCK cell monolayers. Type-specific ELISA in MDCK cells currently appears to have the broadest applicability among assays which have been validated by genotypic analysis.

Genotypic assays

RNA sequence analyses of numerous influenza A viruses have found that resistance results from single nucleotide substitutions in amino acids 26, 27, 30, 31 or 34 of the M2 protein[9,10]. Most resistant isolates contain a single amino acid change, although mixed populations with different resistance mutations and variants with dual mutations have been described[12,21]. Several different amino acid changes have been recognized at certain positions (e.g. Ala → Val or Thr at position 30). Usually, genotypic changes have been determined by sequence analysis of RNA segment 7 by the dideoxynucleotide chain termination method using ^{32}P-labeled oligonucleotide primers. Recently, Klimov *et al.*[34] have described detection of resistant variants by reverse transcription polymerase chain reaction amplification of the M gene coding for the transmembrane domain of M2, followed by restriction analysis with a series of enzymes that distinguish between nucleotide sequences corresponding to wild-type or resistance mutations at individual codons of interest (26, 27, 30 or 31). Genotypic analysis has also provided a marker for epidemiologic studies of virus transmission.

DRUG RESISTANCE IN ANIMAL MODELS OF INFLUENZA

Experimental murine influenza

Early studies assessed the potential for the emergence of resistance in experimentally induced infections in mice[5,28,35]. These studies utilized a mouse-adapted human strain, A/Singapore/1/57 (H2N2) virus. Pheno-typic resistance was determined by the quantitative hemadsorption assay. Oxford *et al.*[35] found that partial resistance was detectable after one passage and complete after three passages in mice. The resistance phenotype was associated with 100-fold or greater reductions of susceptibility *in vitro*. This resistance was stable with passage in the absence of amantadine *in vitro*. In other studies, Oxford and Potter[28] found that the emergence of resistance usually required two or three passages in mice. This selection for resistance required treatment of mice with large amantadine doses (150 mg/kg/day intraperitoneally and in drinking water); it did not occur with 10- or 100-fold lower doses. Earlier studies by Grunert *et al.*[2] had failed to detect the emergence of resistance after passage of influenza A/Swine/S15 virus seven times in mice treated intraperitoneally with 30 mg/kg amantadine. Oxford and Potter[28] also found that the resistant H2N2 variant induced lung lesions in mice irrespective of the presence or absence of amantadine treatment. Thus, the resistance phenotype was expressed *in vivo* as well as in cell culture. Moreover, the resistant variant appeared to replicate and produce disease as well as the parental strain. These studies indicated that highly resistant variants, which appeared to be virulent and stable, could emerge rapidly in experimentally infected mice and that the degree of selective drug pressure appeared to be an important variable.

Experimental avian influenza

Considerable work on drug resistance has been performed in an experimental chicken model of influenza[21,36,37]. This avian model utilizes a virulent A/chicken/Penn/1370/83 (H5N2) virus that replicates primarily in the gastrointestinal and respiratory tracts of infected birds and subsequently spreads to multiple organs, typically causing fatal disease. Webster *et al.*[36] and Beard *et al.*[37] found that therapeutic administration of amantadine (0.01% in drinking water) starting one or two days and, to a lesser extent three days, after infection reduced mortality. These workers also found that prophylactic drug administration begun at the time of viral challenge prevented the early onset of illness, but also reduced humoral immune responses. Beard *et al.*[37] also found that late deaths occurred in about 40% of birds, and this was associated in one instance with the recovery of resistant virus. This may have resulted from the emergence of resistant virus or its transmission from other amantadine-treated birds to susceptible contacts. The resistant variant was as virulent as the sensitive parental virus when inoculated into birds, and amantadine administration did not reduce its lethality[37]. Resistance emergence has been documented during amantadine prophylaxis with another H5 subtype virus[27a].

Subsequently, Bean et al.[21] showed that drug-resistant virus was shed in respiratory secretions as early as two days, and in feces by three days, after initiating amantadine treatment of infected birds (0.1% or ~4 mg/kg/day in drinking water). The duration of shedding resistant variants extended up to 14 days after inoculation. Despite the recovery of resistant variants, amantadine treatment was therapeutically effective. These variants had M2 amino acid substitutions at positions 27 Ile → Thr or Ser, 30 Ala → Thr or Ser, and/or 31 Ser → Asn of the M2 protein, similar to human variants. These workers also determined the relative virulence of resistant strains by inoculating selected sensitive and resistant isolates into birds receiving no treatment[21]. All isolates of resistant or sensitive strains caused infection and illness, and the resistant ones ranged from being partially to fully virulent, as judged by mortality rates (17–83%), compared to those observed following inoculation of sensitive strains (34–83%). In a confirmation of *in vitro* resistance they also showed that mortality due to infection by one resistant variant was not affected by amantadine administration.

Under conditions designed to reflect natural virus transmission in flocks, Webster et al.[36] found that all birds receiving amantadine or rimantadine prophylaxis (0.01% in drinking water) and remaining in close contact with drug-treated infected birds, became infected. Of these 50% became ill and 36% developed fatal infections caused by drug-resistant virus during the second and third weeks after exposure. In comparison, all untreated contacts of untreated birds infected with sensitive virus had illness and died within one week of exposure. The untreated infected donors also died, whereas drug-treated infected donor birds recovered with treatment. These results indicated transmission of resistant virus from treated infected birds to contacts; the possible importance of drug prophylaxis for contact birds was not assessed independently. However, the net outcomes suggested that drug use was superior to no therapy. In addition, Webster et al.[36] found that immunization at the time of exposure did not reduce mortality when used alone in contacts, but it was protective when used in conjunction with amantadine prophylaxis. This was probably due to an initial drug-related delay in viral transmission until an immune response to vaccine could provide protection, or possibly due to interference between the sensitive and resistant populations[27a].

Bean et al.[21] assessed the ability of drug-resistant virus to compete with sensitive wild-type virus for transmission in the absence of selective drug pressure. Birds shedding resistant virus were mixed with those shedding wild-type virus and with non-infected, untreated contact birds. After three days the latter group was removed and placed with another group of non-infected contacts; this process was repeated for three additional exposures.

In three of four experiments extending over a two-week period, resistant virus could still be recovered from some or all of the final group of contact birds. Thus, resistant strains of the H5N2 subtype of avian influenza virus retained resistance during multiple passages *in vivo*. An obvious selective advantage for transmission in the absence of selective drug pressure was not apparent for either wild-type or resistant virus[21]. In summary, these studies with experimental avian influenza showed that drug-resistant strains emerged rapidly during treatment, were transmissible to contacts, were genetically stable, and were capable of competing with wild-type virus for transmission in the absence of selective drug pressure. Moreover, such resistant variants remained pathogenic.

Experimental ferret influenza

As discussed above, drug-resistant viruses appear to retain virulence in animal model studies involving direct inoculation of resistant avian or mouse-adapted human strains. Sweet *et al.*[38] assessed the virulence in ferrets of resistant isolates of the H3N2 subtype of human influenza A virus. These variants contained defined amino acid changes at positions 27, 30 or 31 of the M2 protein[38]. When inoculated intranasally, the drug-resistant viruses replicated to the same extent and induced the same magnitude of fever and nasal cellular inflammatory responses in the ferrets as their drug-sensitive parental strains. No obvious differences in replicative capacity or virulence were found between the wild-type viruses and the corresponding resistant variants.

Genotype-related differences in resistant variants

In general, the results of animal model studies indicate that drug-resistant variants are transmissible to susceptible hosts and replicate and induce disease with efficiencies comparable to those of parental drug-sensitive virus. These findings suggest that viral virulence is not linked directly to amantadine resistance[21]. However, limited information has been developed about the characteristics and replication fitness of specific genotypes conferring resistance. Studies of amantadine-resistant variants of certain H7 avian viruses *in vitro* have shown that certain mutations in M2 (e.g. 30 Ala → Thr or 31 Ser → Asn), which do not affect the growth properties of resistant variants of H3 human or H5 avian viruses, do affect replication in cell culture and are associated with reversion to wild-type or selection of a compensatory M2 mutation during extended passage in the absence of the drug[9]. Thus, particular resistance mutations may not be equally tolerated by different influenza A strains.

DRUG RESISTANCE IN HUMAN INFLUENZA

Surveillance of epidemic human strains

During nearly three decades of limited amantadine and rimantadine use in humans, naturally occurring epidemic strains of influenza A viruses have generally remained sensitive to inhibition by these drugs. Contemporary pandemic strains have been drug sensitive[29,30], and surveys of epidemic isolates have found infrequent evidence of drug resistance in viruses recovered from untreated patients (Table 4.2). Certain highly passaged laboratory strains of H1N1 subtype virus (e.g. A/PR/8/34, A/WSN/33) are resistant; however, the mechanism by which resistance was acquired is unclear. Although the parental strains were initially isolated before the use of the drugs, these viruses are phenotypically resistant and contain sequence changes in the M2 gene that confer resistance (position 31 Ser → Asn)[39]. In addition, an unpublished report indicates that multiple H1N1 subtype strains initially isolated during 1933–1945, decades before the use of amantadine, also had drug resistance associated with position 31 Ser → Asn mutations in M2[40]. However, animal influenza viruses recovered during this time have not contained this M2 mutation[39]. If these observations of circulation of resistant variants are confirmed, they would suggest that some resistant viruses may be capable of extensive transmission in the absence of selective drug pressure.

More recently, several reports of resistant viruses recovered from non-drug exposed persons have appeared, although they have not been substantiated by genotypic analysis[19,20]. In unpublished studies employing both phenotypic and genotypic assays, Ziegler et al.[18] found that 0.8% of 855 clinical isolates recovered from untreated patients during the 1990–1992 influenza seasons were resistant. Houck et al.[17] described a nursing home resident who developed illness due to a resistant variant (position 31 Ser → Asn) without any recognized exposure to either amantadine or rimantadine. These findings also suggest the potential for a low frequency of de novo resistance among influenza A viruses. The failure to recover naturally occurring drug-resistant strains more often indicates that drug resistance does not confer any selective advantage. Whether it reduces viral fitness for survival on a sustained basis in the human population has not been established.

Emergence of resistance during treatment

Several studies have determined the frequency of recovery of drug-resistant virus from individuals receiving rimantadine treatment for

Table 4.2 Susceptibility testing of contemporary epidemic strains of influenza A virus

Assay	Period of collection	Subtype	No. tested isolates	Inhibitory concentration[a] (μg/ml)	Percent sensitive
Quantitative hemadsorption[28]	1968	H3N2	30	0.02–0.26	100
Plaque inhibition[29]	1975–77	H1N1	7	0.1 –0.3	100
Hemadsorption reduction[20]	1980	H3N2	21	0.01–1.0	90.5
ELISA[b][31]	1978–88	H1N1	65	0.1	100
		H3N2	181	0.1 –1.0	97.2[c]
ELISA[b][14]	1987–89	H1N1	11	0.1	100
		H3N2	107	0.1 –1.0	85.1[c]
ELISA[32]	1988–90	H1N1	28	0.02–0.1	100
		H3N2	77	<0.01–0.5	100
ELISA[b][18]	1991–93	Not specified	855	1.0	99.2

[a] The range of reported inhibitory concentrations depended on the assay method utilized. Some assays used several fixed concentrations
[b] Phenotypic resistance confirmed by sequencing of M2 gene
[c] Resistant isolates recovered from family members receiving rimantadine for treatment or prophylaxis

infection with the H3N2 subtype of influenza A virus. Hall *et al.*[11] found that 27% of 37 rimantadine-treated children, and 45% of those who were virus positive after the fourth treatment day, shed a resistant virus. Hayden *et al.*[14] found that 29% of adults or children receiving rimantadine therapy shed resistant virus on the fifth day of treatment. In elderly institutionalized adults, 11% of 26 rimantadine recipients and 27% of those shedding virus four days or later into therapy, had drug-resistant isolates (R. Betts, personal communication). In ambulatory adults with uncomplicated influenza, Hayden *et al.*[41] found that shedding of resistant virus was often detectable by the third day of rimantadine treatment. Several instances of resistance emergence with 48 hours of initiating treatment have been documented[17,41]. These findings indicate that resistant variants can replace sensitive strains rapidly during treatment, and that the recovery of resistant viruses is frequently associated with therapeutic use of these drugs in both children and adults.

In children Hall *et al.*[11] found that shedding of resistant virus may continue for up to seven days, whereas Hayden *et al.*[14] found that those who shed resistant virus on the fifth treatment day were negative for virus by the tenth treatment day. However, these trials have not definitively assessed the duration of shedding of resistant virus and the potential risk period for transmitting infection due to such strains. Although immunocompetent hosts have not had shedding of resistant variants documented after 10 days, prolonged shedding of resistant virus has been found in several immunocompromised transplant patients, one of whom shed virus for several months while on amantadine[34].

It is unknown to what extent virus (strain or subtype), host (age, immunosuppression) and possibly drug (dose, duration of exposure) factors contribute to the emergence of drug-resistant viruses. Kubar *et al.*[42] noted that the percentage of drug-resistant variants isolated in the former Soviet Union was 4.7% for H1N1 subtype viruses but 40.1% for H3N2 subtype viruses. Higher levels and prolonged duration of viral replication probably enhance the likelihood of selecting resistant variants, but the risk factors for shedding of resistant variants have not been defined. In particular, the variables of treatment dose or duration have not been studied in clinical trials, and no direct comparisons of the frequency of resistance emergence have been made between amantadine and rimantadine, although it has occurred during use of both drugs.

Emergence of resistant virus in humans, as in animals, during treatment has not been linked to clinical deterioration in studies to date. Hall *et al.*[11] found that rimantadine-treated children experienced significantly greater reductions in fever and illness severity during the first three days of treatment than those receiving acetaminophen. When the rimantadine recipients who shed resistant virus were compared to those who did not, the illness severity scores tended to be higher later in therapy in those shedding resistant virus, but the differences were considered too small to be clinically discernable. Hayden *et al.*[41], found that rimantadine recipients shedding resistant virus, who accounted for approximately one-third of rimantadine-treated patients, tended to have slower resolution of illness than rimantadine recipients who did not shed resistant virus. No worsening of illness was observed in association with recovery of resistant virus. Kubar *et al.*[42] also reported that the therapeutic response to rimantadine was independent of recovery of resistant or sensitive virus. These studies indicate that rimantadine retains a net therapeutic benefit compared to placebo, despite recovery of resistant virus from a portion of treated patients during the late stages of illness[41]. It remains unclear whether a causal relationship exists between the recovery of resistant virus and prolongation of illness.

Transmissibility of resistant strains in families

Family-based studies have assessed whether amantadine or rimantadine given as prophylaxis for 10 days prevents the development of influenza A virus illness in household contacts exposed to ill family members. In the initial trial conducted during an H2N2 subtype epidemic, Galbraith *et al.*[43] found complete protection of household contacts against influenza A illness with amantadine prophylaxis when ill index cases did not receive concurrent treatment. The same investigators found only 20% protective efficacy during an H3N2 subtype pandemic in the following year[44]. In the second trial both the epidemic strain, against which most contacts had low antibody titers, and the study design, which incorporated treatment of the ill index cases, were different. During an H1N1 subtype epidemic Bricaire *et al.*[45] found that postexposure prophylaxis with rimantadine provided 69% protection against clinical influenza in a study in which ill index cases were not treated. In contrast, during an H3N2 subtype epidemic Hayden *et al.*[14] found that laboratory-proven influenza virus illness occurred in about one-third of either placebo or rimantadine households, and in about one-fifth of contacts in such households. The calculated efficacy of rimantadine for postcontact prophylaxis was only 3%, and secondary illnesses caused by apparent transmission of drug-resistant virus were found in five rimantadine-treated families, in four of which the ill index case was a young child.

Although these studies are not directly comparable, the results suggest that the presence of a treated index case was an important variable in regard to reduced postcontact prophylactic efficacy. Both rimantadine[45] and amantadine[43] appear to be effective for postexposure prophylaxis in families when index cases are not treated. In contrast, the reduced efficacy observed in studies employing treatment of index cases[14,44] supports the conclusion that transmission of resistant virus can occur when these drugs are used concurrently for both treatment of ill index cases and prophylaxis of contacts. However, the effect of treatment of index cases on postexposure prophylactic efficacy has not been directly assessed in trials involving random assignment of index cases and separate assignment of contacts to receive drug or placebo. Employing another strategy, Couch et al.[41] found that treatment of ill index cases with amantadine or rimantadine, without prophylaxis of contacts, reduced the likelihood of secondary, laboratory-documented infection by 32% in untreated family contacts. However, this trial did not determine whether family contacts who developed infection after exposure to drug-treated index cases had resistant virus.

Transmissibility of resistant strains in nursing homes

Transmission of resistant influenza viruses has been implicated by the recovery of resistant virus from prophylaxis failures in several nursing home outbreaks in which amantadine was used for both prophylaxis and treatment[15-17,47]. In studying two nursing home outbreaks, Mast et al.[15] found that clinical influenza developed in 10% of 191 amantadine prophylaxis recipients in one home and 4% of 338 in another. Influenza-specific illness was documented in approximately 2% of each prophylaxis group, and six cases of prophylaxis failure were proved to have resistant virus. Five of these cases resided in one home and included three patients living in contiguous rooms and sharing the same dining facility, who developed influenza over a five-day period. These three prophylaxis failures had infection with a resistant virus containing a relatively uncommon mutation in the M2 protein (position 27 Val $\rightarrow$ Ala). In another nursing home outbreak, Degelau et al.[16] found that 7% of 126 residents developed the illness despite amantadine prophylaxis, and three patients had infection with resistant virus. All three had pneumonia, and one unimmunized patient died following infection. Exposure to treated index cases was implicated in the prophylaxis failures. The isolation of treated index cases in another home was associated with the absence of late prophylaxis failures[16]. Breakthrough illness associated with recovery of resistant virus has been documented as late as the second week after initiating prophylaxis. Recently, Houck et al.[17] found prophylaxis failures in several nursing homes using amantadine, in one of which 5% of recipients had clinical influenza and 2% drug-resistant infections, although transmission of resistant virus was not documented. The novel observation of this study was the recovery of a resistant virus from one resident before any drug use at the facility.

Virulence in humans

Patients who have developed influenza associated with the recovery of resistant virus despite receiving drug prophylaxis have generally had typical influenzal illness[14-17,31]. In families, the contact cases with drug-resistant infection experienced illnesses that were influenzal in character and associated with fever and restricted activity[14]. Several nursing home residents have had lower respiratory tract complications[15-17]. Illness due to infection by resistant variants has been recognized with five different M2 protein substitutions (Table 4.3), but it is uncertain whether any particular M2 mutation is associated with altered virulence. The frequency and spectrum of illness following infection by resistant variants is uncertain, partly because those with milder degrees of illness may not have been cultured for virus in some studies. No obvious difference in viral pathogenicity has yet been found for drug-resistant human influenza viruses but, importantly, no evidence suggests that infections due to resistant viruses are more severe than those caused by wild-type strains.

Genotype-related differences in resistant variants

The relationship between particular mutations in M2 and the biologic characteristics of drug-resistant human influenza viruses has been little

Table 4.3 *M2 mutations in drug-resistant influenza A (H3N2) viruses recovered from untreated persons or from those receiving amantadine or rimantadine for prophylaxis or treatment*

	M2 protein substitution				
No. of persons[a]	26 Leu → Phe	27 Val → Ala	30 Ala → Thr	30 Ala → Val	31 Ser → Asn
Treatment[12,14,17,34,41]	1	1	2	3	16
Prophylaxis failure					
Household[14]	0	0	0	1	4
Nursing home[15-17,47]	2	3	1	1	7
No drug exposure[19]	0	0	0	0	8
Total	3	4	3	5	35

[a] The total number of persons studied was 48. This listing includes two treated patients who had two different mutations recognized in serial samples[34]

studied. Resistance appears to be a stable property, as human variants of various genotypes remain resistant after multiple passages *in vitro* in the absence of drug pressure. Clinical studies have generally found that once shedding of resistant virus develops, subsequent isolates are also resistant[11,14,34,41]. However, a switch from one resistance genotype to another has been found in two immunocompromised hosts being treated with amantadine[34]. This raises the possibility that certain resistance genotypes are more replication competent.

As shown in Table 4.3, the most common mutation detected, particularly during therapeutic use, has been Ser → Asn at position 31. This is also the most common mutation among resistant viruses recovered from both family members and nursing home residents failing drug prophylaxis. However, prophylaxis failures have also been associated with recovery of viral isolates with resistance mutations at other positions in M2. Overall, 70% of 50 sequenced resistant human isolates from 48 patients receiving treatment, prophylaxis or no drug exposure, have had the position 31 Ser → Asn change. These findings, and the earlier observation that H1N1 subtype viruses with position 31 Ser → Asn mutations may have circulated for an extended period[40], suggest that this resistance genotype may be the most fit with regard to transmission.

Changes at each of four positions in M2 have been associated with influenza-like illness, but insufficient data exist to determine whether any particular type of mutation is associated with a lower risk of transmission or reduced pathogenicity. As indicated above, studies of human influenza A/H3N2 viruses with different M2 changes (positions 27, 30 or 31) in ferrets found that the resistant variants were as virulent as the corresponding drug-sensitive parental isolates[38].

Epidemiologic issues

The public health importance of drug resistance in influenza viruses remains uncertain. These viruses appear to possess the biologic characteristics associated with clinically important resistance, but little information is available to judge their actual impact. Monto and Arden[48], Hayden and Couch[24] and others have voiced opinions regarding the implications of resistance and indications for restrictions on drug use. In this regard, Kubar *et al.*[43] have concluded that the efficacy of rimantadine was undiminished in the former Soviet Union despite two decades of use. Some experts have proposed that amantadine and rimantadine be restricted to use during a pandemic or major epidemic for which vaccines were not available, to prophylactic administration only, or to use in high-risk individuals only. However, marked restrictions because of theoretical concerns would negate the proven prophylactic and therapeutic value of these drugs[26,49] and would not guarantee that resistant viruses would not emerge. Further studies are needed to understand the impact of the emergence of drug-resistant viruses and to develop methods to reduce the likelihood of their transmission. Immunization remains the principal means of influenza prevention.

The apparent transmission of drug-resistant influenza virus has been recognized to occur in certain epidemiologic situations involving close contact between treated ill persons and those receiving prophylaxis. As discussed previously by Belshe *et al.*[12,31] and Hayden and Couch[24], the seasonal epidemiology of influenza infections includes immune selection of antigenic variants and the disappearance of previously circulating strains. This process would serve to reduce the likelihood of resistant epidemic strains emerging and disseminating widely, partly because such viruses would probably need alterations in the genes coding for the hemagglutinin and the M2 protein. Although it is unlikely, if an M gene coding for resistance emerged or was introduced into a geographic location where a new epidemic strain developed, resistant virus could disseminate widely in theory. However, it is unknown whether resistant human influenza viruses would be stable and able to compete with wild-type virus for transmission in nature without selective drug pressure, although these features have been documented in short-term studies of experimental avian influenza[21], and possibly in naturally resistant human H1N1 subtype strains[40]. It is also unknown what degree of selective drug pressure would be necessary to cause substantial transmission of resistant viruses during a community epidemic.

The emergence of drug-resistant influenza viruses during an epidemic could pose clinical problems under conditions when such viruses could infect those at increased risk of complications. In particular, nosocomial transmission of resistant virus is a concern for susceptible high-risk contacts in hospitals and chronic care facilities. When nursing home outbreaks have been managed by both mass chemoprophylaxis and treatment of ill patients and staff, transmission of resistant virus appears to have resulted in prophylaxis failures in some instances[15-17,47]. However, the extent of this problem is unclear. To reduce the spread of infection and possible transmission of resistant virus, isolation and cohorting of ill persons appears important. The Advisory Committee on Immunization Practices[50] has recommended that contact between persons taking amantadine or rimantadine for prophylaxis and those taking the drug for treatment be minimized in closed institutional populations. In an outbreak situation, Gomolin *et al.*[51] have recommended that residents with influenzal illness be confined to their rooms for at least three days, that non-ill residents be discouraged from leaving their unit of the facility, that facility-wide or multiunit activities be postponed for at least three days or decentralized, and that ill visitors be excluded from the home. In addition, ill care workers need to be restricted from direct patient contact and, if possible, well staff should avoid working in multiple units[51].

The risk of infection in families relates predominantly to exposure to infected children. Available evidence suggests that avoiding treatment of ill index cases, in particular young children, would markedly reduce the risk of transmission of resistant virus to contacts[14]. The apparent prolongation of viral shedding observed in young children treated with rimantadine[11] may contribute to their higher risk of transmitting resistant virus in families. A study to determine whether an abbreviated course of treatment can provide clinical benefit and reduce the likelihood of shedding of resistant variants is currently in progress in children. Although no higher risk of illness is present in households where the drugs are used for both prophylaxis and therapy, concurrent treatment of young children and prophylaxis of contacts is probably not warranted. In particular, to minimize the possibility of illness due to resistant virus in high-risk susceptible contacts, they should receive prophylaxis without treatment of ill index cases. Another approach is to treat the ill index case without providing prophylaxis to the contacts. This approach provides therapeutic benefit to the treated individual, avoidance of drug side effects in contacts, and a possible reduction in transmission owing to the antiviral effects of the drugs[46]. Because this strategy could also be associated with transmission of resistant virus, illnesses in some contacts might not be amenable to therapy with these drugs.

SUMMARY

Amantadine- and rimantadine-resistant viruses have been recovered from up to 30% of children and adults treated for acute H3N2 subtype influenza. Treatment is accompanied by clinical benefits, despite the recovery of resistant virus from some treated patients. Failures of drug prophylaxis with illness due to apparent transmission of resistant virus have occurred in household contacts receiving rimantadine and nursing home residents receiving amantadine. Limited clinical data indicate that resistant viruses can emerge rapidly during drug therapy, as early as two to three days into treatment, that resistant viruses are stable, and that they cause typical influenza in contacts. It is unknown whether resistant human viruses are capable of competing with wild-type ones during multiple cycles of transmission in the absence of selective drug pressure. The available data indicate that the risks of emergence of resistant virus do not outweigh the documented benefits of drug prophylaxis and therapy in most circumstances. However, the emergence of drug-resistant influenza viruses appears to pose potential clinical problems in certain epidemiologic situations involving close contact with treated patients. Continued surveillance of the drug susceptibility of isolates needs to be maintained.

REFERENCES

1. Neumayer EM, Haff RF, Hoffmann CE. Antiviral activity of amantadine hydrochloride in tissue culture and in ovo. *PSEBM* 1965;119:393–6.
2. Grunert RR, McGahen JW, Davies WL. The *in vivo* antiviral activity of 1-adamantanamine (amantadine). *Virology* 1965;26:262–9.
3. Schild GC, Sutton RNP. Inhibition of influenza viruses *in vitro* and *in vivo* by 1-adamantanamine hydrochloride. *Br J Exp Pathol* 1965;46:263–73.
4. Cochran KW, Maassab HF, Tsunoda A, Berlin BS. Studies on the antiviral activity of amantadine hydrochloride. *Ann N Y Acad Sci* 1965;130:432–9.
5. Oxford JS, Logan IS, Potter CW. Passage of influenza strains in the presence of aminoadamantane. *Ann N Y Acad Sci* 1970;173:300–13.
6. Appleyard G. Amantadine resistance as a genetic marker for influenza viruses. *J Gen Virol* 1977;36:249–55.
7. Lubeck MD, Schulman JL, Palese P. Susceptibility of influenza A viruses to amantadine is influenced by the gene coding for M protein. *J Virol* 1978;28:710–16.
8. Hay AJ, Kennedy NTC, Skehel JJ, Appleyard G. The matrix protein gene determines amantadine sensitivity of influenza viruses. *J Gen Virol* 1979;42:189–91.
9. Hay AJ, Grambas S, Bennett MS. Resistance of influenza A viruses to amantadine and rimantadine. In: A Kumar, ed. *Advances in Molecular Biology and Targeted Treatment for AIDS*. New York: Plenum Press, 1991:345–53.
10. Hay AJ. The action of adamantanamines against influenza A viruses: inhibition of the M2 ion channel protein. *Semin Virol* 1992;3:21–30.
11. Hall CB, Dolin R, Gala CL et al. Children with influenza A infection: treatment with rimantadine. *Pediatrics* 1987;80:275–82.
12. Belshe RB, Smith MH, Hall CB, Betts R, Hay AJ. Genetic basis of resistance to rimantadine emerging during treatment of influenza virus infection. *J Virol* 1988;62:1508–12.
13. Thompson J, Fleet W, Lawrence E et al. A comparison of acetaminophen and rimantadine in the treatment of influenza A infection in children. *J Med Virol* 1987;21:249–55.
14. Hayden FG, Belshe RB, Clover RD et al. Emergence and apparent transmission of rimantadine-resistant influenza A virus in families. *New Engl J Med* 1989;321:1696–702.
15. Mast EE, Harmon MW, Gravenstein S et al. Emergence and possible transmission of amantadine-resistant viruses during nursing home outbreaks of influenza A (H3N2). *Am J Epidemiol* 1991;134:988–97.
16. Degelau J, Somani SK, Cooper SL, Guay DRP, Crossley KB. Amantadine-resistant influenza A in a nursing facility. *Arch Intern Med* 1992;152:390–2.

17. Houck P, Hemphill M, LaCroix S, Hirsh D, Cox N. Amantadine-resistant influenza A in nursing homes: identification of a resistant virus prior to drug use. *Arch Intern Med* 1995;155:533–7.
18. Ziegler T, Hemphill M, Ziegler M.-L, Klimov A, Cox N. Rimantadine resistance of influenza A viruses: an international surveillance. Presented at 7th ISAR Conference, Charleston, SC, March 1994.
19. Pemberton RM, Jennings R, Potter CW, Oxford JS. Amantadine resistance in clinical influenza A (H_3N_2) and (H_1N_1) virus isolates. *J Antimicrob Chemother* 1986;18(Suppl B):135–40.
20. Heider H, Adamczyk B, Presber HW *et al*. Occurrence of amantadine- and rimantadine-resistant influenza A virus strains during the 1980 epidemic. *Acta Virol* 1981;2–5:395–400.
21. Bean WJ, Threlkeld SC, Webster RG. Biologic potential of amantadine-resistant influenza A virus in an avian model. *J Infect Dis* 1989;159:1050–6.
22. Hayden FG. Significance of rimantadine resistance in influenza A viruses. *J Resp Dis* 1989;10(Suppl 12A):S62–S67.
23. Hayden FG, Hay AJ. Emergence and transmission of influenza a viruses resistant to amantadine and rimantadine. In: Holland J, ed. *Current Topics in Microbiology and Immunology*, vol. 176: *Genetic Diversity of RNA Viruses*. Berlin: Springer-Verlag, 1992:119–30.
24. Hayden FG, Couch RB. Clinical and epidemiological importance of influenza A viruses resistant to amantadine and rimantadine. *Rev Med Virol* 1992;2:89–96.
25. Hayden FG. Amantadine and rimantadine resistance in influenza A viruses. *Curr Opin Infect Dis* 1994;7:674–7.
26. Tominack RL, Hayden FG. Rimantadine hydrochloride and amantadine hydrochloride use in influenza A virus infections. In: Knight V, Gilbert B, eds. *Infectious Disease Clinics of North America*. Philadelphia: Saunders, 1987:459–78.
27. Appleyard G, Maber HB. A plaque assay for the study of influenza virus inhibitors. *J Antimicrob Chemother* 1975;1(Suppl):49–53.
27a. Wainwright PO, Perdue ML, Brugh M, Beard CW. Amantadine resistance among hemagglutinin subtype 5 strains of avian influenza virus. *Avian Dis* 1991;35:31–9
28. Oxford JS, Potter CW. Aminoadamantane-resistant strains of influenza A2 virus. *J Hyg Camb* 1973;71:227–36.
29. Hayden FG, Cote KM, Douglas RG Jr. Plaque inhibition assay for drug susceptibility testing of influenza viruses. *Antimicrob Agents Chemother* 1980;17:865–70.
30. Browne MJ, Moss MY, Boyd MR. Comparative activity of amantadine and ribavirin against influenza virus *in vitro*: possible clinical relevance. *Antimicrob Agents Chemother* 1983;23:503–5.
31. Belshe RB, Burk B, Newman F, Cerruti RL, Sim IS. Resistance of influenza A virus to amantadine and rimantadine: results of one decade of surveillance. *J Infect Dis* 1989;159:430–5.
32. Valette M, Allard JP, Aymard M, Millet V. Susceptibilities to rimantadine of influenza A/H1N1 and A/H3N2 viruses isolated during the epidemics of 1988 to 1989 and 1989 to 1990. *Antimicrob Agents Chemother* 1993;37:2239–40.
33. Kendal AP. Short communication. Reference viruses for use in amantadine sensitivity testing of human influenza A viruses. *Antiviral Chem Chemother* 1991;2:115–18.

34. Klimov AI, Rocha E, Hayden FG *et al.* Prolonged shedding of amantadine-resistant influenza A viruses by immunodeficient patients: detection by PCR-restriction analysis. *J Infect Dis* 1995;172:1352–5.
35. Oxford JS, Logan IS. *In vivo* selection of an influenza A2 strain resistant to amantadine. *Nature* 1970;226:82–3.
36. Webster RG, Kawaoka Y, Bean WJ, Beard CW, Brugh M. Chemotherapy and vaccination: a possible strategy for the control of highly virulent influenza virus. *J Virol* 1985;55:173–6.
37. Beard CW, Brugh M, Webster RG. Emergence of amantadine-resistant H5N2 avian influenza virus during a simulated layer flock treatment program. *Avian Dis* 1987;31:533–7.
38. Sweet C, Hayden FG, Jakeman KJ, Grambas S, Hay AJ. Virulence of rimantadine-resistant human influenza A (H3N2) viruses in ferrets. *J Infect Dis* 1991;164:969–72.
39. Ito T, Gorman OT, Kawaoka Y, Bean WJ, Webster RG. Evolutionary analysis of the influenza A virus M gene with comparison of the M1 and M2 proteins. *J Virol* 1991;5491–8.
40. Bean WJ Jr. Unselected amantadine resistance in human influenza virus and its long-term survival in nature. Presented at the American Society for Virology, 11th Annual Meeting, July 11–15, 1992.
41. Hayden FG, Sperber SJ, Belshe RB *et al.* Recovery of drug-resistant influenza A virus during therapeutic use of rimantadine. *Antimicrob Agents Chemother* 1991;35:1741–7.
42. Kubar OI, Brjantseva EA, Nikitina LE, Zlydnikov DM. The importance of virus drug-resistance in the treatment of influenza with rimantadine. *Antiviral Res* 1989;11:313–16.
43. Galbraith AW, Oxford JS, Schild GC, Watson GI. Protective effect of 1-adamantanamine hydrochloride on influenza A2 infections in the family environment. A controlled double-blind study. *Lancet* 1969;2:1026–8.
44. Galbraith AW, Oxford JS, Schild GC, Watson GI. Study of 1-adamantanamine hydrochloride used prophylactically during the Hong Kong influenza epidemic in the family environment. *Bull WHO* 1969;41:677–82.
45. Bricaire F, Hannoun C, Boissel JP. Prevention of influenza A: effectiveness and tolerance of rimantadine hydrochloride. *Presse Med* 1990;19:69–72.
46. Couch RB, Kasel JA, Glezen WP *et al.* Influenza: its control in persons and populations. *J Infect Dis* 1986;153:431–40.
47. Roumillat F, Rocha E, Regnery H, Wells D, Cox N. Emergence of amantadine-resistant influenza A viruses in nursing homes during the 1989–1990 influenza season [abstract P34–42]. In Abstracts of the VIIIth International Congress of Virology, Berlin, 1990:321.
48. Monto AS, Arden NH. Implications of viral resistance to amantadine in control of influenza A. *Clin Infect Dis* 1992;15:362–7.
49. Douglas RG Jr. Drug therapy. Prophylaxis and treatment of influenza. *New Engl J Med* 1990;322:443–50.
50. Centers for Disease Control and Prevention. Prevention and control of influenza: recommendations of the Advisory Committee on Immunization Practices (ACIP). *MMWR* 1995;44–(no. RR–3).
51. Gomolin IH, Leib HB, Arden NH, Sherman FT. Control of influenza outbreaks in the nursing home: guidelines for diagnosis and managements. *J Am Geriatr Soc* 1995;43:71–4.

HERPES SIMPLEX VIRUS AND VARICELLA ZOSTER VIRUS

5

Nucleosides and Foscarnet—Mechanisms

DONALD M. COEN

INTRODUCTION

Herpes simplex virus (HSV) types 1 and 2 and varicella zoster virus (VZV) cause disease, which is usually troublesome in the normal population but can be devastating or fatal, in immunocompromised individuals. Herpesviruses, particularly HSV and VZV, have provided fertile ground for the development of antiviral therapies and thereby for the study of antiviral drug resistance. In particular, drug resistance has been very well explored in HSV, which is an excellent genetic system and whose drug targets can be assayed biochemically with relative ease.

The basic mechanism of HSV and VZV drug resistance has been reviewed[1-7]. This chapter will attempt to update and expand upon certain aspects covered in earlier reviews. The chapter begins with an overview of the HSV and VZV replication cycles. It will then review the mechanisms of action of antiviral drugs, beginning with the nucleoside acyclovir and finishing with the pyrophosphate analog, foscarnet. The most space will be devoted to those drugs that are or will be seeing clinical use. The mechanisms of resistance to these drugs will be outlined concurrently, as they are tied very closely to the mechanisms of action. Indeed, perhaps the best way to determine the overall mechanism of action of an antiviral drug is via drug resistance. The isolation of virus mutants resistant to a drug strongly implies that the drug acts at least in part via a virus-specific process. Once a drug-resistant virus mutant is isolated, a virus-encoded drug target that contributes to antiviral

Antiviral Drug Resistance. Edited by Douglas D. Richman © 1996 John Wiley & Sons Ltd

selectivity can be identified by defining the gene in which mutation to drug resistance has occurred. Moreover, a reasonable case can be made that the maximum degree of resistance observed can tell us how selective an antiviral drug is, and how important a given gene product is for selectivity. In the case of HSV and VZV these principles are illustrated by two kinds of drug targets: a deoxypyrimidine kinase, usually known as thymidine kinase (TK), and the catalytic subunit of a viral DNA polymerase (Pol).

The chapter will then discuss other HSV and VZV gene products that can affect drug susceptibility, the frequency of drug resistance, the relationships of drug-resistance mutations and the structure and function of the drug targets, cross-resistance to other drugs, and the effects of drug-resistance mutations on pathogenicity in animal models. As VZV is a less tractable system than HSV in almost every way, more has been learned more quickly with the HSV system than the VZV system. This is reflected in what follows.

REPLICATION CYCLE

HSV is a large enveloped virus containing a ~150 kilobase pair (kbp) double-stranded DNA. Following entry of the virus into the cell, the DNA enters the nucleus and circularizes[8,9]. The virus then expresses immediate early (α) proteins, whose functions include the induction of expression of the early (β) and late (γ) genes[10]. The early genes mainly encode numerous proteins involved in viral DNA replication[11]. They come in two varieties: proteins such as Pol and the single-stranded DNA-binding protein ICP8, which directly participate in DNA replication and are absolutely essential for virus replication; and proteins such as TK and ribonucleotide reductase (RR), which help make the deoxynucleoside triphosphate precursors for DNA replication. These latter proteins are not essential for virus replication in cells in culture or in certain cells in mammalian hosts. Upon DNA replication expression of the late genes, which are primarily involved in assembly of the virus particle and egress from the cell, becomes maximal.

The VZV genome is ~125 kbp. VZV is highly cell associated so that it is difficult to inoculate cells at high multiplicities to permit a synchronous infection. As a result, it has been difficult to analyze the VZV replication cycle. However, it seems likely that the classes of genes, their functions and their expression are similar to those of HSV. The available evidence mainly supports this hypothesis. It is certainly well established that VZV encodes homologs of most HSV proteins, including Pol and TK[12].

ACYCLOVIR

Acyclovir (ACV) is the antiviral drug against which all others are compared. It is relatively more potent against HSV than against VZV, but its mechanisms against both viruses are essentially identical. ACV consists of a guanine base attached to an acyclic moiety, which is essentially a broken sugar ring (Figure 5.1). It can be thought of as deoxyguanosine missing the CHOH moiety at the 3' position and the CH_2 moiety at the 2' position.

Like most antiherpesvirus drugs (and many other antiviral drugs), ACV is a nucleoside analog whose mechanism entails two steps[13]: activation by phosphorylation so that the activated drug resembles the normal deoxynucleoside triphosphate (dNTP) substrate of DNA polymerases; and inhibition of viral DNA polymerase. Selectivity is then dependent upon how much more efficiently viral enzymes phosphorylate the drug than do

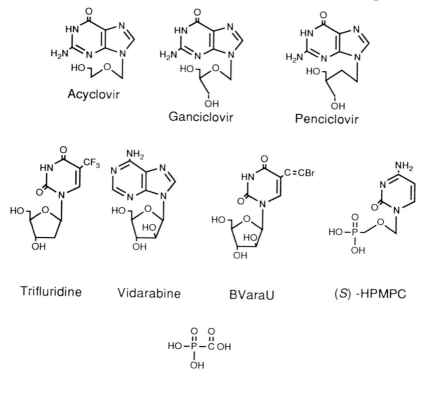

Figure 5.1 Structures of antiviral drugs discussed in this chapter

cellular enzymes, and how much more potently viral DNA synthesis is inhibited than are cellular functions. ACV is selective at both steps (Figure 5.2). It is activated by the HSV and VZV TKs. Thus, HSV- and VZV-infected cells contain much more phosphorylated ACV than do uninfected cells. Some phosphorylation does occur in uninfected cells, but only 1–3% of that found in HSV-infected cells. Thus phosphorylation by TK accounts for much of the antiviral selectivity of ACV.

The ACV monophosphate (ACV-MP) produced by phosphorylation of acyclovir is then converted to ACV di- and triphosphates (ACV-DP and ACV-TP), probably exclusively by cellular enzymes. The ACV-TP then serves as an inhibitor of herpesvirus DNA polymerases. Moreover, it is a more potent inhibitor of these viral polymerases than it is of cellular DNA polymerases[14]. The details of the inhibition of HSV DNA polymerase by ACV-TP *in vitro* include binding, incorporation into primer template, obligatory chain termination and the formation of a 'dead-end' complex[15]. Regardless of whether all of these steps are important *in vivo*, selective inhibition of viral DNA polymerase is a crucial component of ACV action.

Acyclovir resistance mechanisms

One of the ways that we know that the above two-component pathway for ACV selectivity is correct comes from the isolation and analysis of viral mutants that are resistant to ACV. All ACV-resistant mutants to date contain mutations in either the *tk* gene, the *pol* gene or both (Figure 5.2). Because TK is not essential for virus replication in cell culture,

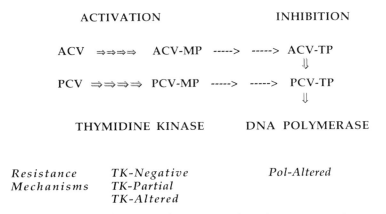

Figure 5.2 *Mechanisms of action and resistance of acyclovir (ACV) and penciclovir (PCV) against HSV and VZV. See text for details*

mutations that completely (TK-negative, TK⁻) or partially inactivate the enzyme (TK-partial) do not prohibit virus replication. One can also find mutations that alter TK to prevent ACV phosphorylation while permitting thymidine phosphorylation (TK-altered). Some mutants are both TK-partial and TK-altered, i.e. they exhibit reduced activity but are more impaired for acyclovir phosphorylation than for thymidine phosphorylation. The differences between these various kinds of mutants, which are not always easy to detect, can loom large in terms of their pathogenic properties in animal models (see below).

Mutations in the *pol* gene result in higher concentrations of ACV-TP being required for inhibition of Pol (Pol-altered). These mutations are especially important in verifying the above mechanism, because at therapeutic concentrations phosphorylated forms of ACV could conceivably act by inhibiting any number of components of cellular metabolism. Indeed, this sort of non-selective action occurs for other antivirals, but for ACV appears to occur only at very high concentrations. An additional interesting point relevant to selectivity is that *pol* mutations that confer resistance to acyclovir and other drugs lie mainly within regions conserved among viral and cellular enzymes (see below). This implies that these drugs act selectively by exploiting relatively subtle differences between viral and cellular polymerases.

The resistance mutations in the *tk* and *pol* genes confirm the quantitative selectivity of ACV and the quantitative contributions of TK and Pol to selectivity[16]. A double ACV-resistant mutant exhibits ≥1000-fold resistance (measured by dividing the 50% effective dose against the mutant by the 50% effective dose against its wild-type parent). Certain mutations in either the *tk* or the *pol* genes can confer ≥100-fold resistance alone. These quantitative aspects contrast with those for other drugs (see below). These quantitative aspects can also affect the impact of resistance in the clinic. This issue is discussed in Chapter 6.

OTHER NUCLEOSIDE ANALOGS

Ganciclovir

Although ganciclovir is now used primarily for cytomegalovirus, it was initially developed as a potential anti-HSV (and anti-VZV) agent, where it exhibits similar potency to ACV. Like ACV, ganciclovir is a guanine linked to an acyclic sugar-like molecule and lacks a 2' CH_2 moiety (see Figure 5.1). However, it contains the 3' CHOH moiety that is missing in ACV. The mechanism of ganciclovir is very similar to that of ACV, with mainly quantitative differences. It is more efficiently activated by HSV

TK than is ACV; correspondingly, greater reductions in TK activity are required to confer ganciclovir resistance than acyclovir resistance[17]. TK-altered mutants can exhibit substantial resistance to ganciclovir[18]. Ganciclovir triphosphate is less potent an inhibitor of the viral DNA polymerases than is ACV-TP, and it is not an obligatory chain terminator. There have been reports of ganciclovir resistance associated with *pol* mutants of HSV[18]. This indicates that ganciclovir is likely to be selective against HSV at the step of Pol inhibition. Even so, the maximum resistance observed was only four- to five-fold, which is consistent with less selectivity at this step than for acyclovir.

Famciclovir/Penciclovir

Famciclovir, which was approved in the US in 1994 for the treatment of the VZV disease herpes zoster (shingles), is the diacetyl 6-deoxy analog of penciclovir (PCV, see structure in Figure 5.1), which is the active drug. It too is a guanine analog. Like ganciclovir, it contains the 3' CHOH moiety that is missing in ACV, but instead of the ether oxygen at the top of the sugar ring it has a CH_2 group. The mechanism of PCV (Figure 5.2) is also quantitatively similar to that of ganciclovir[19]. It is more efficiently activated by HSV and VZV TK than is acyclovir, and thus various TK mutants are resistant. However, PCV-TP is less potent an inhibitor of the viral DNA polymerases than is ACV-TP. Thus, there is less selectivity at the polymerase step. Pol-altered mutants are correspondingly only modestly (~four-fold) resistant to PCV[20,21].

Trifluoridine (TFT)

This older drug, which resembles a natural nucleoside (dT) (see Figure 5.1) much more closely than does ACV, is a much less selective antiviral than is ACV. The mechanism has been reviewed[22]. TFT is phosphorylated not only by viral TK but also by its cellular counterpart. Some selectivity arises from the higher levels of thymidine kinase activity found in virus-infected cells, so that TK-deficient HSV mutants are less susceptible to inhibition by TFT in cells that express relatively low levels of cellular thymidine kinase[23]. TFT is converted to its respective triphosphate predominantly, if not exclusively, by cellular enzymes, and TFT triphosphate can serve both as an inhibitor of and a substrate for Pol. This step appears to be somewhat selective, as Pol-altered mutants that are resistant to TFT have been reported[18,24,25]. However, it seems likely that TFT acts at least in part non-selectively, by inhibiting a variety of cellular pathways (e.g cellular thymidylate synthase[26]), thereby rendering the host cell less able to support virus growth.

Vidarabine (araA)

This compound, like acyclovir, is a purine (adenine) attached to a deoxyribose analog, in this case the sugar arabinose (see Figure 5.1). Its mechanism has been reviewed[27]. Unlike acyclovir and TFT, it is not phosphorylated by a viral enzyme; rather, cellular enzymes are solely responsible for its conversion to the triphosphate (Figure 5.3). Thus, TK-HSV mutants are fully sensitive to araA[23]. Selectivity seems to be due largely, and perhaps entirely, to inhibition of viral Pol by araATP, and/or its incorporation as a substrate by viral Pol at concentrations lower than those for cellular enzymes (Figure 5.3). This conclusion derives principally from the demonstration that araA-resistance mutations map within the viral *pol* gene[28,29] (Figure 5.3). Even then, such resistance is rather slight, indicating that this is not a very selective compound.

Bromovinylarauracil [BVaraU (sorivudine)]

This (Figure 5.1) and several related compounds are especially interesting for a wrinkle in their mechanism of action, which has been reviewed[30]. Like ACV, it is phosphorylated to the monophosphate by HSV and VZV TK far more efficiently than by cellular enzymes. However, unlike the cases of the other nucleoside analogs discussed above, cellular enzymes are inefficient at converting BVaraU-monophosphate to the diphosphate. However, HSV-1 (but not HSV-2) and VZV TK have a thymidylate kinase activity that efficiently carries out this reaction. Thus, HSV-1 *tk* mutants that can phosphorylate thymidine but not thymidylate are highly resistant to this class of compounds[17]. Cellular enzymes convert the diphosphate

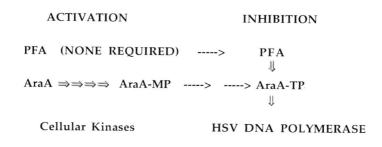

Figure 5.3 Mechanisms of action and resistance of vidarabine (araA) and foscarnet (PFA) against HSV and VZV. See text for details

forms to the triphosphates, which are inhibitors of herpesvirus DNA polymerases[31]. Whether inhibition of viral Pol is selective remains to be demonstrated definitively, as no mutation conferring resistance to this class of compounds has yet been mapped convincingly to the *pol* gene[25].

Cidofovir

Phosphonomethylalkyl derivatives of purines and pyrimidines, of which cidofovir (HPMPC) is a prototype (see Figure 5.1), represent another twist on the mechanisms of action of nucleoside analogs against HSV. HPMPC enters cells with reasonable efficiency, despite being in effect already phosphorylated. HPMPC is then phosphorylated further. The diphosphorylated form of HPMPC is an analog of dCTP and is a more potent inhibitor of HSV Pol than of cellular Pol α[32]. The genetics of resistance supports this mechanism. Thus, TK-negative HSV mutants remain sensitive to HPMPC; indeed, it appears that *tk* mutants are hypersensitive to HPMPC owing to a reduction in the dCTP pools, which normally depend on TK[33]. For at least one phosphonomethylalkyl compound HSV Pol appears to be a selective target, as *pol* mutants are modestly resistant[34].

FOSCARNET

Foscarnet (phosphonoformic acid, PFA; see structure in Figure 5.1) is an analog of pyrophosphate, which is a product of polymerization of nucleic acids. Unlike the other drugs described above it does not require activation by either cell or viral enzymes, but rather inhibits Pol directly (see Figure 5.3). Inhibition is not competitive with deoxynucleoside triphosphates; rather, it appears that PFA acts as a product analog, evidently by binding to the site normally occupied by pyrophosphate and preventing normal pyrophosphate release so that the polymerase cannot complete the catalytic cycle[35,36]. Selectivity arises from the viral Pol being more sensitive than cellular enzymes, which is confirmed by the existence of PFA-resistant *pol* mutants (see Figure 5.3)[37,38]. Resistance is due to an altered polymerase which is less susceptible to PFA inhibition. PFA is not as selective as ACV; correspondingly, the highest degree of resistance observed is about 20-fold.

OTHER GENES AFFECTING DRUG SUSCEPTIBILITY

At least two other genes can affect susceptibility to the drugs discussed in this chapter. The first encodes the large subunit of the ribonuclease reductase (RR). HSV or VZV mutations that knock this gene out confer increased susceptibility (hypersensitivity) to polymerase inhibitors, including ACV, ganciclovir and PFA[39-41]. The mechanism responsible for this is likely to be the depletion of dNTPs normally generated by the RR. For drugs that mimic dNTPs, this would then lead to less competition for binding. Consistent with this, drugs that have been developed to inhibit herpesvirus RRs synergize with acyclovir[41-43]. For drugs such as PFA, which do not inhibit competitively with dNTPs, depletion of dNTPs is nevertheless expected to increase potency, albeit to a lesser extent. This is in fact what is observed[39]. Although not yet tested, mutations that inactivate the small subunit of RR would also be expected to confer drug hypersensitivity. Conversely, one can imagine that mutations that lead to greater RR activity might confer drug resistance. This has not been reported for HSV, but an RR overexpressing virus has been described for vaccinia virus[44].

A second locus for drug hypersensitivity is the HSV gene encoding the single-stranded DNA-binding protein ICP8. Mutations in this gene can confer hypersensitivity to PAA (phosphonoacetic acid) and the polymerase inhibitor aphidicolin[45]. The mechanism for this is not certain, but an appealing possibility is that the mutations alter the ability of ICP8 to interact with polymerase, leading to its becoming more sensitive to the drugs. In the absence of a clear-cut mechanism it is difficult to know whether mutations in the *ICP8* gene could confer drug resistance.

FREQUENCY OF MUTATION TO DRUG RESISTANCE

Drug-resistance mutations occur fairly frequently in HSV during passage in cell culture. Most laboratory and clinical isolates contain ACV-resistant mutants at a level of about 0.01–0.1%; approximately the same frequencies apply to PFA- and araA-resistant mutants, despite their arising in only one rather than two genes[2]. For ACV resistance, many of these mutants are TK negative or express very low levels of TK activity; it is more difficult to obtain TK-altered or *pol* mutants in cell culture. The assays used to measure mutant frequencies are designed to eliminate 'breakthrough' plaques that are actually drug sensitive, and therefore may tend to miss the latter class of mutants, which can be less resistant but more pathogenic (see below). An important clinical issue, however, is what kinds of mutants are most likely to be selected *in vivo*. One effort to assess this involved selection at relatively low doses during passage of HSV in mice, and yielded drug-resistant pathogenic virus[46].

The relatively high frequency of drug-resistant mutants (although low compared to viruses with RNA genomes) found with HSV is due at least in part to the activities of viral gene products. One is the DNA polymerase. Certain *pol* mutants exhibit mutation frequencies more than 100 times lower than wild-type virus (antimutator phenotype[47]). The mutants assessed thus far exhibit improved nucleotide selection rather than increased editing of incorrectly incorporated bases[48]. When *tk* mutations generated by a wild-type polymerase were sequenced, roughly half were transition missense mutations and half were the addition or deletion of a base or two (frameshift mutations). In contrast, a *pol* mutant gave rise only to frameshift mutations[49]. Three other viral functions have been assayed for effects on mutation frequency: TK, deoxyuridine triphosphatase (dUTPase) and uracil DNA glycosylase (UDG)[50]. Of these, the presence of TK seems to increase the mutation frequency as *tk* mutants have a modest antimutator phenotype. The dUTPase has the opposite effect: dUTPase-negative mutants exhibit a mutator phenotype. UDG mutants have no or only a slight mutator phenotype. The effects of these enzymes on mutation frequencies can be readily rationalized in terms of their effects on nucleotide, especially dUTP pools. An interesting implication of these studies is that many *tk* and *pol* drug-resistant mutants are less likely to revert because they have an antimutator phenotype, i.e. drug resistance is more likely to be stable.

The frequency of drug-resistance mutation is difficult to assess in VZV, but it is fairly easy to isolate drug-resistant mutants from stocks of laboratory or clinical isolates[51]. Analysis of such mutants has revealed both missense and frameshift mutations[52].

LOCATIONS OF MUTATIONS AND EFFECTS ON FUNCTION

Sequencing viral genes to identify drug-resistance mutations can be useful for several purposes. One is to understand the mechanisms of drug resistance. A second is to understand basic biological mechanisms utilized by the virus such as gene expression. A third is to lay the foundation for rapid procedures to diagnose resistance, if there are few enough relevant mutations (this appears unlikely for HSV and VZV). A fourth is to identify amino acids that are involved directly or indirectly in recognition of the drugs and the substrates that they mimic. The most useful mutants for this purpose are those that express functional enzymes with altered specificity. In the case of HSV and VZV, these are TK-altered and Pol-altered mutants. When the drug used mimics or competes for binding with the natural substrate, mutations that confer resistance or hypersensitivity to that drug can be expected to alter the binding site for the substrate, either directly or indirectly.

TK mutations

Because TK is not essential for virus replication in cells or in certain locations in mammalian hosts, nonsense, frameshift and missense mutations that confer drug resistance can conceivably arise almost anywhere in the HSV or VZV *tk* gene and confer a TK⁻ phenotype. In HSV, Hwang and Chen[49] found some evidence for 'hot spots' of mutation in homopolymeric runs of Cs or Gs, but it is clear from a vast literature that many mutations will give rise to drug resistance. As yet, the number of mutants analyzed thus far is not sufficient to identify which residues can be altered to permit TK activity and which cannot.

Interestingly, nonsense and frameshift mutations that might be expected to inactivate TK do not necessarily do so. For example, a nonsense mutation between the first and second methionine codons in the HSV *tk* gene permits the synthesis of a truncated TK at about 5%, the level found for the wild-type polypeptide, owing evidently to initiation of translation at the second methionine codon[53]. The truncated polypeptide retains TK activity with a specific activity similar to the wild type, resulting in a TK-partial phenotype (~5%) which, however, scores as TK negative in many TK assays[17]. A second example in HSV involves a single base insertion that shifts the translational reading frame upstream of residues critical for TK activity[54]. This results not only in the synthesis of the expected truncated polypeptide, but also in low levels of full-length TK polypeptide and some TK enzyme activity. This can be ascribed to frameshifting, wherein the translational machinery compensates for the insertion mutation – 2% of the time. This virus also can score as negative for TK activity in an enzyme assay. These examples illustrate the difficulties in distinguishing TK-negative from TK-partial mutants by genotypic or enzymatic assays.

One interesting set of mutants is more resistant to drugs such as BVaraU than drugs such as ACV, and result from decreased thymidylate kinase activity. One of these is a truncation of the first 45 residues[17,53], suggesting that certain N-terminal residues are critical for phosphorylation of thymidylate but not thymidine.

TK-altered mutations would be expected to exhibit a much narrower spectrum of locations. Indeed, of the half dozen or so such mutations reported[51,55−59], about half lie within a small portion of the *tk* gene which encodes a conserved segment (roughly, residues 162–188 in HSV-1; 163–189 in HSV-2; and 129–155 in VZV). The suggestion[55] that this segment forms the nucleoside binding site was based in part on these mutations.

This suggestion has now been confirmed. The three-dimensional structure at 3.0 Å of an N-terminally truncated TK from HSV-1 co-crystallized with thymidine and ATP has been reported[60], as have structures at higher resolution of the full-length enzyme complexed with either thymidine or ganciclovir[61]. From these studies it is evident that nucleosides and nucleoside analogs interact with residues identified from mutational studies as the nucleoside-binding site. This structure and higher resolution solutions should help provide a framework for understanding the effects of specific mutations on the activities of this enzyme towards various natural substrates and antiviral drugs.

Pol mutations

Because Pol is essential for viral replication, all drug-resistant *pol* mutants express an enzyme that is less inhibited by drug than is the wild-type enzyme (Pol-altered) (see Figures 5.2 and 5.3). Although these mutations occupy numerous sites in the *pol* gene, the vast majority lie within about one-quarter of the gene, stretching from its midpoint towards its 3' end. Within this region, the mutations cluster in specific segments that encode motifs which are conserved among the large family of α-like DNA polymerases[62]. This family includes the eukaryotic replicative polymerases α, δ and ε. These conserved motifs include segments found in nearly every α-like polymerase, termed regions I–III, V and VII. An additional motif containing mutations was originally termed region A[63], but following the sequencing of mammalian DNA-polymerase δ was recognized to be a segment termed δ-region C[64], which is shared among cellular polymerases δ and ε and certain viral enzymes The locations of *pol* mutations from HSV and VZV drug-resistant mutants are shown in Table 5.1. As the drugs mimic and/or compete for binding with dNTPs and pyrophosphate, the mutations are expected to alter amino acids that are within or impinge on the binding sites for the drugs and the natural ligands. Regions II and III contain the greatest clustering of mutations and are therefore considered most likely to interact directly with drugs and natural ligands. Mutational and enzymological analyses of other α-like DNA polymerases support the idea that regions II and III are critical for dNTP binding[65]. An interesting question is how does each conserved region contribute to the different stages in the mechanism of ACV-TP inhibition of viral polymerase? Enzymological analyses of mutant DNA polymerases may answer this question.

The sequence data also indicate that the portion of Pol that contains substrate-binding sites and thus polymerase activity extends at least as far as the most distant drug-resistance mutations (>360 amino acids). This distance might be even greater when mutations identified by isolation of suppressors of drug-hypersensitivity mutations are included[66]. Some of these affect residues roughly 700 amino acids away

Table 5.1 Altered drug sensitivity affecting conserved regions of HSV and VZV DNA polymerases. From reference 62 with permission

	δ Region C (includes EXOIII & Region A)	Region II
Consensus	XXXXLSSYKLNXVA..XXXEXARXXGIPhXRXhXXGQQ	YNGGXXhXPXXG..VhhDhNSLYPSIMX
HSV wild type	531	696
	DKIKLSSYKLNAVA..ELSAVARLAGINITRTIYDGQQ	YQGARVLDPTSG..VVFDFASLYPSIIQ
HSV mutations	A	
	N K V	H G
		V N*
VZV mutations	K D	Y
		T

	Region III	Region I
Consensus	XQhhhkLXXNShYGXXGXXX..XXhhhXXhXXXGRX	hXhIYGDTDSIFV
HSV wild type	806	880
	QQAAIKVVCNSVYGFTGVQH..CLNVAATVTTIGRE	MRIIYGDTDSI FV
HSV mutations	M S* C M	S S FV
		A* CM
		Y
		L
VZV mutations	S	

	Region VII	Region V
Consensus	XKKXYhhX	KXXXKGXXXXRXXXX
HSV wild type	937	949
	AKKKYIGV	KMLIKGVDLVRKNNC
HSV mutations	H	K

For each conserved region, the first line provides a consensus sequence showing residues shared among many family members in single letter code, with X indicating no clear consensus and h indicating a hydrophobic residue. In one case, where two amino acids predominate, both are indicated. The second line provides the wild-type HSV sequence with the number of the first residue shown. Portions of the sequence omitted are indicated as '..'. Below these are indicated residues found in *pol* mutations from viruses exhibiting altered drug sensitivity. Note that in a few cases it has not yet been demonstrated that the mutation observed actually causes the altered drug sensitivity phenotypes. HSV mutations[62]; VZV mutations, K. Biron, personal communication. * Apart from mutations that have been tested in the authentic context of the virus genome, several mutations that affect drug sensitivity of HSV Pol *in vitro* have been identified. These include substitutions of the S in region II not only to the N asterisked, but also to A,D,E,H,I,K,Q and T; and substitutions of the N in region III not only to the S asterisked, but also to A,D,E,G,L,Q,V and Y[75]. Also, the S to A substitution that is italicized in region I was only tested *in vitro*[76]

from the most distal drug-resistance mutation. These and other data argue that HSV Pol is not as modular as first thought. Rather, it appears that its polymerase activity requires contributions from nearly the entire length of the polypeptide. Clearly, a three-dimensional structure of a herpesvirus Pol would aid interpretation of the phenotypes of these mutants.

CROSS-RESISTANCE

Experience with drug-resistant bacteria has highlighted the importance of having alternative antimicrobial agents for any given pathogen. This is becoming important for antiviral agents as well. For HSV and VZV (Table 5.1), *tk* mutants of all three classes remain sensitive to drugs such as PFA and HPMPC that do not require phosphorylation by TK. TK-negative and TK-partial mutants are generally resistant to any drug like PCV that does require phosphorylation. It is harder to predict how the TK-altered and *pol* mutants will behave, as they can vary widely in terms of cross-resistance. As things currently stand, one can imagine a double mutant that would be resistant to all currently available anti-HSV drugs. If the *tk* mutation in this double mutant were TK-altered, then the virus might retain considerable pathogenicity (see below).

PATHOGENICITIES OF DRUG-RESISTANT MUTANTS

Animal models of viral disease

In the human host productive replication by HSV and VZV can be manifested by lesions at various sites, most typically the skin or eyes.

Table 5.2 *Cross-resistance profiles of different classes of HSV and VZV drug-resistant mutants to selected antiviral drugs*

Type of mutant	Resistant to	Sensitive to
TK negative	ACV, PCV, GCV, BVaraU	PFA, AraA, HPMPC
TK altered or partial	Depends*	PFA, AraA, HPMPC
Polymerase altered	Depends*	Depends*
TK, polymerase double	Possibly all	Possibly none

*Certain TK-altered or TK-partial mutants can be cross-resistant to all nucleoside analogs that require TK for activation, or they can be resistant to only one or two of these. Similarly, certain polymerase-altered mutants can be resistant to any of the antiviral drugs, whereas others might be resistant to only one

However, like all herpesviruses, HSV and VZV share the property of latency; that is, after the symptoms of primary infection are gone, viral genomes persist in a relatively quiescent state in cellular reservoirs protected from immune surveillance. From this state of latency HSV and VZV can reactivate to cause recurrent disease. The reservoirs for HSV and VZV are ganglia of the peripheral nervous system, which is a common characteristic of the alphaherpesvirinae subfamily of the Herpesviridae to which HSV and VZV belong.

Considerable effort has gone into developing animal models for both the disease manifestations of these viruses and for latency. Unfortunately, thus far, it has been very difficult to establish suitable animal models for VZV disease and latency. However, there are numerous models of HSV disease and latency. This has led to much study of the effects of HSV mutations, including those that confer drug resistance, on pathogenesis. For the purpose of brevity only two kinds of studies, using immunocompetent mice, will be reviewed here. The first involves lethal infection of the central nervous system (neurovirulence). The second, which better mimics the natural course of most infections of humans involves inoculation at a peripheral site, such as the footpad, snout or cornea. The virus replicates at the peripheral site, gains access to nerve terminals and is transported back to neuronal cell bodies in sensory ganglia. In animal models at least, the virus replicates acutely in ganglia. Over several days acute replication ceases and the virus establishes a latent infection in neurons, where no infectious virus can be detected in ganglion homogenates. The latent virus can, however, be reactivated, most commonly by explant of the ganglia. The relevance of either assay for HSV disease and latency in humans is not certain. It should now be possible, however, to correlate the behavior of drug-resistant clinical isolates in such animal models and the clinical course associated with the isolates.

Behavior of drug-resistant mutants

Almost all drug-resistant HSV mutants exhibit some degree of attenuation in these assays of pathogenesis (Table 5.1[1,7]). TK-negative mutants are generally the most attenuated. They are somewhat deficient for lethal infection of the CNS and for replication at certain peripheral sites. They can establish latent infections following peripheral inoculation, albeit with lower efficiency. Most strikingly, there is little or no replication of virus in ganglia acutely and no reactivation from latency following normal explant procedures. These ganglionic defects can definitely be ascribed to a *tk* mutation[67]. There have been reports of viruses described as TK negative yet exhibiting ganglionic replication or reactivation or

Table 5.3 *Effects of drug-resistance mutations on neurovirulence, replication at the periphery, and reactivation from latency in mice*[a]. *Reproduced from reference 7 by permission of Elsevier Science*

Type of virus	Relative neuro-virulence[b]	Replication at periphery[c]	Reactivation from latency[d]
Wild type	100%	100%	70–100%
TK negative	0.01–3	10–100	0
TK partial	3–100	20–100	10–100
TK altered	10	100	50–100
Polymerase	1–10	20–100	50–100

[a] The ranges reflect different behaviors of different mutants in each class due to molecular differences among the mutants, different wild-type parental strains, or differing routes of inoculation
[b] The amount of virus required to kill 50% of mice (LD_{50}) following intracerebral inoculation of the wild type is set at 100%. Mutant viruses with, for example, tenfold higher LD_{50} values, are expressed as 10% etc.
[c] Replication at the peripheral site of inoculation, expressed as a percentage of the wild-type titer
[d] Percent of sensory ganglia from animals infected with the given mutant that reactivate virus following explant

both; however, these may be due to those viruses not being truly TK negative but expressing some TK owing to leaky or reverting mutations. Indeed, certain nonsense and frameshift mutants that mainly synthesize truncated TK polypeptides and can appear TK negative in certain enzyme assays, can express low levels of TK that are sufficient for ganglionic replication and reactivation[17,54].

As implied, TK-partial mutants are attenuated but can replicate acutely in ganglia and reactivate from latency. Generally speaking, the more TK activity expressed by the mutant, the more ganglionic replication and reactivation. TK-altered and *pol* mutants are variably attenuated for lethal CNS infection, but most replicate robustly at the periphery and in the ganglia, and reactivate from latency. Thus, these two classes of mutants include the most pathogenic drug-resistant mutants. The *pol* mutants are interesting in part because of their variability, with some being much more attenuated than others.

Only a few double mutants have been assayed for drug resistance. So far, combining TK-negative or TK-partial and *pol* mutations yields considerably more attenuation than either mutation alone[24,68]. However, not all combinations have been assayed. It may be that certain combinations of *pol* and TK-altered mutations could permit considerable pathogenicity.

This picture becomes even more complicated when mixtures of drug-resistant mutants with each other or with drug-sensitive virus are considered. Experimentally constructed mixtures of such viruses can complement each other for pathogenicity or drug resistance or both in mice[46,69-73]. Selection for drug resistance in mice yields even more complex mixtures that are especially resistant to therapy[46,71]. It is possible that *pol* mutations might play an especially important role in such mixtures because such mutations are co-dominant, that is, they allow both resistant and sensitive viruses to replicate in the same cell during drug treatment[74]. At least one heterogeneous mixture from a patient retained full neurovirulence and latency competence in mice[75] (Pelosi and Coen, unpublished observations). It is therefore appealing to hypothesize that virus heterogeneity may play an important role in clinically significant drug resistance. This hypothesis implies that it is important to consider heterogeneity in assays of drug susceptibilities of virus isolated from patients. Further study of such isolates will be required to test the importance of virus heterogeneity in the clinic.

SUMMARY

The basic mechanisms by which HSV and VZV become resistant to currently available antiviral drugs and the consequences of drug resistance in laboratory settings are well understood. The HSV system in particular permits the study of drug resistance from a change in nucleotide sequence to the effects of that change on pathogenesis and drug therapy in an animal model. The mechanisms of resistance illuminate the mechanisms of action of the drugs. Thus far, all mutants resistant to these drugs contain mutations in the viral *tk* or *pol* genes or both, but mutations at other loci can affect drug susceptibility. Mutation to drug resistance occurs at a fairly high frequency and resistance is a stable phenotype, due in part to the properties of the TK and Pol enzymes. The locations of *tk* and *pol* mutations have shed light on the structure–function relationships of TK and Pol. The phenotypic properties of drug-resistant mutants in terms of cross-resistance and pathogenicity may have important implications for drug resistance in the clinic. Among the important questions remaining is the correlation of the genotypes and phenotypes of drug-resistance mutants with clinical outcome (see Chapter 6).

Acknowledgments

I thank K. Biron for communicating results prior to publication. Grant support from the NIH (AI19838, AI26126, AI24010, AI26077) is gratefully acknowledged.

98   D. M. Coen

REFERENCES

1. Larder BA, Darby G. Virus drug resistance: mechanisms and consequences. *Antiviral Res* 1984;4:1–42.
2. Coen DM. General aspects of virus drug resistance with special reference to herpes simplex virus. *J Antimicrob Chemother* 1986;18B:1–10.
3. Coen DM. The implications of resistance to antiviral agents for herpesvirus drug targets and drug therapy. *Antiviral Res* 1991;15:287–300.
4. Chatis PA, Crumpacker CS. Resistance of herpesviruses to antiviral drugs. *Antimicrob Agents Chemother* 1992;36:1589–95.
5. Coen DM. Drug resistance in herpesviruses. *Int Antiviral News* 1993;1:98–9.
6. Field AK, Biron KK. 'The end of innocence' revisited: resistance of herpesviruses to antiviral drugs. *Clin Microbiol Rev* 1994;7:1–13.
7. Coen DM. Acyclovir-resistant, pathogenic herpesviruses. *Trends Microbiol* 1994;2:481–5.
8. Poffenberger KL, Roizman B. A non-inverting genome of a viable herpes simplex virus 1: presence of head-to-tail linkages in packaged genomes and requirements for circularization after infection. *J Virol* 1985;53:587–95.
9. Garber DA, Beverley SM, Coen DM. Demonstration of circularization of herpes simplex virus DNA following infection using pulsed field gel electrophoresis. *Virology* 1993;197:459–62.
10. Roizman B, Sears A. Herpes simplex viruses and their replication. In: Fields BN *et al.*, eds. Field's 3rd edn. *Virology*. New York: Lippincott-Raven, 1996:2231–95.
11. Challberg MD, Kelly TJ. Animal virus DNA replication. *Ann Rev Biochem* 1989;58:671–717.
12. Davison AJ, Scott JE. The complete DNA sequence of varicella-zoster virus. *J Gen Virol* 1986;67:1759–1816.
13. Elion GB. History, mechanism of action, spectrum and selectivity of nucleoside analogs. In: Mills J, Corey L, eds. *Antiviral Chemotherapy: New Directions for Clinical Application and Research*. New York: Elsevier, 1986:118–37.
14. Martin JL, Brown CE, Matthews-Davis N, Reardon JE. Effects of antiviral nucleoside analogs on human DNA polymerases and mitochondrial DNA synthesis. *Antimicrob Agents Chemother* 1994;38:2743–9.
15. Reardon JE, Spector T. Herpes simplex virus type 1 DNA polymerase: mechanism of inhibition by acyclovir triphosphate. *J Biol Chem* 1989;264:7405–11.
16. Furman PA, Coen DM, St. Clair MH, Schaffer PA. Acyclovir-resistant mutants of herpes simplex virus type 1 express altered DNA polymerase or reduced acyclovir phosphorylating activities. *J Virol* 1981;40:936–41.
17. Coen DM, Irmiere AF, Jacobson JG, Kerns KM. Low levels of herpes simplex virus thymidine–thymidylate kinase are not limiting for sensitivity to certain antiviral drugs or for latency in a mouse model. *Virology* 1989;168:221–31.
18. Larder BA, Darby G. Susceptibility to other antiherpes drugs of pathogenic variants of herpes simplex virus selected for resistance to acyclovir. *Antimicrob Agents Chemother* 1986;29:894–8.
19. Vere Hodge RA, Cheng Y-C. The mode of action of penciclovir. *Antiviral Chem Chemother* 1993;4 (Suppl. 1):13–24.
20. Ertl P, Snowden W, Lowe D, Miller W, Littler E. A comparative study of the in vitro and in vivo antiviral activities of acyclovir and penciclovir. *Antiviral Chem Chemother* 1995;6:89–97.

21. Chiou HC, Kumura K, Hu A, Kerns KM, Coen DM. Penciclovir-resistance mutations in the herpes simplex virus DNA polymerase gene. *Antiviral Chem Chemother* 1995;6:281–8.
22. Prusoff WH, Mancini WR, Lin T-S *et al*. Physical and biological consequences of incorporation of antiviral agents into virus DNA. *Antiviral Res* 1984;4:303–15.
23. Field H, McMillan A, Darby G. The sensitivity of acyclovir-resistant mutants of herpes simplex virus to other antiviral drugs. *J Infect Dis* 1981;143:281–5.
24. Darby G, Churcher MJ, Larder BA. Cooperative effects between two acyclovir resistance loci in herpes simplex virus. *J Virol* 1984;50:838–46.
25. Coen DM, Fleming HE Jr, Leslie LK, Retondo MJ. Sensitivity of arabinosyladenine-resistant mutants of herpes simplex virus to other antiviral drug and mapping of drug hypersensitivity mutations to the DNA polymerase locus. *J Virol* 1985;53:477–88.
26. Reyes P, Heidelberger C. Fluorinated pyrimidines XXVI. Mammalian thymidylate synthetase: its mechanism of action and inhibition by fluorinated nucleotides. *Mol Pharmacol* 1965;1:14–30.
27. North TW, Cohen SS. Aranucleosides and aranucleotides in viral chemotherapy. In: Shugar D, ed. *International Encyclopedia of Pharmacology and Therapeutics: Viral Chemotherapy* (Pt 1). Oxford: Pergamon, 1984:303–40.
28. Coen DM, Furman PA, Gelep PT, Schaffer PA. Mutations in the herpes simplex virus DNA polymerase gene can confer resistance to 9-β-D-arabinofuranosyladenine. *J Virol* 1982;41:909–18.
29. Fleming HE Jr, Coen DM. Herpes simplex virus mutants resistant to arabinosyladenine in the presence of deoxycoformycin. *Antimicrob Agents Chemother* 1984;6:382–7.
30. De Clercq E, Walker RT. Synthesis and antiviral properties of 5-vinyl-pyrimidine nucleoside analogs. *Pharmacol Ther* 1984;26:1–44.
31. Ruth JL, Cheng Y-C. Nucleoside analogues with clinical potential in antivirus chemotherapy. The effect of several thymidine and 2'-deoxycytidine analogue 5'-triphosphates on purified human (α, β) and herpes simplex virus (types 1,2) DNA polymerases. *Mol Pharmacol* 1981;20:415–22.
32. Merta A, Votruba I, Rosenberg I *et al*. Inhibition of herpes simplex virus DNA polymerase by diphosphates of acyclic phosphonylmethoxyalkyl nucleotide analogues. *Antiviral Res* 1990;13:209–18.
33. Mendel DB, Barkhimer DB, Chen MS. Biochemical basis for increased susceptibility to cidofovir of herpes simplex viruses with altered or deficient thymidine kinase activity. *Antimicrob Agents Chemother* 1995;39:2120–2.
34. Foster SA, Cerny J, Cheng Y-C. Herpes simplex virus-specified DNA polymerase is the target for the antiviral action of 9-(2-phosphonylmethoxyethyl)adenine. *J Biol Chem* 1991;266:238–44.
35. Erikkson B, Larsson A, Helgstrand E, Johansson N-G, Oberg B. Pyrophosphate analogues as inhibitors of herpes simplex virus type 1 DNA polymerase. *Biochim Biophys Acta* 1980;607:53–64.
36. Ostrander M, Cheng Y-C. Properties of herpes simplex virus type 1 and type 2 DNA polymerase. *Biochim Biophys Acta* 1980;609:232–45.
37. Erikkson B, Oberg B. Characteristics of herpes virus mutants resistant to phosphonoformate and phosphonoacetate. *Antimicrob Agents Chemother* 1979;15:758–62.
38. Sacks SL, Wanklin RJ, Reece DE *et al*. Progressive esophagitis from acyclovir-resistant herpes simplex: clinical roles for DNA polymerase mutants and viral heterogeneity? *Ann Intern Med* 1989;111:893–9.

39. Coen DM, Goldstein DJ, Weller SK. Herpes simplex virus ribonucleotide reductase mutants are hypersensitive to acyclovir. *Antimicrob Agents Chemother* 1989;33:1395–9.

40. Mineta T, Rabkin SD, Martuza RL. Treatment of malignant gliomas using ganciclovir-hypersensitive, ribonucleotide reductase-deficient herpes simplex viral mutant. *Cancer Res* 1994;54:3963–6.

41. Heineman TC, Cohen JI. Deletion of the varicella-zoster virus large subunit of ribonucleotide reductase impairs growth of virus *in vitro*. *J Virol* 1994;68:3317–23.

42. Spector T, Averett DR, Nelson DJ *et al*. Potentiation of antiherpetic activity of acyclovir by ribonucleotide reductase inhibition. *Proc Natl Acad Sci USA* 1985;82:4254–7.

43. Liuzzi M, Déziel R, Moss N *et al*. A potent peptidomimetic inhibitor of HSV ribonucleotide reductase with antiviral activity *in vivo*. *Nature* (London) 1994;372:695–8.

44. Slabaugh M, Roseman N, Davis R, Mathews C. Vaccinia virus-encoded ribonucleotide reductase: sequence conservation of the gene for the small subunit and its amplification in hydroxyurea-resistant mutants. *J Virol* 1988;62:519–27.

45. Chiou HC, Weller SK, Coen DM. Mutations in the herpes simplex virus major DNA-binding protein gene leading to altered sensitivity to DNA polymerase inhibitors. *Virology* 1985;145:213–26.

46. Field HJ. Development of clinical resistance to acyclovir in herpes simplex virus-infected mice receiving oral therapy. *Antimicrob Agents Chemother* 1982;21:744–52.

47. Hall JD, Coen DM, Fisher BL *et al*. Generation of genetic diversity in herpes simplex virus. An antimutator phenotype maps to the DNA polymerase locus. *Virology* 1984;132:26–37.

48. Hall JD, Furman PA, St. Clair MH, Knopf CW. Reduced *in vivo* mutagenesis by mutant herpes simplex DNA polymerase involves improved nucleotide selection. *Proc Natl Acad Sci USA* 1985;82:3889–93.

49. Hwang CBC, Chen HJ-H. An altered spectrum of herpes simplex virus mutations mediated by an antimutator DNA polymerase. *Gene* 1995;152:191–3.

50. Pyles RB, Thompson RL. Mutations in accessory DNA replicating functions alter the relative mutation frequency of herpes simplex virus type 1 strains in cultured murine cells. *J Virol* 1994;68:4514–24.

51. Biron KK, Fyfe JA, Noblin JE, Elion GB. Selection and preliminary characterization of acyclovir-resistant mutants of varicella zoster virus. *Am J Med* 1982;73(Acyclovir Symp):383–6.

52. Lacey SF, Suzutani T, Powell KL, Purifoy DJM, Honess RW. Analysis of mutations in the thymidine kinase genes of drug-resistant varicella-zoster virus populations using the polymerase chain reaction. *J Gen Virol* 1991;72:623–30.

53. Irmiere AF, Manos MM, Jacobson JG, Gibbs JS, Coen DM. Effect of an amber mutation in the herpes simplex virus thymidine kinase gene on polypeptide synthesis and stability. *Virology* 1989;168:210–20.

54. Hwang CBC, Horsburgh B, Pelosi E *et al*. A net +1 frameshift permits synthesis of thymidine kinase from a drug-resistant herpes simplex virus mutant. *Proc Natl Acad Sci USA* 1994;91:5461–5.

55. Darby G, Larder BA, Inglis MM. Evidence that the 'active centre' of the herpes simplex virus thymidine kinase involves an interaction between three distinct regions of the polypeptide. *J Gen Virol* 1986;67:753–8.

56. Sawyer MH, Inchauspe G, Biron KK *et al*. Molecular analysis of the pyrimidine deoxyribonucleoside kinase gene of wild-type and acyclovir-resistant strains of varicella-zoster vimus. *J Gen Virol* 1988;69:2585–93.

57. Roberts GB, Fyfe RK, Gaillard RK, Short SA. Mutant varicella-zoster virus thymidine kinase: correlation of clinical resistance and enzyme impairment. *J Virol* 1991:6407–13.

58. Talarico CL, Phelps WC, Biron KK. Analysis of the thymidine kinase genes from acyclovir-resistant mutants of varicella-zoster virus isolated from patients with AIDS. *J Virol* 1993;67:1024–33.

59. Kost RG, Hill EL, Tigges M, Straus SE. Brief report: recurrent acyclovir-resistant genital herpes in an immunocompetent patient. *New Engl J Med* 1993;329:1777–82.

60. Wild K, Bohner T, Aubry A, Folkers G, Schulz GE. The three-dimensional structure of thymidine kinase from herpes simplex virus type 1. *FEBS Lett* 1995;368:289–92.

61. Brown DG, Visse R, Sandhu G *et al*. Crystal structures of the thymidine kinase from herpes simplex virus type-1 in complex with deoxythymidine and ganciclovir. *Nature Struct Biol* 1995;2:876–80.

62. Coen DM. Viral DNA polymerases. In: DePamphilis M, ed. *DNA Replication in Eukaryotic Cells*. Cold Spring Harbor: Cold Spring Harbor Laboratory Press, 1996.

63. Gibbs JS, Chiou HC, Bastow KF, Cheng Y-C, Coen DM. Identification of amino acids in herpes simplex virus DNA polymerase involved in substrate and drug recognition. *Proc Natl Acad Sci USA* 1988;85:6672–6.

64. Zhang J, Chung DW, Tan C-K *et al*. Primary structure of the catalytic subunit of calf thymus DNA polymerase δ: sequence similarities with other DNA polymerases. *Biochemistry* 1991;30:742–50.

65. Wang TSF. Cellular DNA polymerases. In: DePamphilis M, ed. *DNA Replication in Eukaryotic Cells*. Cold Spring Harbor: Cold Spring Harbor Laboratory Press, 1996.

66. Wang Y, Woodward S, Hall JD. Use of suppressor analysis to identify DNA polymerase mutations in herpes simplex virus which affect deoxynucleoside triphosphate substrate specificity. *J Virol* 1992;66:1814–16.

67. Jacobson JG, Ruffner KL, Kosz-Vnenchak M *et al*. Herpes simplex virus thymidine kinase and specific stages of latency in murine trigeminal ganglia. *J Virol* 1993;67:6903–8.

68. Jacobson J, Kramer M, Rozenburg F, Hu A, Coen DM. Synergistic effects on ganglionic herpes simplex virus infections by mutations or drugs that inhibit the viral polymerase and thymidine kinase. *Virology* 1995;206:263–8.

69. Tenser RB, Ressel S, Dunstan ME. Herpes simplex virus thymidine kinase expression in trigeminal ganglion infection: correlation of enzyme activity with ganglion virus titer and evidence of *in vivo* complementation. *Virology* 1981;112:328–41.

70. Tenser RB, Edris WA. Trigeminal ganglion infection by thymidine kinase-negative mutants of herpes simplex virus after *in vivo* complementation. *J Virol* 1987;61:2171–4.

71. Field H, Lay E. Characterization of latent infections in mice inoculated with herpes simplex virus which is clinically resistant to acyclovir. *Antiviral Res* 1984;4:43–52.

72. Sedarati F, Javier RT, Stevens JG. Pathogenesis of lethal mixed infection in mice with two nonneuroinvasive herpes simplex virus strains. *J Virol* 1988;62:3037–9.

73. Ellis MN, Waters R, Hill EL *et al*. Orofacial infection of athymic mice with defined mixtures of acyclovir-susceptible and acyclovir-resistant herpes simplex virus type 1. *Antimicrob Agents Chemother* 1989;33:304–10.

74. Coen DM, Schaffer PA. Two distinct loci confer resistance to acycloguanosine in herpes simplex virus type 1. *Proc Natl Acad Sci USA* 1980;77:2265–9.

75. Matthews JT, Terry BJ, Field AK. The structure and function of the HSV replication proteins: defining novel antiviral targets. *Antiviral Res* 1993;20:89–114.

76. Dorsky DI, Plourde C. Resistance to antiviral inhibitors caused by mutation S889A in the highly conserved 885-GDTDS motif of the herpes simplex virus type 1 DNA polymerase. *Virology* 1993;195:831–5.

6
Nucleosides and Foscarnet—Clinical Aspects

SHARON SAFRIN

CLINICAL MANIFESTATIONS OF ANTIVIRAL RESISTANCE IN HERPES SIMPLEX

Introduction

Resistance to antiviral agents in herpes simplex virus (HSV) was reported in 1965, when *in vitro* resistance to the new pyrimidine nucleoside 5-iodo-2-deoxyuridine (IUDR), was described[1]. IUDR became widely used as a topical treatment for herpes keratitis[2], but descriptions of treatment failure associated with *in vitro* resistance to the drug soon appeared[3]. Resistance to acyclovir (9-(2-hydroxyethoxymethyl)guanine) was reported in the initial description by Elion *et al.*[4] of its mechanism of action, accompanied by a demonstration that mutations in the virus thymidine kinase conferred resistance. Thus, recognition of *in vitro* resistance to acyclovir was virtually simultaneous with discovery of the compound. Resistance to acyclovir can be selected for quite readily in tissue culture, e.g. with a single passage of HSV in BHK cells in the presence of 10 times the 50% effective dose (ED$_{50}$) of acyclovir[5]. However, although clinical isolates with demonstrable resistance to acyclovir *in vitro* were recovered from patients in the earliest clinical trials of acyclovir[6,7], descriptions of progressive or refractory HSV infections despite therapy with acyclovir were only sporadically reported in patients with severe immunodeficiency until the advent of the AIDS epidemic. Two reports in 1982 described the lack of response to therapy with acyclovir in immunodeficient children with

Antiviral Drug Resistance. Edited by Douglas D. Richman © 1996 John Wiley & Sons Ltd

orofacial HSV infection[8,9], and rare reports over the ensuing decade described immunocompromised patients with hematologic malignancies or after organ transplantation that had acyclovir-resistant HSV infection[10-15]. Beginning in 1987, however, numerous case reports and case series of non-healing infections despite treatment with acyclovir in patients with advanced HIV infection began to appear in the literature[16-27].

Epidemiology and clinical presentation

To date, over 100 patients with acyclovir-resistant HSV infection have been reported in the English medical literature; all patients have been severely immunocompromised. The single exception is a report by Kost *et al.*[28] (see below).

Although the perirectal area has been the most frequently reported area of involvement with resistant HSV infection, particularly in patients with AIDS, numerous other sites have been described as well, including the orofacial region, the genitals, fingers, the lungs, the esophagus and the brain[10,12,15,16,19,21,22,25]. Lesions are most often deeply ulcerative confluencies causing pain and disfigurement. Spontaneous resolution of such lesions over time has not been reported, probably owing to the lack of recovery of immune function in patients with AIDS. Fortunately, lesions are most often localized rather than disseminated; visceral dissemination and central nervous system involvement have been only rarely reported[12,22].

In a single report of an HIV-negative immunocompetent man with an acyclovir-resistant HSV infection, increasingly frequent recurrences of genital herpes occurred despite the use of maximal doses of oral acyclovir for suppression or treatment[28]. This patient, however, admitted to having had three new sexual partners in the recent past, two of whom had HIV infection. Thus the occurrence of direct transmission of the resistant virus appeared likely. Additionally, he never developed a chronic non-healing lesion, as described in severely immunocompromised patients.

Determination of *in vitro* resistance in isolates of HSV

There are many different assays for antiviral susceptibility testing of isolates of HSV currently in use, including the plaque reduction assay[29,30], the neutral red dye uptake assay[29] and a DNA hybridization assay[31]. The plaque reduction assay entails determination of the degree of inhibition of virus growth by enumeration of the number of plaques present at different concentrations of a given antiviral drug. The dye uptake assay uses a semi-automated method to quantify spectrophotometrically the uptake of neutral red dye by viable cells. Drug activity is measured as a reduction in HSV cell death. The DNA hybridization assay quantifies viral DNA after exposure to an antiviral agent using a radio-iodinated DNA probe specific for HSV-1 and HSV-2.

Clinical lesions caused by HSV tend to be composed of heterogeneous mixtures of viral phenotypes, both susceptible (i.e. wild type) and resistant (i.e. mutants)[15,33]. Therefore, the use of clinically derived isolates rather than laboratory-generated clonal populations would appear to be important in the critical comparison of antiviral susceptibility testing assays. However, comparative studies of the three major assays have typically utilized laboratory-derived strains of acyclovir-resistant HSV[29] or mixtures of acyclovir-susceptible and -resistant isolates generated by *in vitro* reconstruction experiments[32]. One study comparing plaque reduction with the Hybriwix (Diagnostic Hybrids Inc., Athens, Ohio, USA) DNA hybridization assay did utilize a small number of acyclovir-resistant patient isolates[31], and found a good correlation between the two. A more recent study utilized 30 clinical isolates of varying susceptibility patterns to acyclovir and foscarnet for a three-way comparison of these assays[34]. The results showed that ID_{50} values (i.e. the concentration of drug required to inhibit virus growth by $\geqslant 50\%$) were higher using the dye uptake and plaque reduction assays than from the DNA hybridization assay, with four- and two-fold differences on average, respectively[34].

This same study also evaluated the correlation between *in vitro* susceptibility result and clinical response to therapy with either acyclovir or foscarnet[34]. This analysis suggested a slightly greater proportion of concordancies of the dye uptake assay results with therapeutic response when compared with the other two assays. However, this observation was felt to require validation through the testing of larger numbers of isolates. All three assays were felt to be suboptimal owing to a long turnaround time, the requirement for technician expertise and expense. More rapid and reproducible tests, with objective rather than subjective endpoints, are clearly needed.

A separate study examined the correlation between susceptibility testing results using the plaque reduction assay and clinical response to acyclovir or foscarnet therapy in 243 clinical isolates collected from 115 HIV-infected patients[35] (Table 6.1). The predictive value of an *in vitro* susceptibility result showing resistance to acyclovir for failure to heal in response to acyclovir therapy was 95%; for foscarnet the predictive value of a resistant result for failure to heal was 88%[35]. Possible explanations for instances of discordance between *in vitro* susceptibility result and therapeutic response are numerous: imprecision of the assay, inadequacy of host immune responses that ultimately result in failure of

Table 6.1 *Association of* in vitro *susceptibility results with response to antiviral therapy in patients with outbreaks of HSV*

| | Response to antiviral therapy[*] | | | | | |
| | Acyclovir | | | Foscarnet | | |
	Complete healing	Partial healing	Failure to heal	Complete healing	Partial healing	Failure to heal
In vitro result[†]						
Susceptible	24	8	7	55	12	0
Resistant	2	2	72	0	1	7
Total	26	10	79	55	13	7

[*] Complete healing was defined as re-epithelialization, partial healing as lack of increase in size of lesion without full re-epithelialization, and failure to heal as enlargement of the lesion(s)
[†] Definitions of resistance, using the plaque reduction assay in Vero cells, were $ID_{50} \geq 2\mu g/ml$ for acyclovir and $ID_{50} \geq 100\ \mu g/ml$ for foscarnet

the lesion to heal despite therapy with an agent to which the virus is susceptible, or the sampling of a clinical lesion while the predominant phenotypic population is in transition, from susceptible to resistant.

A variety of more rapid methods of susceptibility testing have been evaluated, including two enzyme-linked immunosorbent assays[36,37]. Although their rapidity and use of an objective standardized endpoint are appealing, each needs further evaluation using a larger number of specimens, with clinical validation of *in vitro* susceptibility results.

Management of resistant HSV infections

As delineated in the previous chapter, three mechanisms of resistance in HSV have been described: deficiency or absence of thymidine kinase activity, alteration in substrate specificity of the virus-specified thymidine kinase, and alteration in the substrate specificity of the viral DNA polymerase[38,39]. Although the great majority of acyclovir-resistant mutants from clinical lesions have deficient thymidine kinase activity[19,21], resistant clinical mutants with either the thymidine kinase-altered or DNA polymerase-altered phenotypes have occasionally been recovered as well[14,15,40-43]. Although thymidine kinase mutants are typically cross-resistant with agents which depend on thymidine kinase-mediated activation (e.g. ganciclovir, famciclovir), they will have preserved susceptibility to agents such as foscarnet or vidarabine. In contrast, a DNA polymerase mutant may be cross-resistant with foscarnet and vidarabine, and will therefore be more difficult to treat.

There are several antiviral agents with activity against HSV currently available in the United States that might serve as alternative therapies for the patient failing to respond to acyclovir. Continuous infusion of acyclovir, with serial adjustment in dosing to target serum levels of 20–80 μmol/l, induced healing in five immunocompromised patients who were unresponsive to intermittent therapy with acyclovir for durations of 13–28 days[44,45]. Although healing occurred in one patient after only eight days of therapy, the other four patients required six weeks of continuous acyclovir infusion therapy. The fact that *in vitro* resistance to acyclovir may be overcome by constant high levels of acyclovir in the serum is of great interest; however, this approach is likely to be impractical for the majority of patients with HSV infections which are refractory to standard doses of acyclovir, owing to the lack of availability of serum acyclovir levels in most clinical laboratories, to the requirement for an infusion pump, and to the relatively long duration of therapy necessary to effect healing.

Ganciclovir is a nucleoside analog currently licensed for the treatment of cytomegalovirus infections. It is an agent with excellent *in vitro* activity against HSV, with intracellular levels of ganciclovir triphosphate in HSV-infected cells which are 10 times greater than those of acyclovir triphosphate. The affinity of ganciclovir for the viral and cellular kinases necessary for triphosphorylation is greater than that of acyclovir, and the half-life of ganciclovir triphosphate is longer in infected cells[46]. ID_{50} values for HSV-1 and HSV-2 are approximately the same for ganciclovir and acyclovir, since a lower affinity of the virus DNA polymerase for ganciclovir triphosphate than for acyclovir triphosphate in effect neutralizes the above advantages of ganciclovir[46]. More importantly, the cross-resistance of ganciclovir with acyclovir demonstrated in clinical isolates of HSV[19,21] renders the substitution of ganciclovir for acyclovir in a patient who is failing to respond to acyclovir unlikely to succeed.

The nucleoside analog vidarabine is activated through phosphorylation by cellular rather than virus kinases, and thus retains activity against thymidine kinase-deficient mutants of HSV[19,21]. However, initial reports of its use to treat acyclovir-resistant HSV infection did not suggest efficacy[10,16,22,25,47], despite *in vitro* susceptibility. Furthermore, in a randomized comparison with foscarnet (discussed below), vidarabine was markedly inferior as therapy for acyclovir-resistant HSV infection in patients with AIDS, failing to induce healing in any of six patients and causing neurologic manifestations of toxicity in three[21].

Foscarnet is a pyrophosphate analog with *in vitro* activity against all of the human herpesviruses, acting to directly inhibit the virus DNA polymerase without requirement for activation through phosphorylation, and thus retaining activity against thymidine kinase-deficient mutants[19,21]. Preliminary case reports and case series suggested its efficacy as therapy for patients with acyclovir-resistant HSV infection[23-25]. In 1991, intravenous foscarnet (40 mg/kg every 8 hours) was compared with intravenous vidarabine (15 mg/kg once daily) for this indication in a randomized multicenter trial[21] (Table 6.2). The study was terminated prematurely owing to the inferior efficacy and excessive toxicity of vidarabine, revealing a shorter time to complete healing of lesions (median 13.5 vs. 38.5 days; $P = 0.001$) and cessation of virus shedding (median 6 vs. 17 days; $P = 0.006$) in patients receiving foscarnet using an intention-to-treat analysis. In this study, although adverse reactions in association with the administration of foscarnet were not uncommon, including proteinuria, hyperphosphatemia, gastrointestinal intolerance and hypocalcemia[21], none were dose-limiting. As noted above, no patient receiving vidarabine achieved complete healing. Interestingly, however, only two of the five patients crossing over to receive foscarnet thereafter achieved complete healing of their lesion(s); in the other three patients healing was partial rather than complete.

Limitations to the use of foscarnet include its broad spectrum of potential toxicities (including azotemia, seizures, penile ulcerations, hyper- and hypophosphatemia, hypocalcemia and anemia), its requirement for parenteral administration using an infusion pump, and the need for frequent laboratory monitoring and serial titration of the dosage during administration. In addition to these practical limitations, a recent report has documented the emergence of resistance to foscarnet in a total of six AIDS patients who had received the drug either intermittently or as a chronic suppressive regimen[30]. In these patients in vitro resistance to foscarnet was correlated with lack of therapeutic response. Interestingly, although five of the six patients had documented in vitro resistance to acyclovir in early clinical isolates, in vitro susceptibility to acyclovir had re-emerged in several, allowing for successful treatment of the foscarnet-resistant HSV lesions with the addition or substitution of acyclovir therapy[30]. These data imply that withdrawal of the selection pressure induced by chronic exposure to a drug may result in reversion of the virus to its original drug-susceptible phenotype.

The identification of a topical alternative therapy would clearly hold great appeal, and several have been evaluated to date. Trifluorothymidine (TFT) is a nucleoside analog currently marketed as an ophthalmic solution for the treatment of herpes keratitis. The drug is triphosphorylated intracellularly to its active compound by cellular enzymes, independent of the virus-specified thymidine kinase[48]; as such it retains activity against TK-deficient mutants of HSV[49]. Topical application of TFT, either alone or in combination with interferon-α, has been reported to effect healing in several patients with acyclovir-resistant

Table 6.2 Results of a randomized trial comparing foscarnet with vidarabine for treatment of acyclovir-resistant HSV infection in patients with AIDS[21]

Treatment assignment	Location of lesion	Size of lesion (cm²)	CD4 count (cells/mm³)	Virus type	Total days of initial treatment	Therapeutic outcome*	Total days of crossover treatment	Therapeutic outcome* +
Vidarabine	perirectal	16 800	10	2	10	fail	14.7	heal
Vidarabine	perirectal, genital	9950	18	2	9	fail	0	
Vidarabine	perirectal	6000	4	2	10	fail	24	partial
Vidarabine	perirectal, genital	10 259	9	2	16	fail	31.7	partial
Vidarabine	perirectal	2995	35	2	10	fail	20.3	heal
Vidarabine	perirectal	69 700	unknown	2	10	fail	38.3	partial
Foscarnet	perirectal, genital	15	38	2	12.3	heal		
Foscarnet	orofacial	1800	9	2	10.3	heal	0	
Foscarnet	perirectal	7968	3	2	13	heal	0	
Foscarnet	orofacial	1200	48	1	12	heal	0	
Foscarnet	perirectal	9600	1	2	24.3	heal	0	
Foscarnet	genital	33 750	15	2	19.7	heal	0	
Foscarnet	perirectal, genital	3254	20	2	19.3	heal	0	
Foscarnet	genital, orofacial	2625	49	2	14	heal	0	

* Failure to heal signifies enlargement of the lesion despite antiviral therapy, healing denotes complete re-epithelialization of the lesion(s), and partial response is defined by shrinkage in size of the lesion(s) without complete healing
+ All patients crossing over from vidarabine received therapy with foscarnet

HSV infection[50,51]. In a trial conducted by the AIDS Clinical Trials Group of the National Institute for Allergy and Infectious Diseases, topical TFT solution was applied thrice daily to acyclovir-unresponsive lesions of HSV in a total of 24 HIV-infected patients and covered with polysporin ointment. Fifty-eight percent of patients had a 50% or greater reduction in the surface area of the lesion at a median of 2.4 weeks[52] (also H. Kessler, personal communication). Lesion pain resolved completely in 45% of patients at a median of five weeks, and complete healing was observed in 29% of patients at a median of 7.1 weeks. One-third of patients developed new lesions during study drug therapy. Fewer lesions at the time of study entry, as well as an orofacial location, were associated with a greater likelihood of response to therapy. Although the proportion of patients achieving complete healing was clearly less than that achieved in clinical trials with foscarnet[21], it is important to note that a majority of patients experienced substantial symptomatic relief, as well as shrinkage of lesions, within a relatively short time. It is encouraging that a topical therapy, devoid of adverse effects, is able to accomplish this, and it may serve as a useful option in many patients with acyclovir-resistant HSV lesions. It is important, however, that both the patient and the physician expect to use the therapy for a prolonged period, potentially without effecting a cure, and with the expectation that new herpetic lesions may develop during therapy. Attempts are under way to reformulate trifluorothymidine into a gel or ointment preparation rather than a solution for this indication; conceivably the efficacy of therapy will increase as a result of this modification alone.

Compounds that inhibit HSV ribonucleotide reductase appear to potentiate the activity of acyclovir *in vitro*[53] and in animal models[54], even against acyclovir-resistant HSV mutants. The ribonucleotide reductase inhibitor BW 348U87 was combined in a 3% cream formulation with 5% acyclovir and applied topically up to six times daily to acyclovir-resistant HSV lesions in 10 patients with AIDS[55]. Although a decrease in total surface area of the lesion was noted in seven patients within the first two weeks of therapy, complete healing (i.e. re-epithelialization) was observed in only one patient, at 28 days. In addition, five patients developed new lesions during therapy. Although the reasons for ultimate failure in the majority of patients despite *in vitro* susceptibility are unclear, the drug in its current formulation will not be a useful alternative to patients with resistant HSV lesions.

SP-303 is a naturally occurring bioflavonoid derived from plant products that inhibits the penetration of herpesvirus into cells[56] and retains *in vitro* activity against acyclovir-resistant clinical isolates of HSV[57,58]. Nine AIDS patients with acyclovir-unresponsive muco-cutaneous HSV infection applied SP-303 ointment thrice daily[59].

Although four patients sustained a transient decrease in lesion size, no patient achieved complete healing after receiving 10–41 days of therapy. Also, although three patients showed a quantitative decrease in virus burden during study drug therapy, no patient ceased to shed virus. Seven patients complained of transient burning or pain at the site of study drug application, and six developed new lesions at contiguous sites. Therefore this compound is not recommended, in its current formulation, for the treatment of acyclovir-resistant HSV infection.

An algorithm for the management of immunocompromised patients with acyclovir-unresponsive HSV infection has been proposed by a panel of experts[60]. If HSV lesions fail to show shrinkage in size after three to five days of therapy with standard doses of oral acyclovir (i.e. 200–400 mg five times daily), or if new lesions are continuing to form, an increase in the dose of oral acyclovir to 800 mg five times daily is recommended. Use of maximal doses of oral acyclovir in this setting might either combat a partial resistance to acyclovir, if present, or overcome malabsorptive problems, resulting in higher serum levels of the drug. The administration of intermittent intravenous acyclovir therapy at 5 mg/kg every eight hours in this setting has not been shown to be of additional benefit[21]. If the patient continues to show no sign of therapeutic response after high-dose oral therapy for five to seven days, then alternative therapy for presumed acyclovir-resistant HSV infection should be instituted. In addition, the clinical isolate should be referred for susceptibility testing, in order to document *in vitro* acyclovir resistance and to evaluate susceptibility to alternative antiviral therapies. This will become increasingly important as options for alternative therapies grow. At present rational choices for alternative therapy are limited to three options: intravenous foscarnet therapy, topical trifluorothymidine application, or enrolment of the patient in a clinical trial of experimental therapies. As summarized above, administration of intravenous foscarnet therapy, in doses of 40 mg/kg every eight hours[21,23-25] or 60 mg/kg every 12 hours[27], might be expected to result in complete healing after approximately 14 days[21], whereas the use of topical trifluorothymidine thrice daily might require considerably longer but have no associated toxicities.

In 1994, two clinical trials were initiated to evaluate alternative therapies in AIDS patients with HSV lesions that are refractory to therapy with oral acyclovir. In one, patients are randomized to receive either 0.3% topical cidofovir gel, 1.0% topical cidofovir gel, or placebo. Cidofovir ((S)-1-[3-hydroxy-2-(phosphonylmethoxy)propyl]-cytosine; previously called HPMPC) is a nucleotide analog (i.e. a nucleoside monophosphate) that circumvents the need for activation by the virus-specified thymidine kinase and thus retains activity against acyclovir-resistant mutants of HSV both *in vitro*[26,61] and in animal models[62]. Several recent case reports have described the successful healing of acyclovir-resistant HSV lesions following either topical[63,64] or intravenous[65] administration of the drug. A prolonged intracellular half-life of the drug permits relatively infrequent administration, an additional advantage to its potential use for this indication[62].

The second clinical trial is evaluating 1% foscarnet cream in an open-label study design. Given its benefit when administered intravenously for the indication of acyclovir-resistant HSV infection[21,23,25], the evaluation of a topical formulation of foscarnet with potentially fewer toxicities seems appropriate and important.

Several new agents with activity against HSV have been licensed or are currently under active clinical investigation. These include famciclovir, valacyclovir and 1-β-D-arabinofuranosyl-E-5-(2-bromovinyl)uracil (BV-araU; sorivudine). Famciclovir is a prodrug of the nucleoside analog penciclovir, with *in vitro* activity against HSV-1, HSV-2 and varicella zoster virus[66]. It was licensed for the treatment of zoster in the United States in 1994, and evaluation of the drug as a therapy for genital herpes is ongoing. Preliminary reports comparing patient-initiated famciclovir versus placebo for the treatment of recurrent genital herpes describe a significant decrease in the times to complete healing, to loss of symptoms and to cessation of virus shedding in those taking famciclovir[67]. Famciclovir requires thymidine kinase-dependent phosphorylation for activation, however, and displays cross-resistance with acyclovir *in vitro*[68]. Valacyclovir is a prodrug of acyclovir. Although administration of valacyclovir orally results in serum levels of acyclovir that are three to five times higher than those after ingestion of oral acyclovir[69], it is unlikely to be of use against acyclovir-resistant disease. BV-araU is a uracil derivative with potent activity against varicella zoster virus (see below). It has activity against HSV-1 but not HSV-2, and requires phosphorylation by the virus-specified thymidine kinase[70]. Therefore, cross-resistance with acyclovir is to be expected.

In patients with acyclovir-resistant HSV infection in whom therapy results in complete re-epithelialization, recurrent disease remains a serious risk. Several reports have noted that recurrent HSV lesions following healing of an acyclovir-resistant lesion are often susceptible to acyclovir, implying that the original virus latent in the paraspinous ganglion has persisted, despite the mutations occurring peripherally[21]. In one prospective study, seven of 10 first recurrences which occurred at the site of the healed resistant lesion were susceptible to acyclovir, whereas three were acyclovir-resistant[21]. However, each of eight patients having second recurrences at that same site had lesions which were resistant to acyclovir. Overall, the median time to recurrence of acyclovir-resistant HSV following healing of the initial resistant lesion was 41 days (range two to 173 days)[21]. Despite the fact that the risk of recurrence is high, there are no data currently available to address the issue of optimal maintenance therapy with either acyclovir or foscarnet once the initial resistant lesion has healed.

CLINICAL MANIFESTATIONS OF ANTIVIRAL RESISTANCE IN VARICELLA ZOSTER VIRUS INFECTIONS

Introduction

As with HSV, varicella zoster virus (VZV) selectively phosphorylates acyclovir by a viral thymidine kinase, and acyclovir triphosphate blocks virus replication through inhibition of the viral DNA polymerase[46]. Acyclovir, however, is less active *in vitro* against VZV than against HSV: ID_{50} values are two to four times higher than against HSV-2 and HSV-1[46]. As with HSV, drug-resistant mutants of VZV are readily isolated in tissue culture by serial passage in the presence of acyclovir[71]. However, clinically significant acyclovir-resistant VZV infection has been less frequently reported than acyclovir-resistant HSV infection, with only about 20 patients described in the English-language literature[35,72-79] (Table 6.3).

Epidemiology and clinical presentation

Acyclovir-resistant VZV infection was first reported in a four-year-old girl with congenital HIV infection[72]. As with acyclovir-resistant HSV infection, all affected patients have been severely immuno-compromised. However, patients with acyclovir-resistant VZV infection have all had advanced HIV disease rather than other forms of immunosuppression.

Acyclovir-resistant VZV lesions tend to be sparse in number, but may be widely disseminated cutaneously. In the original description by Pahwa and colleagues in 1988[72], and in subsequent reports[73-75,77,78], hyperkeratotic verrucous lesions were noted that persisted despite therapy with acyclovir. Ulcerative indurated lesions of acyclovir-resistant VZV have also been described[35,75,76]. The clinical appearance of mucocutaneous lesions may not, therefore, reliably reflect their susceptibility phenotype, and hyperkeratosis may be more indicative of chronicity than of resistance[74]. A report of a patient with meningoradiculitis[79] represents the only description of a viscerally disseminated infection caused by acyclovir-resistant VZV.

Table 6.3 *HIV-infected patients with acyclovir-resistant VZV infection*

Age (years)	CD4 count (mm³)	Duration of lesion(s) (months)	Attempted therapies	Therapeutic outcome +	Reference
2		14	PO ACV, IV ACV, VID	fail	71
27		14	IV ACV	fail	75
26		2	PO ACV, IV ACV	fail	73
31		5	PO ACV, IV ACV, VID	fail	73
31		5	PO ACV, IV ACV, VID	fail	76
32		6	PO ACV, IV ACV, VID	fail	72
34		3	IV ACV, PO ACV, GCV	fail	72
34		14	PO ACV, GCV	fail	72
7		4	PO ACV, IV ACV	fail	72
40	4	4	PO ACV, IV ACV, FOS	heal (FOS)	74
28	3	5	PO ACV, IV ACV, FOS	fail	74
26	80	5	PO ACV, IV ACV, FOS	partial (FOS)	74
47	30	1	PO ACV, IV ACV, FOS	heal (FOS)	74
45	4	3.5	PO ACV, FOS	heal (FOS)	74

PO, oral; IV, intravenous; ACV, acyclovir; VID, vidarabine; FOS, foscarnet; GCV, ganciclovir
+ failure to heal signifies enlargement of the lesion despite antiviral therapy, healing denotes complete re-epithelialization of the lesion(s), and partial response is defined by shrinkage in size of the lesion(s) without complete healing

Diagnosis of *in vitro* resistance

As with HSV, resistance to acyclovir in VZV is conferred by mutations of either the thymidine kinase or DNA polymerase[80]. Alteration of the substrate specificity of the viral thymidine kinase, resulting in a decreased rate of nucleoside phosphorylation, appears to be more commonly found in clinical isolates of resistant VZV than of resistant HSV[73,75,79]. Clinical isolates deficient in thymidine kinase have also been described[73–74,77,81], as have rare strains with cross-resistance to both acyclovir and foscarnet that presumably contain DNA polymerase mutations[72,75].

DNA hybridization[58,73,75,77,81] and plaque reduction[72,78,79] assays are the most commonly utilized methods of susceptibility testing. PCR-based amplification and sequencing of specific regions of the thymidine kinase gene has also been used to more rapidly identify mutations associated with acyclovir resistance[81]. An enzyme-linked immunosorbent assay requiring only three days has also been described[82]. The presence of both cell-associated and cell-free virus within clinical samples not only causes greater difficulty in isolating the virus in the laboratory than with HSV, but may result in differing susceptibility testing results, according to whether cell-associated or cell-free virus is tested[83].

Management of acyclovir-resistant VZV infections

There are no reports in the medical literature of controlled clinical trials of therapies for acyclovir-resistant HSV infection, reflecting the rarity of the condition. Foscarnet has been reported to effect healing of lesions in several case reports[78], and in four of five patients in one case series[75]. Preservation of *in vitro* susceptibility to foscarnet in acyclovir-resistant mutants of VZV has also been demonstrated[73,75,77,79]. However, as noted above, the use of foscarnet is limited by its requirement for parenteral administration by infusion pump, the associated expense, and the spectrum of potential toxicities.

As with acyclovir-resistant HSV, clinical response to vidarabine in patients with acyclovir-resistant VZV has been disappointing. Despite *in vitro* susceptibility against clinical isolates of acyclovir-resistant mutants of VZV[73,79], therapeutic attempts have so far met with failure[72–74,77].

Are there other alternative therapies worth considering? Trifluoro-thymidine has *in vitro* activity against VZV and is not dependent on the viral thymidine kinase to catalyze intracellular activation[48]. One report described its successful use in a 20 cm^2 acyclovir-resistant ulcer caused by thymidine kinase-deficient VZV, following thrice daily application for a total of 16 weeks[84]; another reported complete healing of painful hyperkeratotic acyclovir-resistant VZV lesions of the right leg and left hip in a patient with AIDS following a three-month course of therapy, with topical application of 1% TFT four times daily combined with intralesional therapy with interferon-α-2b twice weekly[85]. As noted above, reformulation of the current liquid formulation into a cream, ointment or gel, if accomplished, may result in enhanced penetration as well as improved ease of application. Another potential future option may be that of cidofovir, which is active against thymidine kinase-deficient strains of acyclovir-resistant VZV mutants *in vitro*[86]. Although not currently under study, topical formulations of both cidofovir and foscarnet (see above) merit evaluation as alternative therapies for acyclovir-resistant VZV infection.

A consensus statement discussing the optimal approach to the immunocompromised patient with acyclovir-unresponsive VZV infection proposed that those with recurrent episodes of zoster, felt to be at highest risk for the development of resistant VZV infection, be treated promptly with intravenous acyclovir (7.5–10 mg/kg every 8 h)[60]. Failure of lesions to respond after seven to 10 days of therapy is highly sugges-tive of acyclovir resistance, and should be managed as such. It is important to note that resistance to acyclovir has been documented in at least two patients having a first (rather than recurrent) episode of zoster[75,76], suggesting that resistance should be considered in any severely immunocompromised patient with an unexpectedly poor response to acyclovir therapy, regardless of prior history of zoster.

There are several new agents with *in vitro* activity against VZV: famciclovir, valacyclovir and BV-araU. Famciclovir, used in doses of 500 mg three times daily[87], typically shows cross-resistance with acyclovir; however, rare clinical isolates of acyclovir-resistant VZV have retained *in vitro* susceptibility to famciclovir[58]. Similarly, occasional clinical isolates of acyclovir-resistant VZV have retained *in vitro* susceptibility to BV-araU[58], despite expected cross-resistance due to thymidine kinase dependency. Cross-resistance of valacyclovir, a prodrug of acyclovir, with acyclovir is invariable; whether resistance can be overcome with higher serum levels remains to be investigated.

In contrast to patients in the general population, AIDS patients have a higher frequency of recurrent episodes of zoster[88]. Similarly, acyclovir-resistant lesions of VZV may also recur[75,84]. Of four patients followed after resolution of acyclovir-resistant VZV infection, two had recurrences of zoster seven and 14 days later, respectively[75]. In both instances *in vitro* testing demonstrated susceptibility to acyclovir. However, although one patient had healing in response to therapy with intravenous acyclovir, the other did not despite 12 days of high-dose oral acyclovir therapy (i.e. 800 mg five times daily). Prompt institution of antiviral therapy is warranted if lesions recur. If using acyclovir, intravenous rather than oral therapy should be considered to overcome poor oral bioavailability and to achieve the high levels of the drug necessary to inhibit varicella zoster virus[89].

REFERENCES

1. Sery TW, Nagy RM. A stable mutation of herpes virus resistance to IUDR. *Invest Ophthalmol* 1965;4:947–54.
2. Kaufman HE, Nesburn AB, Maloney ED. IDU therapy of herpes simplex. *Arch Ophthalmol* 1962;67:583–7.
3. Jawetz E, Coleman VR, Dawson CR, Thygeson P. The dynamics of IUDR action in herpetic keratitis and the emergence of IUDR resistance *in vivo*. *Ann N Y Acad Sci* 1970;173:282–91.

4. Elion GB, Furman PA, Fyfe JA *et al.* Selectivity of action of an antiherpetic agent, 9-(2-hydroxyethoxymethyl) guanine. *Proc Natl Acad Sci USA* 1977;79:5716–20.
5. Field HJ, Darby G, Wildy P. Isolation and characterization of acyclovir-resistant mutants of herpes simplex virus. *J Gen Virol* 1980;49:115–24.
6. McLaren C, Corey L, Dekket C, Barry DW. *In vitro* sensitivity to acyclovir in genital herpes simplex viruses from acyclovir-treated patients. *J Infect Dis* 1983;148:868–75.
7. Wade JC, McLaren C, Meyers JD. Frequency and significance of acyclovir-resistant herpes simplex virus isolated from marrow transplant patients receiving multiple courses of treatment with acyclovir. *J Infect Dis* 1993;148:1077–82.
8. Sibrack CD, Gutman LT, Wilfert CM *et al.* Pathogenicity of acyclovir-resistant herpes simplex virus type 1 from an immunodeficient child. *J Infect Dis* 1982;146:673–82.
9. Crumpacker CS, Schnipper LE, Marlowe SI *et al.* Resistance to antiviral drugs of herpes simplex virus isolated from a patient treated with acyclovir. *New Engl J Med* 1982;306:343–6.
10. Vinckier F, Boogaerts M, De Clerck D, De Clercq E. Chronic herpetic infection in an immunocompromised patient: report of a case. *J Oral Maxillofac Surg* 1987;45:723–8.
11. Bean B, Fletcher C, Englund J, Lehrman SN, Ellis MN. Progressive mucocutaneous herpes simplex infection due to acyclovir-resistant virus in an immunocompromised patient: correlation of viral susceptibilities and plasma levels with response to therapy. *Diagn Microbiol Infect Dis* 1987;7:199–204.
12. Ljungman P, Ellis MN, Hackman RC, Shepp DH, Meyers JD. Acyclovir-resistant herpes simplex virus causing pneumonia after marrow transplantation. *J Infect Dis* 1990;162:244–8.
13. Westheim AI, Tenser RB, Marks JG Jr. Acyclovir resistance in a patient with chronic mucocutaneous herpes simplex infection. *J Am Acad Dermatol* 1987;5:875–80.
14. Parker AC, Craig JIO, Collins P, Oliver N, Smith I. Acyclovir-resistant herpes simplex virus infection due to altered DNA polymerase. *Lancet* 1987;2:1461.
15. Sacks SL, Wanklin RJ, Reece DE *et al.* Progressive esophagitis from acyclovir-resistant herpes simplex. Clinical roles for DNA polymerase mutants and viral heterogeneity. *Ann Intern Med* 1989;111:893–9.
16. Norris SA, Kessler HA, Fife KH. Severe progressive herpetic whitlow caused by an acyclovir-resistant virus in a patient with AIDS. *J Infect Dis* 1987;157:209–10.
17. Youle MM, Hawkins DA, Collins P *et al.* Acyclovir-resistant herpes in AIDS treated with foscarnet. *Lancet* 1988;2:341–2.
18. Causey DM. Foscarnet treatment of acyclovir-resistant herpes simplex proctitis in an AIDS patient. Abstract 3589. IV International Conference for AIDS 1988; Stockholm, Sweden.
19. Erlich KS, Mills J, Chatis P *et al.* Acyclovir-resistant herpes simplex virus infections in patients with the acquired immunodeficiency syndrome. *New Engl J Med* 1989;320:293–6.
20. Birch CJ, Tachedjian G, Doherty RR, Hayes K, Gust ID. Altered sensitivity to antiviral drugs of herpes simplex virus isolates from a patient with the acquired immunodeficiency syndrome. *J Infect Dis* 1990;162:731–4.

21. Safrin S, Crumpacker C, Chatis P *et al.* and the AIDS Clinical Trials Group. A controlled trial comparing foscarnet with vidarabine for acyclovir-resistant mucocutaneous herpes simplex in the acquired immunodeficiency syndrome. *New Engl J Med* 1991;325:551–5.

22. Gateley A, Gander RM, Johnson PC *et al.* Herpes simplex virus 2 meningo-encephalitis resistant to acyclovir in a patient with AIDS. *J Infect Dis* 1990;161:711–15.[73,73,]

23. Erlich KS, Jacobson MA, Koehler JE *et al.* Foscarnet therapy for severe acyclovir-resistant herpes simplex virus type-2 infections in patients with the acquired immunodeficiency syndrome (AIDS): an uncontrolled trial. *Ann Intern Med* 1989;110:710–13.

24. Chatis PA, Miller CH, Schrager LE, Crumpacker CS. Successful treatment with foscarnet of an acyclovir-resistant mucocutaneous infection with herpes simplex virus in a patient with acquired immunodeficiency syndrome. *New Engl J Med* 1982;320:297–300.

25. Safrin S, Assaykeen T, Follansbee S, Mills J. Foscarnet therapy for acyclovir-resistant mucocutaneous herpes simplex virus infection in 26 AIDS patients: preliminary data. *J Infect Dis* 1990;161:1078–84.

26. Bevilacqua F, Marcello A, Toni M *et al.* Acyclovir resistance/susceptibility in herpes simplex virus type-2 sequential isolates from an AIDS patient. *JAIDS* 1991;4:967–9.

27. Hardy WD. Foscarnet treatment of acyclovir-resistant herpes simplex virus infection in patients with acquired immunodeficiency syndrome: preliminary results of a controlled, randomized, regimen-comparative trial. *Am J Med* 1992;92(Suppl 2A):30S–35S.

28. Kost RG, Hill EL, Tigges M, Straus SE. Brief report: recurrent acyclovir-resistant genital herpes in an immunocompetent patient. *New Engl J Med* 1993;329:1777–82.

29. McLaren C, Ellis MN, Hunter GA. A colorimetric assay for the measurement of the sensitivity of herpes simplex viruses to antiviral agents. *Antiviral Res* 1983;3:223–34.

30. Safrin S, Kemmerly S, Plotkin B *et al.* Foscarnet-resistant herpes simplex virus infection in patients with AIDS. *J Infect Dis* 1994;169:193–6.

31. Swierkosz EM, Scholl DR, Brown JL, Jollick JD, Gleaves CA. Improved DNA hybridization method for detection of acyclovir-resistant herpes simplex virus. *Antimicrob Agents Chemother* 1987;31:1465–9.

32. Ellis MN, Waters R, Hill EL *et al.* Orofacial infection of athymic mice with defined mixtures of acyclovir-susceptible and acyclovir-resistant herpes simplex virus type 1. *Antimicrob Agents Chemother* 1989;33:304–10.

33. Parris DS, Harrington JE. Herpes simplex virus variants resistant to high concentrations of acyclovir exist in clinical isolates. *Antimicrob Agents Chemother* 1982;22:71–7.

34. Safrin S, Phan L, Elbeik T. A comparative evaluation of three methods of antiviral susceptibility testing of clinical herpes simplex virus isolates. *Clin Diagn Virol* 1995;4:81–91.

35. Safrin S, Elbeik T, Phan L *et al.* Correlation between response to acyclovir and foscarnet therapy and *in vitro* susceptibility result for isolates of herpes simplex virus from human immunodeficiency virus-infected patients. *Antimicrob Agents Chemother* 1994;38:1246–50.

36. Weinberg A, Bate BJ, Masters HB *et al.* In vitro activities of penciclovir and

acyclovir against herpes simplex virus types 1 and 2. *Antimicrob Agents Chemother* 1993;36:2037–8.

37. Leahy BJ, Christiansen KJ, Shellam G. Standardisation of a microplate in situ ELISA (MISE-test) for the susceptibility testing of herpes simplex virus to acyclovir. *J Virol Meth* 1994;48:93–108.

38. Coen DM, Schaffer PA. Two distinct loci confer resistance to acycloguanosine in herpes simplex virus type 1. *Proc Natl Acad Sci USA* 1980;77:2265–9.

39. Schnipper LE, Crumpacker CS. Resistance of herpes simplex virus to acycloguanosine: role of viral thymidine kinase and DNA polymerase loci. *Proc Natl Acad Sci USA* 1980;77:2270–3.

40. Ellis MN, Keller PM, Fyfe JA *et al.* Clinical isolate of herpes simplex virus type 2 that induces a thymidine kinase with altered substrate specificity. *Antimicrob Agents Chemother* 1987;31:1117–25.

41. Nugier F, Collins P, Larder BA *et al.* Herpes simplex virus isolates from an immunocompromised patient who failed to respond to acyclovir treatment express thymidine kinase with altered substrate specificity. *Antiviral Chem Chemother* 1991;2:295–302.

42. Collins P, Larder BA, Oliver NM *et al.* Characterization of a DNA polymerase mutant of herpes simplex virus from a severely immunocompromised patient receiving acyclovir. *J Gen Virol* 1989;70:375–82.

43. Hwang CBC, Ruffner KL, Coen DM. A point mutation within a distinct conserved region of the herpes simplex virus DNA polymerase gene confers drug resistance. *J Virol* 1992;66:1774–6.

44. Fletcher CV, Englund JA, Bean B *et al.* Continuous infusion of high-dose acyclovir for serious herpesvirus infections. *Antimicrob Agents Chemother* 1989;33:1375–8.

45. Engel JP, Englund JA, Fletcher CV, Hill EL. Treatment of resistant herpes simplex virus with continuous-infusion acyclovir. *JAMA* 1990;263:1662–4.

46. Elion GB. Mechanism of action, spectrum and selectivity of nucleoside analogs. In: Mills J, Corey L, eds. *Directions for Clinical Application and Research.* New York: Elsevier, 1986:118–37.

47. Siegal FP, Lopez C, Hammer GS *et al.* Severe acquired immunodeficiency in male homosexuals, manifested by chronic perianal ulcerative herpes simplex lesions. *New Engl J Med* 1981;305:1439–44.

48. Heidelberger C. On the molecular mechanism of the antiviral activity of trifluorothymidine. *Ann N Y Acad Sci* 1974:317–24.

49. Field H, McMillan A, Darby G. The sensitivity of acyclovir-resistant mutants of herpes simplex virus to other antiviral drugs. *J Infect Dis* 1981;143:281–5.

50. Murphy M, Morley A, Eglin RP, Monteiro E. Topical trifluridine for mucocutaneous acyclovir-resistant herpes simplex II in AIDS patient. *Lancet* 1992;340:1040.

51. Birch CJ, Tyssen DP, Tachedjian G *et al.* Clinical effects and *in vitro* studies of trifluorothymidine combined with interferon-α for treatment of drug-resistant and -sensitive herpes simplex virus infections. *J Infect Dis* 1992;166:108–12.

52. Kessler HA, Weaver D, Benson CA *et al.* ACTG 172: treatment of acyclovir-resistant (ACV-R) mucocutaneous herpes simplex virus (HSV) infection in patients with AIDS: open label pilot study of topical trifluridine (TFT). Abstract 82, Infectious Diseases Society of America; Anaheim, CA, 1992.

53. Spector T, Harrington JA, Morrison RW Jr *et al*. 2-acetylpyridine5-[(dimethylamino)thiocarbonyl]-thiocarbonohydrazone(A111OU), a potent inactivator of ribonucleotide reductases of herpes simplex and varicella-zoster viruses and a potentiator of acyclovir. *Proc Natl Acad Sci USA* 1989;86:1051–5.

54. Lobe DC, Spector T, Ellis MN. Synergistic topical therapy by acyclovir and A111OU for herpes simplex virus induced zosteriform rash in mice. *Antiviral Res* 1991;15:87–100.

55. Safrin S, Schacker T, Delehanty J, Hill E, Corey L. Topical treatment of infection with acyclovir-resistant mucocutaneous herpes simplex virus with the ribonucleotide reductase inhibitor 348U87 in combination with acyclovir. *Antimicrob Agents Chemother* 1993;37:975–9.

56. Barnard DL, Huffman JH, Meyerson LR, Sidwell RW. Mode of inhibition of respiratory syncytial virus by a plant flavonoid, SP-303. *Chemotherapy* 1993;39:212–17.

57. Barnard DL, Smee DF, Huffman JH, Meyerson LR, Sidwell RW. Antiherpes-virus activity and mode of action of SP-303, a novel plant flavonoid. *Chemotherapy* 1993;39:203–11.

58. Talarico CL, Phelps WC, Biron KK. Analysis of the thymidine kinase genes from acyclovir-resistant mutants of varicella-zoster virus isolated from patients with AIDS. *J Virol* 1993;67:1024–33.

59. Safrin S, McKinley G, McKeough M, Robinson D, Spruance SL. Treatment of acyclovir-unresponsive cutaneous herpes simplex virus infection with topically applied SP-303. *Antiviral Res* 1994;25:185–92.

60. Balfour HH Jr, Benson C, Braun J *et al*. Management of acyclovir-resistant herpes simplex and varicella-zoster virus infections. *JAIDS* 1994;7:254–60.

61. De Clercq E. Virus-drug resistance: thymidine kinase-deficient (TK-) mutants of herpes simplex virus. Therapeutic approaches. *Ann 1st Super Sanita* 1987;23:841–8.

62. De Clercq E, Holy A. Efficacy of (S)-1-(3-hydroxy-2-phosphonylmethoxy-propyl)cytosine in various models of herpes simplex virus infection in mice. *Antimicrob Agents Chemother* 1991;35:701–6.

63. Snoeck R, Andrei G, De Clercq E *et al*. A new topical treatment for resistant herpes simplex infections. *New Engl J Med* 1993;329:968–9.

64. Snoeck R, Andrei G, Gerard M *et al*. Successful treatment of pro-gressive mucocutaneous infection due to acyclovir- and foscarnet-resistant herpes simplex virus with (S)-1-(3-hydroxy-2-phosphonylmethoxypropyl)cytosine(HPMPC). *Clin Infect Dis* 1994;18:570–8.

65. Lalezari JP, Drew WL, Glutzer E *et al*. Treatment with intravenous (S)-1-[3-hydroxy-2-(phosphonylmethoxy)propyl]-cytosine of acyclovir-resistant mucocutaneous infection with herpes simplex virus in a patient with AIDS. *J Infect Dis* 1994;170:570–2.

66. Boyd MR, Safrin S, Kern ER. Penciclovir: a review of its spectrum of activity, selectivity, and cross-resistance pattern. *Antiviral Chem Chemother* 1993; 4(Suppl 1):3–11.

67. Sacks SL, Aoki FY, Diaz-Mitoma F *et al*. and The Canadian Cooperative Study Group. Patient-initiated treatment (tx) of recurrent genital herpes (RGH) with oral famciclovir (FCV): a Canadian, multicenter, placebo-(PLB)-controlled, dose-ranging study. Abstract H4, the 34th ICAAC; Orlando, Florida, 1994.

68. Safrin S, Phan L. *In vitro* activity of penciclovir against clinical isolates of

acyclovir-resistant and foscarnet-resistant herpes simplex virus. *Antimicrob Agents Chemother* 1993;37:2241–3.

69. Jacobson MA, Gallant J, Wang LH *et al.* Phase I trial of valaciclovir, the L-valyl ester of acyclovir, in patients with advanced human immunodeficiency virus disease. *Antimicrob Agents Chemother* 1994;38:1534–40.

70. Yokota T, Konno K, Mori S *et al.* Mechanism of selective inhibition of varicella zoster virus replication by 1-β-D-arabinofuranosyl-E-5-(2-bromovinyl)uracil. *Mol Pharmacol* 1989;36:312.

71. Biron KK, Fyfe JA, Noblin JE, Elion GB. Selection and preliminary characterization of acyclovir-resistant mutants of varicella-zoster virus. *Am J Med* 1982;73:383–6.

72. Pahwa S, Biron K, Lim W *et al.* Continuous varicella-zoster infection associated with acyclovir resistance in a child with AIDS. *JAMA* 1988;260:2879–82.

73. Jacobson MA, Berger TG, Fikrig S *et al.* Acyclovir-resistant varicella zoster virus infection after chronic oral acyclovir therapy in patients with the acquired immunodeficiency syndrome (AIDS). *Ann Intern Med* 1990;112:187–91.

74. Hoppenjans WB, Bibler MR, Orme RL, Solinger AM. Prolonged cutaneous herpes zoster in acquired immunodeficiency syndrome. *Arch Dermatol* 1990;126:1048–50.

75. Safrin S, Berger TG, Gilson I *et al.* Foscarnet therapy in five patients with AIDS and acyclovir-resistant varicella-zoster virus infection. *Ann Intern Med* 1991;115:19–21.

76. Janier M, Hillion B, Baccard M *et al.* Chronic varicella zoster infection in acquired immunodeficiency syndrome. *J Am Acad Dermatol* 1988;18:584–5.

77. Linnemann CC, Biron KK, Hoppenjans WG, Solinger AM. Emergence of acyclovir-resistant varicella zoster virus in an AIDS patient on prolonged acyclovir therapy. *AIDS* 1990;4:577–9.

78. Smith KJ, Kahlter DC, Davis C *et al.* Acyclovir-resistant varicella zoster responsive to foscarnet. *Arch Dermatol* 1991;127:1069–71.

79. Leport C, Puget S, Pepin JM *et al.* Meningoradiculoneuritis due to acyclovir-resistant varicella-zoster virus in a patient with AIDS. *J Infect Dis* 1993;168:1330–1.

80. Shiraki K, Ogino T, Yamanishi K, Takahashi M. Isolation of drug resistant mutants of varicella-zoster virus: cross resistance of acyclovir resistant mutants with phosphonoacetic acid and bromodeoxyuridine. *Biken J* 1983;26:17–23.

81. Boivin G, Edelman CK, Pedneault L *et al.* Phenotypic and genotypic characterization of acyclovir-resistant varicella-zoster viruses isolated from persons with AIDS. *J Infect Dis* 1994;170:68–75.

82. Berkowitz FE, Levin MJ. Use of an enzyme-linked immunosorbent assay performed directly on fixed infected cell monolayers for evaluating drugs against varicella-zoster virus. *Antimicrob Agents Chemother* 1985;28:207–10.

83. Shiraki K, Ochiai H, Namazue J *et al.* Comparison of antiviral assay methods using cell-free and cell-associated varicella-zoster virus. *Antiviral Res* 1992;18:209–14.

84. Ives V, Stanat SC, Biron KK, Harris S. Successful treatment of acyclovir-resistant zoster with topical trifluorothymidine (TFT). Abstract 292. Second National Conference on Human Retroviruses, Washington DC, 1995.

85. Rossi S, Whitfeld M, Berger T. The treatment of acyclovir-resistant herpes

zoster with trifluorothymidine and interferon alfa. *Arch Dermatol* 1995;131:24–6.

86. Ho HT, Woods KL, Bronson JJ *et al.* Intracellular metabolism of the antiherpes agent (S)-1-[3-hydroxy-2-(phosphonylmethoxy)propyl]cytosine. *Mol Pharmacol* 1991;41:197–202.

87. Degreef H, Famciclovir Herpes Zoster Clinical Study Group. Famciclovir, a new oral antiherpes drug: results of the first controlled clinical study demonstrating its efficacy and safety in the treatment of uncomplicated herpes zoster in immunocompetent patients. *Int J Antimicrob Agents* 1994;4:241–6.

88. Colebunders R, Mann JM, Francis H *et al.* Herpes zoster in African patients: a clinical predictor of human immunodeficiency virus infection. *J Infect Dis* 1988;157:314–18.

89. Dorsky DI, Crumpacker CS. Drugs five years later: acyclovir. *Ann Intern Med* 1987;107:859–74.

CYTOMEGALOVIRUS

7
Nucleosides and Foscarnet—Mechanisms

KAREN K. BIRON AND F. BALDANTI

CYTOMEGALOVIRUS: CHARACTERISTICS OF THE VIRUS AND ITS DISEASES

The cytomegaloviruses (CMV) are members of the β subfamily of herpesviruses; human CMV has also been designated as human herpesvirus 5 (HHV5). Among the herpesviruses the cytomegaloviruses are distinctive in their species specificity, cell tropisms and characteristically slow growth in culture[1]. Studies of genomic content and arrangement within the herpesviruses indicate evolutionary divergence of CMV and HHV6 from HSV1, HSV2 (herpes simplex virus) and VZV (varicella zoster virus).

The human CMV genome, a double-stranded linear DNA molecule of 230–240 kb, is the largest of the herpesvirus genomes. It exists in a complex arrangement of four isomers bounded by inverted and direct repeats, similar to the genome arrangement of HSV. Only a fraction of the 208–227 open reading frames (ORFs) encoded by CMV strains have been assigned a functional role, either by direct product identification or by sequence homology with the genomes of HSV, VZV or Epstein–Barr virus (EBV)[2]. The majority of these homologs encode functions required for DNA replication, maturation and virion structure. Several of these represent targets for current or developing therapeutics: the viral DNA polymerase, the helicase–primase, the protease and the putative terminase. CMV is susceptible *in vitro* to several antiviral agents active against HSV and VZV, notably the nucleoside analogs adenine arabinoside, ganciclovir and acyclovir, and the pyrophosphate analogs phosphonoacetate and phosphonoformate (Figure 7.1)[3].

Antiviral Drug Resistance. Edited by Douglas D. Richman © 1996 John Wiley & Sons Ltd

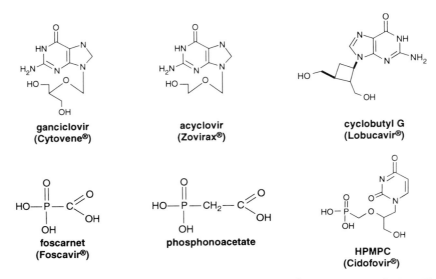

Figure 7.1 Antiviral agents with in vitro activity against human cytomegalovirus. The drug structures and generic and trade names are indicated. These agents are developed by Roche-Syntex (Cytovene), Glaxo Wellcome (Zovirax), Bristol Myers Squibb (Lobucavir), Astra Pharmaceuticals (Foscavir) and Gilead Sciences (Cidofovir)

CMV shares the characteristic abilities of the other herpesviruses to establish persistence or lifelong latency following primary infection, and to reactivate as cell-mediated immunity declines. Whereas the peripheral nervous system harbors latent HSV or VZV, the monocyte precursors[4,5] have been implicated as the sites for latent CMV. The regulation of this process is not yet understood, although the importance of the immune system in restricting CMV is evidenced by its disease epidemiology. The developing fetus is particularly susceptible to the destructive effects of CMV replication, and neonatal CMV infection can result in significant morbidity. CMV infections are a leading cause of life-threatening disease in bone marrow and solid organ transplant patients, and in patients with AIDS. Pneumonitis is a major complication in transplant populations, and disseminated CMV infections occur in almost 100% of end-stage patients with AIDS. Retinitis is the most common manifestation of localized organ infection by CMV, and is present in roughly 20% of patients with AIDS. Once retinitis has developed, patients require lifelong therapy to prevent recurrences and thus preserve vision. Systemic disease may involve many organ systems, resulting in gastroenteritis, hepatitis, pancreatitis and, less commonly, peripheral (polyradiculopathy) and central (encephalitis) nervous systems. The management of CMV disease in the absence of immune restriction is further complicated by the fact that individuals (especially those with certain high-risk behaviors) may be infected with multiple strains of CMV[6,7,22]. These strains can reactivate simultaneously or sequentially, and different virus populations (i.e. strains or drug-resistant phenotypes) may be present at different body sites. Furthermore, these sites may vary in their accessibility to antiviral drugs, complicating the potential for disease breakthrough or the emergence of drug-resistant strains. The dominant factors favoring the emergence of drug-resistant viruses in the immunocompromised patient are high virus load and the requisite chronic or intermittent therapy.

ANTIVIRAL AGENTS AND THE EMERGENCE OF DRUG-RESISTANT CMV

Ganciclovir (Cytovene®) and foscarnet (Foscavir®) are the two agents currently licensed for the treatment of CMV disease. Ganciclovir 9-[2-hydroxy-1-(hydroxymethyl) ethoxymethyl] guanine, is a nucleoside analog with *in vitro* activity against CMV, HSV1 and 2, VZV, EBV, and HHV6[8,9]. Foscarnet (phosphonoformic acid, or PFA) is a pyrophosphate analog with broad-spectrum antiherpetic activity *in vitro* against herpesviruses, the human immunodeficiency virus (HIV) and several other RNA and DNA viruses[10]. Acyclovir, 9-(2-hydroxyethoxymethyl) guanine, is an analog of deoxyguanosine with potent and selective activity against HSV1 and 2, VZV and EBV and moderate activity against CMV[11].

Therapies in various stages of clinical development for treatment of CMV infections include HPMPC (Cidofovir®), a nucleotide analog[12,13]; cyclobutylguanine (cbG, Lobucavir®), another nucleoside analog of deoxyguanosine[14]; and ISIS 2922, a phosphorothioate antisense oligonucleotide directed against CMV IE mRNA (an intravitreal therapy)[15].

Drug-resistant strains of HIV, HSV, VZV and CMV have emerged in immunocompromised patients receiving antiviral therapy, creating the impetus for the characterization of drug-resistant genotypes and efforts to establish rapid diagnostic methods. Ganciclovir and foscarnet are inadequate for effective suppression of CMV because they demonstrate dose-related toxicities and potency limitations. Disease progression results from virus amplification, necessitating chemotherapeutic control. In these patients drug resistance may also limit the effectiveness of chronic suppressive therapy. Reports have linked the presence of ganciclovir-resistant and foscarnet-resistant virus with apparent clinical failures[16-23]. More studies are needed to establish a causal link, as other factors can account for therapeutic failure. However, the presence of drug-resistant virus is a predictor of poor clinical outcome.

Ganciclovir-resistant virus is generally isolated after a minimum cumulative drug exposure of three months, at which time a significant proportion of the recovered isolate is drug resistant *in vitro*. These resistant variants undoubtedly exist as minor components of the virus population at earlier times. Early detection of drug-resistant mutants will be facilitated as sensitive probes for genetic lesions in target genes become more available. The use of conventional cell culture methods to determine drug susceptibility is time-consuming and problematic. The plaque reduction assay has been used most extensively: suggested cut-off values for *in vitro* drug resistance to ganciclovir and foscarnet are >6 μM and $\geqslant 400$ μM, respectively[22-24]. Since between laboratories variation in absolute IC_{50} values occurs, it is reasonable to look for at least a three- to fivefold elevation in IC_{50} values of test isolates compared to susceptible controls included in the same assays as an indication of drug resistance (see Chapter 8). The elevation in IC_{90} or IC_{95} values can also signal the presence of a low proportion of drug-resistant quasi species.

In one study the overall prevalence of ganciclovir resistance in treated retinitis patients was approximately 7.6%; resistant virus was only recovered in those patients who continued to shed virus after approximately 3 months of drug exposure (5 of 13, 38%)[24]. With the availability of alternate therapy in the form of foscarnet, a successful management strategy has been to switch the ganciclovir non-responders to this drug. Recently, strains with *in vitro* resistance to both ganciclovir and foscarnet were recovered from a few of these patients; these strains carried mutations in both the UL97 'ganciclovir kinase' gene and in the viral DNA polymerase gene. Fortunately, these isolates were susceptible to HPMPC, suggesting its potential as a rescue therapy. More effective, less toxic therapeutic agents for CMV are needed, particularly those directed against other viral gene products, such as protease, IE genes or the UL89-encoded terminase. The availability of multiple agents with independent modes of action would facilitate disease management through drug combination or alternating drug regimes.

DRUG MECHANISMS OF ACTION

Ganciclovir and Acyclovir

As a deoxyguanosine analog, ganciclovir blocks herpes viral DNA replication by acting as a competitor of the natural substrate for incorporation by the viral DNA polymerases. This antiviral action requires phosphorylation of ganciclovir to its triphosphate form in virus-infected cells. The rate-limiting step in this conversion is the initial phosphorylation. In normal cells this is catalyzed inefficiently by the 5' acid nucleotidase, which accounts in part for the cytotoxicity of this drug to rapidly growing cells (i.e. marrow progenitors). In cells infected with HSV1 or 2, or with VZV, this monophosphorylation is catalyzed efficiently by the viral-encoded deoxypyrimidine kinase (thymidine kinase, TK)[11]. CMV, however, does not encode an analogous TK gene. There were early reports that cellular deoxyguanosine kinases performed this function in CMV-infected cells[25-27]. This seemed plausible because CMV infection resulted in the stimulation of cytosol deoxycytidine and thymidine kinases. Subsequent genetic studies, however, demonstrated that the preferential monophosphorylation of ganciclovir in CMV-infected cells is controlled, directly or indirectly, by the gene product of the UL97 open reading frame[28-31]. This was determined by genetic mapping of the phosphorylation-deficient phenotype of a ganciclovir-resistant, laboratory-derived mutant[30]. The direct role of this gene product in ganciclovir monophosphorylation was substantiated by its expression in a bacterial system[31]. Sequence homology to known classes of protein kinases and bacterial aminoglycoside phosphotransferases implies that the UL97 gene product is a protein kinase[32-35]. These bacterial enzymes also catalyze the addition of a phosphate to the 5'-OH of a sugar moiety in aminoglycoside antibiotics. It is likely that evolutionary similarity to these bacterial enzymes allows the UL97 gene product as a phosphotransferase to anabolize a nucleoside analog. Comparison of the intracellular levels of ganciclovir anabolites in cells infected with HSV or CMV indicates that the HSV TKs are roughly ten times more efficient than the CMV UL97 enzyme in this process[28].

There is evidence that the UL97 phosphotransferase also contributes to the intracellular activation of acyclovir in CMV-infected cells[36]. The mutant 759'D100, which is deficient in the ability to induce ganciclovir phosphorylation, and which was originally used to identify the UL97 ORF, is also deficient in the intracellular anabolism of acyclovir. Other laboratory-selected ganciclovir-resistant UL97 strains exhibited reduced susceptibility to acyclovir *in vitro*, as did 759'D100[37].

Ganciclovir and acyclovir monophosphates are converted to their diphosphate forms by cellular guanylate kinase[38]. The kinetics of this enzyme favor the phosphorylation of ganciclovir monophosphate over acyclovir monophosphate[38,39]. The triphosphates are ultimately generated by non-specific cellular enzymes, such as phosphoglycerate kinase[40]. Both triphosphate analogs are potent competitive inhibitors for the incorporation of dGMP by the CMV DNA polymerase[41]. The relative potency of acyclovir triphosphate for this reaction is approximately three to 10 times higher than that of ganciclovir triphosphate (apparent k_i acyclovir triphosphate $= 8$ nM, apparent k_i ganciclovir triphosphate $= 22$ nM)[50]. The k_i values of acyclovir triphosphate and ganciclovir triphosphate for mammalian DNA polymerase α were 96 nM and 146 nM, respectively[41,51]. Ganciclovir triphosphate can be incorporated internally into the DNA of dividing cells expressing functional HSV TK[42], although the rate of DNA elongation is slower. Template incorporation and extension studies suggested that the DNA polymerases of HSV2 and CMV encounter translocation difficulties after incorporation of ganciclovir mono-phosphate[43]. By contrast, acyclovir triphosphate is an obligate chain terminator: it lacks the 3'C-OH moiety necessary for chain extension.

Foscarnet

Foscarnet is a pyrophosphate analog that directly inhibits the viral DNA polymerase: it does not require activation by viral-encoded nucleoside kinases or phosphotransferases. As a pyrophosphate mimic, foscarnet interferes with the release of pyrophosphate from deoxynucleotide triphosphate during the substrate incorporation event. Foscarnet inhibits the herpes viral DNA polymerases at concentrations that do not affect cellular DNA polymerases or normal cell growth[44-47]. This mechanism constitutes non-competitive inhibition of the CMV DNA polymerase with respect to the four deoxynucleoside triphosphate substrates; it is uncompetitive inhibition with respect to the template used[46]. Foscarnet inhibits the DNA polymerases of susceptible CMV strains with inhibitory values (50%) of 0.3 μM, compared to IC_{50} values of ~40 μM for the mammalian αDNA polymerase[45].

Phosphonoacetic acid (PAA), a close analog of foscarnet, was originally used for *in vitro* mechanism studies in HSV systems. Foscarnet- or PAA-resistant laboratory strains of HSV and VZV have resulted from DNA polymerase active site alterations associated with single amino acid substitutions.

HPMPC

HPMPC, (5)-1-(3-hydroxy-2-phosphonylmethoxypropyl) cytosine, is effectively a nucleoside monophosphate or phosphonate. This drug only requires the addition of the second and third phosphates to reach the activated antiviral state. These phosphorylations are accomplished by cellular enzymes; therefore HPMPC does not require any viral-encoded TKs or phosphotransferases[13,48,49]. The selectivity of HPMPC is achieved at the level of inhibition of viral DNA polymerase. The diphosphate form (HPMPC-DP) is a competitive inhibitor for the incorporation of deoxycytosine monophosphate by the CMV DNA polymerase. Based on *in vitro* enzyme kinetic studies, HPMPC-DP was predicted to have little effect on DNA repair and mitochondrial DNA synthesis. The k_i value for inhibition of the repair enzyme *pol* β was 520 μM; for the mitochondrial enzyme k_i was 299 μM[49]. Predictably, HPMPC is active against acyclovir-resistant TK mutants of HSV or VZV, and against ganciclovir-resistant strains of CMV that carry UL97 alterations[50].

The efficacy of antiviral nucleoside analogs is also influenced by the persistence of the drug in tissues and plasma and the persistence of the activated antiviral form in virally infected cells. Ganciclovir triphosphate has an intracellular half-life ($t\frac{1}{2}$) of 15–26 hours in CMV- or HSV-infected cells[25,29,51]. Acyclovir triphosphate, however, exhibits an intracellular $t\frac{1}{2}$ of 1–2 hours[11]. These properties probably contribute to the relative efficacy of these two agents in animal models and in humans. HPMPC is unique in its extraordinary persistence in cultured cells[52] and *in vivo*, allowing infrequent dosing (weekly or biweekly) to achieve efficacy.

CMV UL97 AND GANCICLOVIR RESISTANCE

The CMV UL97 protein serves as the ganciclovir kinase in CMV-infected cells; this enzyme activity is essential to the antiviral action of ganciclovir *in vitro*. There is a direct correlation between the intracellular levels of ganciclovir triphosphate in infected cells and the sensitivity of the infecting strain to ganciclovir *in vitro* (Figure 7.2)[50]. Moreover, the majority of ganciclovir-resistant clinical isolates examined are of the ganciclovir-kinase-deficient phenotype that results from mutations in the UL97 gene[50]. The features of the UL97 gene product, which are consistent with a protein kinase, have been described and a considerable database of UL97 gene sequence diversity has accumulated. Resistance mutations have been identified, and one rapid method to detect these

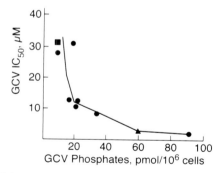

Figure 7.2 *Susceptibility of HCMV strains to ganciclovir compared with the intracellular anabolism of ganciclovir. Infected and uninfected MRC-5 cells were pulse-labeled on day 4 (post-infection) with 25 μM [^{14}C]-ganciclovir for 16 hours. Intracellular anabolites were extracted and quantified using cation exchange chromatography[50]. Susceptibilities of clinical strains to ganciclovir were determined by DNA hybridization assay. Controls included laboratory strain AD169 (▲) and its ganciclovir-resistant laboratory-derived mutant 759'D100 (■). Seven clinical isolates were obtained from L. Drew[24,50]. Reproduced from Field and Biron[68] with permission from ASM Publications*

genotypes in isolated viruses or directly in clinical specimens has been reported.

CMV UL97: a protein kinase homolog

The 2.1 kb gene of the UL97 ORF encodes a 707 amino acid, 78 kDa protein which contains sequence motifs conserved among protein kinases, bacterial aminoglycoside phosphotransferases and guanylyl kinase[32-35]. Homologs exist in all the human herpesviruses examined: HSV UL13, HHV6 15R, VZV gene 47, and the EBV BGLF4[32,33]. The role of the UL97-encoded phosphotransferase or protein kinase homolog in CMV replication or pathogenesis is not known.

The UL97 enzyme may have a functional role analogous to the protein kinase activity recently attributed to the UL13 homolog of HSV by Roizman and colleagues. After constructing a UL13 deletion mutant[53,54], they examined the replication of this UL13-deficient virus in cells and found a pattern of reduced protein synthesis similar to that induced by defects in the HSV α22 gene (a transcriptional transactivator). These results provided indirect evidence that the HSV UL13 gene product is a protein kinase that controls the normal post-translational phosphorylation of the α22, thereby regulating the expression of specific late-structural proteins and the levels of another regulatory protein, the ICPO[54]. The HSV UL13 also has been implicated in the HSV virion host shut-off function, which is dependent upon the UL41 gene, although this effect may not be mediated simply by direct phosphorylation of the UL41 protein by the UL13[55]. The UL13 protein is found in the HSV virion[56], although experimental data suggest that only newly synthesized enzyme performs the transcriptional regulatory function in infected cells[54]. While the UL13 protein appears somewhat dispensable for the replication of HSV *in vitro*, virus lacking UL13 is not virulent in a mouse model of systemic infection[55]. This result suggests that this class of protein kinase homologs represent a valid target for the development of chemotherapeutic agents.

Finally, the product of the VZV gene 47 was recently reported to phosphorylate the early regulatory protein of gene 62[57]. Therefore, this conserved family of protein kinase homologs in the human herpesviruses may have crucial regulatory roles in virus replication. The identification of the natural substrate for the CMV UL97 awaits further research. The herpesviruses share a process of ordered mRNA and protein expression; however, there is no direct counterpart to the HSV α22 in CMV. There is no animal model for the human CMV that could be used to investigate the requirement for functional UL97 in CMV pathogenesis. Indirect evidence that the UL97-encoded enzyme is important for pathogenesis is provided by the absence of null mutants among the 50 clinical strains studied which carry ganciclovir-resistance mutations in UL97. The ability of the CMV UL97 phosphotransferase to recognize and phosphorylate ganciclovir seems rather fortuitous. The HSV UL13 homolog and the VZV gene 47 homolog and not likely to share this ability, since TK negative strains of these two viruses are resistant to ganciclovir and acyclovir *in vitro*.

Sequence diversity in UL97 and mutations associated with ganciclovir resistance

The primary mechanism by which CMV escapes ganciclovir suppression is through selection of UL97 variants. The application of genetic techniques for diagnosis of these variants becomes feasible only if there is limited nucleotide sequence variation in the UL97 of ganciclovir-sensitive isolates and a small number of mutations responsible for drug resistance. Considerable data are accumulating on the sequence diversity in the UL97 gene from a variety of laboratory and clinical studies. Initial restriction analyses of the UL97 gene of 15 clinical and two laboratory strains with MspI and TaqI indicated the existence of only four distinct profiles, one of which predominated (12 of 15 clinical strains) and was represented by Towne vaccine strain but not AD169[58]. Subsequent studies on UL97 nucleotide sequence confirmed that the UL97 gene is highly conserved among clinical strains. Furthermore, ganciclovir resistance results from select mutations in two regions of the gene encoding the catalytic domain. Thus the potential for the application of diagnostic techniques is high.

In a comprehensive study of UL97 sequence, Chou and his collaborators[59] reported the complete sequence alignments of eight clinical strains (three ganciclovir-sensitive, five resistant). The analyses revealed >99% identity at the nucleotide level and >98% homology at the amino acid level[59]. Of 708 total codons in the UL97 polypeptide, only 11 (1.6%) showed sequence change that would alter amino acid sequence. The majority of sequence variation in ganciclovir-sensitive isolates occurred in the NH_2-terminal half of the gene, which encodes the regulatory domain of the enzyme. Amino acid substitutions were predicted at codons 19, 68, 108, 126 and 244. In the part of the gene encoding the catalytic domain, additional sequence information was collected on an additional eight ganciclovir-sensitive isolates and five resistant isolates. Substitutions were noted at codons 449, 460, 469, 594, 595 and 665. The changes in codons 460, 594 and 595 were not found in any sensitive strains. Four mutations were observed at these three codons. The nucleotide changes and resulting amino acid substitutions are summarized in Table 7.1. The role of changes in these three codons in conferring the ganciclovir-resistant phenotype was confirmed by marker transfer experiments in this study. Recombinant AD169 strains carrying

Table 7.1 *UL97 mutations associated with ganciclovir resistance*

UL97 subdomain	Nucleotide change	Codon change	Amino acid substitution	Laboratory strains	Clinical isolates	References
VI	G1380T	ATG→ATT	M460I	3	5	37
	A1378G	ATG→GTG	M460V	0	10	59, 65
VIII	C1560G	CAC→CAG	H520Q	0	2	62, 65
IX	C1772T	GCC→GTC	A591V	0	1	65
	T1774G	TGC→GGC	C592G	0	2	65, 82
	1768–1779 del	(GCG GCC TGC CGC)	A590ACR593 deletion	1	0	30
	1771–1782 del	(GCC TGC CGC)	A591CRA594 deletion	0	1	65
	C1781T	GCC→GTG	A594V	0	10	59, 65
	C1781G	GCC→GGG	A594G	1	0	82
	T1784C	TTG→TCG	L595S	0	11	59, 60, 65
	G1785T	TTG→TTT	L595F	0	1	59, 60, 65
	T1784G	TTG→TGG	L595W	0	1	65
	1783–1785 del	(TTG) del	L595 deletion	0	1	61
	A1787G	GAG→GGG	E596G	0	1	65
XI	C1976T	ACC→ATC	T659I	0	1	60

the individual substitutions encoding Val460, Val594 or Ser595 acquired the ganciclovir phosphorylation-deficient resistant phenotype. The change at codon 665, which was present along with Ser595 in one strain, was not transferred during the recombination event, suggesting that this change was not necessary for the ganciclovir resistance of this isolate. The distribution of UL97 mutations at these three codons in this study set was Met460Val (four isolates), Ala594Val (two isolates), and Leu595Ser (three isolates) or Leu595Phe (one isolate).

Wolf *et al.*[60] also compared the sequence of the UL97 genes in two sensitive and four resistant clinical isolates. Among the sensitive strains there were common silent nucleotide substitutions noted at positions 972, 1368, 1509, 1575, 1657, 1737, 1794, 1902, 2064 and 2106, compared to AD169. Included in the sensitive strains was an isolate encoding the Ala594Val alteration, a change that clearly conferred ganciclovir resistance in the Chou study. Among the isolates with reduced ganciclovir susceptibility, the Leu595Ser substitution was seen in four isolates (two of which were previously included in the Chou study), one Leu595Phe was found, and a novel mutational change of Thr659Ile was observed (Table 7.1). This last mutation was not found in sensitive strains, although marker transfer was not performed to confirm its role in conferring ganciclovir resistance. The resistance mutation of Leu595Phe was validated by marker transfer. Wolf *et al.* then detected the presence of these UL97 mutations directly in plasma samples (10 μl), using PCR amplification and sequence analyses. With this approach, Wolf screened the plasma samples of 10 patients with clinically resistant CMV retinitis. The plasma of eight of these patients carried CMV with UL97 mutations at codons 460, 594, 595 and 659, although corresponding viral isolates were not always available for comparison. Two patient specimens did not encode amino acid substitutions in UL97, and their viral isolates remained susceptible to ganciclovir *in vitro*[60].

The importance of this Leu595 in enabling the UL97 phosphotransferase to catalyze ganciclovir monophosphorylation in infected cells was reinforced by the identification of a Leu595 deletion variant[61]. This phosphorylation-defective variant was recovered from an AIDS patient after more than three months of ganciclovir treatment[22]. The strain was originally present in a mixture of two other unrelated strains in the patient's blood; it emerged during drug therapy, and subsequently was replaced following discontinuation of treatment. The mutation, which consisted of an in-frame deletion of TTG at nucleotide positions 1783–1785, was shown to be present in PBL samples from the patient and was transferred from the isolate to strain AD169. The resulting ganciclovir-resistant recombinant produced cell-free viral titers comparable to those achieved with the parent strain AD169, implying that this Leu595 deletion did not impair virus growth *in vitro*[61]. Similar *in vitro* growth competency had been observed with the 759ʳD100 laboratory-derived mutant that carried a 12 bp deletion encoding AlaAlaCysArg at codon 590–593[29,30]. The HSV UL13 is somewhat non-essential *in vitro*, since the efficiency of growth of the HSV UL13 deletion mutant was only marginally reduced. Cellular enzymes may partially compensate for deficiency in the viral protein kinase function.

An uncommon mutation in the UL97 gene was identified in a CMV strain recovered from a patient with AIDS after prolonged therapy with ganciclovir[62]. The strain carried a point mutation (CAC to CAG) at nucleotide 1560, which encoded a His520Gln. This mutation was not present in the patient's pretherapy isolate. Interestingly, the original post-therapy isolate showed a high degree of *in vitro* ganciclovir resistance, with an IC_{50} of >200 μm, compared to 1.2 μm for the susceptible prether-apy isolate. The recombinant strain AD169, which carried the His520Gln mutation, showed an intermediate level of resistance compared to AD169 (21-fold increase in IC_{50}). These observations are similar to those reported for laboratory-derived, ganciclovir-resistant strains, which carried resistance mutations in both the UL97 and the UL54 (*pol*) genes[30,37,63]. The isolate pair and recombinant virus bearing the UL97 change were all susceptible to foscarnet *in vitro*. The presence of a DNA polymerase point mutation that conferred ganciclovir resistance and HPMPC cross-resistance in the original isolate was subsequently confirmed[64].

Although all of four laboratory-derived, ganciclovir-resistant strains contained both UL97 and polymerase mutations, this event seems uncommon in the clinic. However, this interpretation is based solely on comparisons of the *in vitro* ganciclovir susceptibilities of recombinant strains bearing specific UL97 mutations to that of their original ganciclovir-resistant isolates. A biochemical or genetic examination of the isolate DNA polymerases would be required to confirm this interpretation. Another observation that emerges from studies of laboratory and clinical strains is that CMV *pol* mutations alone confer a somewhat lower degree of *in vitro* ganciclovir resistance than do the UL97 changes. Logically, the presence of mutations in both genes imparts a higher level of *in vitro* resistance. Susceptibility testing against several DNA polymerase inhibitors (par-ticularly HPMPC) is a useful approach to the identification of ganciclovir-resistant strains bearing mutations in UL97 and DNA polymerase genes.

Detection methods for UL97 mutant ganciclovir-resistant genotypes

Based on the prevalence of mutations at codons 460, 594 and 595, Chou[65] designed a simple diagnostic test for these genetic changes that involved

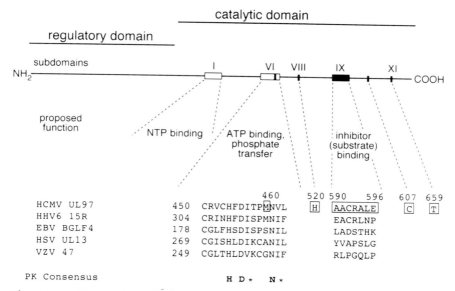

Figure 7.3 *Linear schematic of the UL97 polypeptide, showing the regulatory and catalytic domains. The subdomains, with assigned functions, are designated according to Hanks et al.[34] and Chee et al.[32], and are indicated along the linear polypeptide. The solid areas indicate regions bearing ganciclovir-resistance mutations. The herpesvirus homologies in the subdomains VI and IX are indicated below. The boxed codons in the UL97 sequence are those that are altered in ganciclovir-resistant isolates; their codon position is indicated immediately above. The nucleotide changes and amino acid substitutions are summarized in Table 7.1*

two PCR reactions and digestion with four specific restriction endonucleases. The Met460Val or the Met460I1e mutation disrupted an NlaIII restriction site (CATG). The PCR product used for this reaction extended from nucleotides 1088 to 1619. Similarly, the Ala594Val substitution resulted in the loss of a Hha1 restriction site (GCGC recognition sequence). Three Hha1 sites are normally present in the PCR product, extending from nucleotides 1713 to 1830, which covers codons 572–610 of the UL97 catalytic domain. As there are no naturally occurring restriction sites at the Leu595Ser or Phe mutations, Chou designed a primer that created recognition sites for Taq1 (TCGA) in Leu595Ser mutations, and a recognition site for MseI (TTAA) in Leu595Phe changes[60] (see Figure 7.4). Reconstruction mixtures of wild-type and specific mutant sequences demonstrated that this restriction method could detect the presence of 10% mutant genotype population. Using this PCR restriction enzyme digestion assay as a primary screen for UL97 resistance mutations, Chou subsequently analyzed a set of

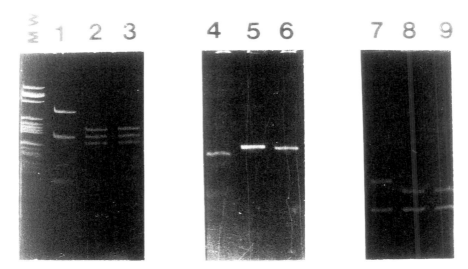

Figure 7.4 *Rapid characterization of the most common UL97 amino acid changes conferring ganciclovir resistance, based on a published method[59]. Lanes 1, 2 and 3, restriction profiles of PCR products obtained with primer pair CPT 1088–1619 and digested with Nla III: in lane 1 the restriction pattern from a ganciclovir-resistant HCMV isolate carrying the Met460Val or Ile change is shown; for comparison the restriction patterns from two ganciclovir-sensitive isolates are shown in lanes 2 and 3. Lanes 4, 5 and 6, restriction profiles of PCR products obtained with primer pair CPT 1713–1830 and digested with Taq1; in lane 4 the restriction pattern from a ganciclovir-resistant HCMV isolate carrying the Leu595Ser change is shown; restriction patterns from two ganciclovir-sensitive isolates are shown in lanes 5 and 6. Lanes 7, 8 and 9, restriction profiles of PCR products obtained with primer pair CPT 1713–1830 and digested with Hha1: in lane 7 the restriction pattern from a ganciclovir-resistant HCMV isolate carrying the Ala594Val change is shown; restriction patterns from two ganciclovir-sensitive isolates are shown in lanes 8 and 9. MW, molecular weight markers*

22 ganciclovir-resistant isolates identified by Drew[65]. Sequence analysis also was performed to confirm the results of positive diagnosis by this rapid restriction digestion technique, and to identify other less common sequence alterations associated with ganciclovir resistance. Interestingly, the prevalence data for distribution of UL97 resistance mutations at codons 460, 594 and 595 from the earlier studies of both Chou and Wolf were confirmed in this expanded study. An important feature of this study was the fact that this analysis was performed directly on low-passage clinical isolates. There was no attempt to separate out genetically pure representatives of mixed populations, as was done in earlier studies for the purposes of quantitative phenotypic, biochemical and genetic studies[50,59]. As a consequence, some resistant isolates contained two or

even three UL97 mutant genotypes. Interestingly, there was no clear additive effect of multiple UL97 mutations on the *in vitro* ganciclovir susceptibilities. The distribution of UL97 genetic lesions in this study was M460V[5], M460I[4], A594V[8], L595S[5], L595W[1], E596G[1], C592G[1], H520Q[1], and one deletion mutant lacking codons 591–594 (ACRA). According to current data, these techniques will detect ~70% of the ganciclovir-resistant genotypes. Chou also detected these mutant genotypes directly in the patient's corresponding plasma samples with this method. Baldanti has applied this screening method in a blinded fashion to a series of isolates recovered from HIV-infected patients treated for retinitis by D. Jabs and colleagues (Figure 7.4). The isolates with UL97 mutations showed reduced *in vitro* susceptibilities to ganciclovir.

The UL97 mutations associated with ganciclovir resistance occur in two regions of the catalytic domain of the UL97 polypeptide (Figure 7.3)[32–35]. The Met460 codon lies in an important element that is a component of the catalytic binding loop, designated as subdomain VI[34]. This element contains a Mg-ATP binding site that is probably involved in the phosphate transfer reaction. This is one of the most highly conserved catalytic motifs among cellular and herpesvirus protein kinases, and is also conserved in bacterial aminoglycoside phosphotransferases. The Met460 codon lies on a short variable region flanked by the relatively invariant residues of the Mg-ATP binding site (HDXL). One proposal suggests that such a unique stretch also participates in substrate recognition[66]. It is pertinent that the HSV and VZV homologs of the CMV UL97 do not contain a corresponding Met, and that these viruses are unable to compensate for the TK-negative phenotype to maintain ganciclovir susceptibility. By contrast, the closely related HHV-6 does contain the analogous Met460; it is also a TK-negative β herpesvirus that is susceptible to ganciclovir inhibition *in vitro*. The Met codon is the only residue substituted in this crucial motif. Cellular protein kinases are generally intolerant of modifications in this Mg-ATP binding site. The consequences of the Met460 substitution on the function of UL97 await determination of the natural substrate and its role in virus replication.

The second region altered in ganciclovir-resistant isolates is designated as subdomain IX. No functional role has been assigned to this region, although it probably participates in substrate recognition. This suggestion is based on the fact that a peptide inhibitor of the bovine cyclic AMP-dependent protein kinase binds in this region, at residues analogous to those altered in ganciclovir-resistant strains[67]. The UL97 amino acids participating in ganciclovir substrate recognition in this subdomain extend from codons 590 to 596, based on mutational analysis.

The His520Gln alteration lies in subdomain VIII. This region contains a conserved triplet sequence that is located at or near the active site of protein kinases. In 45 of 65 aligned protein kinase sequences, the triplet sequence consists of AlaProGlu. The HSV UL13 and VZV 47 contain the triplet ProProGlu, while the equivalent position in CMV contains IleCysAsp at codons 533–535. The His520 is the only residue in this subdomain that is occasionally substituted in response to ganciclovir therapy.

As the clinical use of ganciclovir continues, additional UL97 mutations will be identified. The current database provides a useful snapshot of genetic prevalence, which would support the application of diagnostic methods for the early detection of UL97 variants. There are many unanswered questions about the biological properties of these mutant strains. Do any of these specific mutations alter their tissue tropisms or virulence? How stable would these genetically altered strains be after the removal of drug-selective pressure? There are no suitable animal models of HCMV infection by which to address these issues. Many of these questions could be answered by appropriately designed clinical trials or individual patient monitoring. Laboratory experience with genetically pure populations indicates that none of these deletions or point mutations significantly impairs strains for growth in culture. The recombinant laboratory strain bearing individual changes at 460, 594, 595 or 520, or the deletions at Leu595 and AACR 590–593, all grow to high titers. This becomes important because isolates often must be amplified in culture before characterization. Isolates that are predominately ganciclovir resistant or that are plaque purified appear stable upon multiple passages in the absence of drug. Mixing (competition) experiments would be required to detect a replication advantage of wild type over UL97 variant in the absence of drug-selective pressure. However, one should avoid unnecessary serial passage of clinical isolates before genetic or phenotypic analyses. Detection of mutant genotypes directly in clinical specimens would be ideal.

CMV DNA POLYMERASE AND RESISTANCE TO GANCICLOVIR AND FOSCARNET

The majority of antiherpes or anti-HIV drugs are directed against viral replication enzymes. In the case of herpesvirus therapeutics, these include substrate analogs ganciclovir, acyclovir, HPMPC, lobucavir and the pyrophosphate analog foscarnet. These enzymes are essential for viral multiplication and are distinguished from mammalian cell enzymes, which allows their exploitation as targets for drug development. One would predict that such essential enzymes are constrained in the numbers of mutations permissive for function. The herpes DNA polymerases possess proofreading abilities. Drug-resistant strains of HSV, VZV and CMV altered in their DNA polymerase have arisen following growth in the presence of nucleoside analogs or pyrophosphate analogs *in vitro*. As the viral-encoded nucleoside kinases provide the first avenue of escape in the clinic, there are relatively few HSV or VZV DNA polymerase variants associated with disease progression[68]. The situation with CMV following ganciclovir therapy may be similar: UL97-mediated ganciclovir resistance predominates. However, more widespread use of foscarnet in immunocompromised patients with high CMV load may lead to the increased prevalence of CMV DNA polymerase variants. Information on drug resistance mutations in the HSV and VZV DNA polymerases should be predictive for CMV.

Viral DNA polymerase structure and function

The HCMV DNA polymerase is a product of the HCMV UL54 gene, a 3711-nucleotide gene that encodes a 1237 amino acid protein with a molecular weight of 140 kDa. Comparative sequence analysis revealed that the HCMV UL54 gene shares a high degree of homology with the corresponding DNA polymerase genes of the other herpesviruses[69-71]. In the most conserved regions, UL54 contains motifs present in the eukaryotic, viral, and bacteriophage DNA polymerases of the α-like family. Such similarities suggest a functional role for these regions. Genetic characterization of HSV temperature-sensitive and drug-resistant mutants has allowed the identification of conserved domains with the predicted functions of nucleotide binding, pyrophosphate binding and DNA proofreading and processing (see Chapter 5). These domains occur in the same spatial order in the polymerases of the herpesviruses and are numbered I–VII on the basis of decreasing homology. Between regions IV and II is located a relatively non-conserved region (domain A) that shares similarity with other viral polymerases but not with DNA polymerase α (Figure 7.5). Genetic characterizations of drug-resistant strains of CMV and VZV have also indicated the functional importance of a short stretch of amino acids between regions IV and A, which is similar among the HSV enzymes[72,73]. The tentative assignment of UL54 codons to these conserved regions is as follows: IV (379–421), A (538–598), II (696–742), VI (771–790), III (805–845), I (905–919), VII (962–970) and V (978–988)[73]. The DNA polymerases of all of the herpesviruses exhibit distinctive behavior during chromatographic separation and show enhanced activity when assayed in the presence of high salt concentrations, which has facilitated their biochemical characterization. These herpesvirus enzymes have

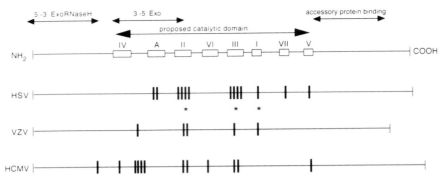

Figure 7.5 *Linear representation of the polypeptides of HSV, VZV and HCMV DNA polymerases. Conserved regions are indicated by boxes I to VI and A. Laboratory and clinical drug-resistant mutants are indicated by vertical lines. The * indicates changes in homologous amino acids. CMV DNA polymerase amino acid changes and resulting drug susceptibility phenotypes are listed in Table 7.2. Adapted from Field and Biron[68]. Reproduced with permission from ASM Publications*

been expressed in reticulocyte transcription–translation systems, in yeast and in baculoviruses, and the consequences of specific mutations on enzyme function and structure have been studied[68,74].

CMV DNA polymerase: drug-resistant genotypes and resulting phenotypes

Resistance of HSV or VZV to nucleoside analogs (acyclovir, ganciclovir, vidarabine) or to the pyrophosphate analogs (phosphonoacetic acid (PAA) or foscarnet) has resulted from single amino acid substitutions in conserved domains of the polymerase polypeptide or, occasionally, outside the conserved domains. In the case of HSV, mutations conferring resistance to acyclovir or PAA have mapped to the DNA-encoding conserved regions A, II, III, I, VII, and V (Figure 7.5). VZV drug resistance mutations have mapped to the DNA-encoding conserved regions I, II, III, and to the small region of herpesvirus polymerase homology between regions IV and A. The resulting drug susceptibility phenotypes are complex and variable[69,74]. Three of the amino acid substitutions in the VZV polymerase occurred at the homologous residues changed in polymerase mutants of HSV resistant to acyclovir and PAA, which mapped in conserved regions I, II and III (Figure 7.5). Thus, although there are a few amino acid residues that are modified relatively frequently among drug-resistant strains of herpesviruses recovered from patients, the broad distribution of mutations in the majority of these HSV and VZV strains makes rapid genetic screening methods impractical. Thus far, the situation with CMV bears out the predictions from the HSV and VZV studies: laboratory and clinical mutants show diverse resistance genotypes.

Four independently derived ganciclovir-resistant laboratory variants of CMV bearing DNA polymerase changes have been reported[62,72]. As previously noted, resistance in these laboratory strains was associated with mutations in both the UL97 and the DNA polymerase genes. These four CMV DNA polymerase mutants showed cross-resistance to HPMPC but were foscarnet sensitive, suggesting different mechanisms of resistance for pyrophosphate analogs. UL54 mutations involved in ganciclovir resistance produced single amino acid substitutions located in regions IV, V and between regions IV and A of the polypeptide (Table 7.2, Figure 7.5). UL97 and UL54 mutations were separated using genetic transfer techniques, and two recombinant HCMV strains carrying only the UL54 substitutions were obtained[63,72]. In the case of one mutant, 759^{r}D100, the DNA polymerase gene carried a single nucleotide change that resulted in a Gly987Ala substitution within conserved region V of the enzyme[63]. Recombinant virus carrying only this DNA polymerase change showed intermediate resistance to ganciclovir (four- to sixfold) and ganciclovir cyclic phosphate (sixfold), and somewhat higher levels of resistance to HPMPC (eight- to 10-fold), HPMPA (~eightfold), and the cytosine equivalent of ganciclovir (DHPC, 12-fold).

Two of the three ganciclovir-resistant laboratory mutants reported by Lurain[78] (strains D 1/3/4 and D 6/3/1) showed a conservative amino acid substitution of Leu501Ile, in the region extending between domains IV and A. The resulting phenotype was foscarnet sensitive, araT hypersensitive and HPMPC resistant. This Leu residue is conserved in the DNA polymerases of all human herpesviruses. The overall homology in this short stretch is not conserved among polymerases other than the herpesviruses. A mutation in the VZV DNA polymerase gene of an isolate recovered from an AIDS patient following foscarnet therapy mapped to this same region[75] (see Figure 7.5). No mutants of HSV have yet been described in this region. However, its functional importance is reinforced by the fact that three additional DNA polymerase mutations of CMV occur in this area. Two of these were laboratory-derived acyclovir-resistant strains, which were cross-resistant to foscarnet but still susceptible to HPMPC.

In Lurain's report, the third ganciclovir-resistant laboratory strain carried a T1893G change that encoded a Phe412Val change. This mutation falls within conserved region IV (Figure 7.5); the mutant strain also showed hypersensitivity to araT. This Phe residue is conserved in all of the human herpesvirus polymerases. Together with region A, region IV lies in the predicted 3'-5'-exonuclease functional domain, as defined by mutagenesis studies of the phage ϕ29 DNA polymerase[76].

Table 7.2 CMV DNA polymerase mutations conferring drug resistance

Selective agent	Strain	Amino acid substitution	Polypeptide conserved region	Drug susceptibility phenotype	References
GCV	GDC^r P53–Lab (759^{r}D100 parent)	G987A	V	GCV^r ACV^s PFA^s HPMPC^r HPMPA^r	63
GCV	D6/3/1–Lab D1/3/4–Lab	L501I	between IV and A	GCV^r ACV^s PFA^s HPMPC^r HPMPA^r	72
GCV	D10/3/2–Lab	F412V	IV	GCV^r ACV^s PFA^s HPMPC^r HPMPA^r	72, 5
None	D16–Clinical	D301N	upstream of IV	GCV^r ACV$^{s\pm}$ PFA^r HPMPC^r HPMPA^r	78
None	D19–Clinical	T503I	between IV and A	GCV^r ACV^s PFA^s HPMPC^r HPMPA^r	78
PFA	PFA^r B300–Lab	ND		GCV^s ACV^r PFA^r HPMPC^s HPMPA^s	79
GCV and PFA	VR 4760–Clinical	V715M	II	GCV^r (UL97 Mut) ACV^r PFA^r HPMPC^s HPMPA^s CbC^s	23
GCV and PFA	VR 5120–Clinical	V715M	II	GCV^r (UL97 Mut) ACV^r PFA^r HPMPC^s HPMPA^s	23
GCV and PFA	VR 4955–Clinical	T700A	II	GCV^r (UL97 Mut) ACV^r PFA^r HPMPC^s HPMPA^s	23
GCV and PFA	VR 5105–Clinical	V781I	VI	GCV^r (UL97 Mut) ACV$^{r?}$ PFA^r HPMPC$^{r?}$ HPMPA$^{r?}$	80, 81

GCV, ganciclovir; PFA, foscarnet

One ganciclovir-resistant clinical strain was recovered from the bronchial brushing of a heart transplant recipient[77]. The ganciclovir-resistant virus represented <1% of the virus population recovered from the patient prior to ganciclovir therapy. The resistant population contained two ganciclovir-resistant variants, each with a single mutation[78]. These may be naturally occurring variants, although there was no information on earlier patient exposure to other antivirals. Both strains of this isolate were cross-resistant to HPMPC and HPMPA, and one of them showed a decreased susceptibility to foscarnet. One mutation resulted in a Thr503Ile substitution, which again falls within the conserved regions IV and A, with a drug susceptibility phenotype similar to that of the laboratory strains. The second mutation, Asp301 Asn, was located upstream of region IV, within a putative 5'-3' exonuclease RNase functional domain (Table 7.2, Figure 7.5).

Foscarnet was more recently introduced into clinical practice, and reports of foscarnet-resistant isolates are still few. Clinical isolates showing resistance to both ganciclovir and foscarnet have also been reported[17,23]. Foscarnet-resistant HCMV strains were predicted to carry mutations in UL54. Experimental data from HSV strains resistant to PAA confirm that single mutations in the polymerase gene are responsible for the drug resistance[68,71]. A laboratory-induced, foscarnet-resistant strain retained sensitivity to both ganciclovir and HPMPC. The responsible mutation was not identified[79]. Very little is currently known about the molecular basis of foscarnet resistance in CMV.

Recently, Baldanti and colleagues[80] identified four CMV isolates from AIDS patients following extensive therapy with both ganciclovir and foscarnet. The clinical isolates were resistant *in vitro* to both drugs. Phenotypic and genetic analysis of the four isolates showed that, in each case, mutations encoding single amino acid changes in conserved regions of both UL97 and UL54 polypeptides were responsible for the dual resistance[80]. Recombinant AD169 strains were generated that individually carried three of the polymerase mutations. Considering the amino acid variations evident among drug-susceptible strains, these authors were able to conclude that foscarnet resistance was the result of single amino acid changes in domain II of the gene (Table 7.1). Two out of the three strains, which were genetically unrelated, showed the identical change of Val715Met. The third isolate contained a mutation which produced a Thr to Ala in codon 700[23].

Sequential isolates from the fourth patient showed a progression first to ganciclovir resistance, and then to both ganciclovir and foscarnet resistance. Sequencing of the UL97 and UL54 genes of these sequential isolates or their plaque-purified derivatives revealed that ganciclovir-resistant virus bearing a UL97 mutation emerged in response to therapy. Following extensive foscarnet therapy the UL97-altered virus acquired a mutation in the DNA polymerase that correlated with disease progression. In clinical practice, ganciclovir is a first-choice drug for the management of HCMV infections, and patients are shifted to foscarnet therapy after ganciclovir-related adverse effects, or clinical and virological failure of ganciclovir treatment. If the UL97 variants predominate in the circulating virus load at the time of therapy change, then the scenario of dual resistance is a real possibility. The UL97 mutation may have accounted for the ganciclovir resistance of the original isolate, since the recombinant strain carrying the foscarnet-resistant polymerase mutation retained ganciclovir susceptibility. However, other ganciclovir resistance mutations in the polymerase of the parent isolate may have existed which were not transferred to the recombinant virus.

A very important feature of these foscarnet-resistant strains was their slower growth in cell cultures[80]. The relationship between the foscarnet-resistance mutations of Ala700 and Met715 and the slow-growth phenotype was confirmed by the slower replication of their recombinant strains compared to AD169 (Ile781 studies in progress). This finding has important implications for the way in which clinical isolates are handled prior to drug-sensitivity testing. The presence of a mixed population of sensitive and foscarnet-resistant strains with this growth impairment could affect the results of susceptibility testing, since the resistant population would be overgrown by the sensitive one in cell culture. Such a mixture is likely to be present in the early phases of the clinical emergence of drug resistance, and a bias in sensitivity testing could delay the timely detection of the foscarnet-resistant strain.

The picture of foscarnet resistance in CMV is incomplete. Investigators are still collecting genetic data on UL54 variation in wild-type clinical strains. The amino acid substitutions common to foscarnet-sensitive and -resistant strains include the following: Phe365Leu, Asp588Asn, Pro628Leu, Ser655Leu, Asn685Ser, Gly874Arg, Ser884insert, Ala885Thr, Ser897Leu, Asn898Asp and Ala1122Thr. Amino acid substitutions associated with PFA-resistance are: Asp301Asn, Glu756Lys, Leu802Met, Thr700Ala, Val715Met, Val781Ile and Ala809Val. The lack of clarity has led several investigators to propose that combinations of mutations are associated with foscarnet resistance. The paucity of data and the lack of marker transfer studies makes it difficult to draw conclusions. What is clear is that it will be difficult to design rapid diagnostic methods for these polymerase variants.

SUMMARY

CMV resistance to ganciclovir will most commonly result from a restricted number of mutations in the UL97 gene. More than 90% of the

UL97 variant genotypes will occur at codons 460 and 520, and within 590–596, and these can be detected directly in patient samples, i.e. blood or cerebrospinal fluid. Furthermore, ganciclovir-resistant genotypes should be detectable as a minor component of the isolate population, based on *in vitro* reconstruction. Genetic diagnostic methods should therefore facilitate patient management by allowing the early, rapid detection of emerging, ganciclovir-resistant genotypes. It will be necessary to establish the predictive value of such findings for patient outcome. These UL97 variants do retain *in vitro* susceptibility to the DNA polymerase inhibitors foscarnet and HPMPC, but may exhibit reduced susceptibility to acyclovir.

The CMV *pol* changes associated with ganciclovir resistance, and probably also foscarnet and HPMPC resistance, consist of single amino acid substitutions. Ganciclovir resistance can result from mutations in both the UL97 and the *pol* genes; this may be less common in the clinic than in the laboratory. Such strains may retain susceptibility to foscarnet. There are not enough data to identify useful markers for foscarnet resistance.

Review of existing data on resistance mutations in all the herpesviruses suggests that testing for the presence of resistance by directly monitoring for mutations in the virion DNA polymerase gene (e.g. by PCR amplification and hybridization) will not be feasible. Because the drug-susceptibility phenotypes resulting from individual genetic changes are complex and variable, a biological test for antiviral susceptibility of CMV strains would be more informative in terms of patient management. The availability of newer therapies directed against other viral enzymes should allow disease management based on clinical response parameters.

REFERENCES

1. Mocarski ES Jr. Cytomegalovirus biology and replication. In: Roizman B, Whitley RJ, Lopez C, eds. *The Human Herpesvirus*. New York: Raven Press, 1993.
2. Chee MS, Bankier AT, Beck S *et al*. Analysis of the protein-coding content of the sequence of human cytomegalovirus strain AD169. *Curr Topics Microbiol Immunol* 1990;154:125–70.
3. Griffiths PD. Progress in the clinical management of herpesvirus infections. *Antiviral Chem Chemother* 1995;6:191–209.
4. Taylor-Wiedeman J, Sissons JGP, Borysiewicz LK, Sinclair JH. Monocytes are a major site of persistence of human cytomegalovirus in peripheral blood mononuclear cells. *J Gen Virol* 1991;72:2059–64.
5. Kondo K, Kaneshima H, Mocarski ES. Human cytomegalovirus latent infection of granulocyte-macrophage progenitors. *Proc Natl Acad Sci USA* 1994;91:11879–83.

6. Drew WL, Sweet ES, Miner RC, Mocarski ES. Multiple infections by cytomegalovirus in patients with acquired immunodeficiency syndrome: documentation by Southern blot hybridization. *J Infect Dis* 1984;150:952–3.

7. Chou S. Differentiation of cytomegalovirus strains by restriction analysis of DNA sequences amplified from clinical specimens. *J Virol* 1990;162:738–42.

8 Cheng YC, Huang ES, Lin JC. Unique spectrum of activity of 9-((1,3-dihydroxy-2-propoxy)methyl)-guanine against herpesviruses *in vitro* and its mode of action against herpes simplex virus type 1. *Proc Natl Acad Sci USA* 1983;80/91:2767–70.

9. Faulds D, Hall RC. Ganciclovir, a review of its antiviral activity, pharmacokinetic properties and therapeutic efficacy in cytomegalovirus infections. *Drugs (US)* 1990;39:597–638.

10. Chrisp P, Clissold SP. Foscarnet – a review of its antiviral activity, pharmacokinetic and therapeutic use in immunocompromised patients with cytomegalovirus retinitis. *Drugs* 1991;41:104–29.

11. Elion GB, Furman PA, Fyfe JA *et al*. Selectivity of action of an antiherpetic agent, 9-(2-hydroxyethoxymethyl)guanine. *Proc Natl Acad Sci USA* 1977;74:5716–20.

12. Bronson JJ, Ghazzouli I, Hitchcock JM, Web RR, Martin JC. Synthesis and antiviral activity of the nucleotide analog (S)-1-(3-hydroxy-2-(phosphonylmethoxy)propyl)cytosine. *J Med Chem* 1989;32:1457–63.

13. Neyts J, Snoeck R, Schols D, Balzarini J, De Clercq E. Selective inhibition of human cytomegalovirus DNA synthesis by (S)-1-(3-hydroxy-2-phosphonylmethoxypropyl)cytosine   [(S)-HPMPC]   and   9-(1,3-dihydroxy-2-propoxymethyl)guanine (DHPG). *Virology* 1990;179:41–50.

14. Norbeck DW, Kern K, Hayashi S *et al*. Cyclobut-A and Cyclobut-G: broad-spectrum antiviral agents with potential utility for the therapy of AIDS. *J Med Chem* 1990;33:1281–5.

15. Polis MA. Promising new treatments for cytomegalovirus retinitis. *JAMA* 1995;273:1457–9.

16. Erice A, Chou S, Biron KK *et al*. Progressive disease due to ganciclovir-resistant cytomegalovirus in immunocompromised patients. *New Engl J Med* 1989;320:289–93.

17. Knox KK, Drobyski WR, Carrigan DR. Cytomegalovirus isolate resistant to ganciclovir and foscarnet from a marrow transplant patient. *Lancet* 1991;337:1292–3.

18. Jacobson MA, Drew WL, Feinberg J *et al*. Foscarnet therapy for ganciclovir-resistant cytomegalovirus retinitis in patients with AIDS. *J Infect Dis* 1991;163:1348–51.

19. Leport C, Puget S, Pepin JM *et al*. Cytomegalovirus resistant to foscarnet: clinicovirologic correlation in patient with human immunodeficiency virus. *J Infect Dis* 1993;168:1329–30.

20. Tokumoto JI, Hollander H. Cytomegalovirus polyradiculopathy caused by a ganciclovir-resistant strain. *Clin Infect Dis* 1993;17:854–6.

21. Crane LR, Ebright JR. Cytomegalovirus polyradiculopathy caused by a ganciclovir-resistant strain [letter]. *Clin Infect Dis* 1994;19:365.

22. Gerna G, Baldanti F, Zavattoni M *et al*. Monitoring of ganciclovir sensitivity of human cytomegalovirus strains coinfecting blood of an AIDS patient by an immediate-early antigen plaque assay. *Antivir Res* 1992;19:333–45.

23. Baldanti F, Underwood MR, Stanat SC *et al*. Single amino acid changes in the DNA polymerase confer foscarnet resistance and slow-growth phenotype,

while in the UL97-encoded phosphotransferase confer ganciclovir resistance in three double resistant HCMV strains recovered from AIDS patients. *J Virol* 1996; 90:1390–5.

24. Drew WL, Miner RC, Busch DF *et al.* Prevalence of resistance in patients receiving ganciclovir for serious cytomegalovirus infection. *J Infect Dis* 1991;163:716–19.
25. Matthews T, Boehme R. Antiviral activity and mechanism of action of ganciclovir. *Rev Infect Dis* 1988;10:490–4.
26. Smee DF. Interaction of 9-(1,3-dihydroxy-2-propoxymethyl)guanine with cytosol and mitochondrial deoxyguanosine kinases: possible role in anti-cytomegalovirus activity. *Mol Cell Biochem* 1985;69:75–81.
27. Lewis RA, Watkins L, St. Jeor S. Enhancement of deoxyguanosine kinase activity in human lung fibroblast cells infected with human cytome-galovirus. *Mol Cell Biochem* 1984;65:67–71.
28. Biron KK, Stanat SC, Sorrell JB *et al.* Metabolic activation of the nucleoside analog 9-{[2-hydroxy-1-(hydroxymethyl)ethoxy]methyl} guanine in human diploid fibroblasts infected with human cytomegalovirus. *Proc Natl Acad Sci USA* 1985;82:2473–7.
29. Biron KK, Fyfe JA, Stanat SC *et al.* A human cytomegalovirus mutant resistant to the nucleoside analog 9-{[2-hydroxy-1-(hydroxymethyl)ethoxy]methyl} guanine (BW B759U) induces reduced levels of BW B759U triphosphate. *Proc Natl Acad Sci USA* 1986;83:8769–73.
30. Sullivan V, Talarico CL, Stanat SC *et al.* A protein kinase homologue controls phosphorylation of ganciclovir in human cytomegalovirus-infected cells. *Nature* 1992;358:162–4.
31. Littler E, Stuart AD, Chee MS. Human cytomegalovirus UL97 open reading frame encodes a protein that phosphorylates the antiviral nucleoside analogue ganciclovir. *Nature* 1992;358:160–2.
32. Chee MS, Lawrence GL, Barrell BG. Alpha-, beta- and gammaherpesviruses encode a putative phosphotransferase. *J Gen Virol* 1989;70:1151–60.
33. Smith RF, Smith TF. Identification of new protein kinase-related genes in three herpesviruses, herpes simplex virus, varicella-zoster virus, and Epstein–Barr virus. *J Virol* 1989;63:450–5.
34. Hanks SK, Quinn AM, Hunter T. The protein kinase family: conserved features and deduced phylogeny of the catalytic domains. *Science* 1988;241:42–52.
35. Brenner S. Phosphotransferase sequence homology. *Nature (Lond)* 1987;329:21.
36. Talarico CL, Stanat SC, Biron KK. Evidence that HCMV-encoded UL97 contributes to the phosphorylation of acyclovir in HCMV-infected cells. 34th Interscience Conference on Antimicrobial Agents and Chemotherapy 1994; Abstract H65.
37. Lurain N, Spafford LE, Thompson KD. Mutation in the UL97 open reading frame of human cytomegalovirus strains resistant to ganciclovir. *J Virol* 1994;68:4427–31.
38. Boehme RE. Phosphorylation of the antiviral precursor 9-(1,3-dihydroxy-2-propoxymethyl)guanine monophosphate by guanylate kinase isozymes. *J Biol Chem* 1984;259:12346–9.
39. Miller WH, Miller RL. Phosphorylation of acyclovir (acycloguanosine) monophosphate by GMP kinase. *J Biol Chem* 1980;255:7204–7.
40. Miller WH, Miller RL. Phosphorylation of acyclovir diphosphate by cellular enzymes. *Biochem Pharmacol* 1982;31:3879–84.

41. Mar EC, Chiou JF, Cheng YC, Huang ES. Inhibition of cellular DNA polymerase α and human cytomegalovirus-induced DNA polymerase by the triphosphates of 9-(2-hydroxy-ethoxymethyl)guanine and 9-(1,3-dihydroxy-2-propoxy-methyl)guanine. *J Virol* 1985;53:776–80.

42. St. Clair MH, Lambe CU, Furman PA. Inhibition by ganciclovir of cell growth and DNA synthesis of cells biochemically transformed with herpesvirus genetic information. *Antimicrob Agents Chemother* 1987;31: 844–9.

43. Reid R, Mar EC, Huang ES, Topal MD. Insertion and extension of acyclic, dideoxy, and ara nucleotides by herpesviridae, human alpha and human beta polymerases. A unique inhibition mechanism for 9-(1,3-dihydroxy-2-propoxymethyl)guanine triphosphate. *J Biol Chem (US)* 1988;263: 3898–904.

44. Sabourin CLK, Reno JM, Boezi JA. Inhibition of eukaryotic DNA polymerases by phosphonoacetate and phosphonoformate. *Arch Biochem Biophys (USA)* 1978;187:96–101.

45. Eriksson B, Oberg B, Wahren B. Pyrophosphate analogues as inhibitors of DNA polymerases of cytomegalovirus, herpes simplex virus and cellular origin. *Biochem Biophys Acta* 1982;696:115–23.

46. Wahren B, Eriksson B. Cytomegalovirus DNA polymerase inhibition and kinetics. *Adv Enzyme Regul* 1985;23:263–74.

47. Crumpacker CS. Mechanism of action of foscarnet against viral polymerases. *Am J Med* 1992;92:3S–7S.

48. Neyts J, De Clercq E. Mechanism of action of acyclic nucleoside phosphonates against herpesvirus replication. *Biochem Pharmacol* 1994;47:39–41.

49. Cherrington JM, Allen JS, McKee BH, Chen MS. Kinetic analysis of the interaction between the diphosphate of (S)-1-(3-hydroxy-2-phosphonyl-methoxypropyl)cytosine, ddGTP, AZTTP, and FIAUTP with human DNA polymerases beta and gamma. *Biochem Pharmacol* 1994;48:1986–8.

50. Stanat SC, Reardon JE, Erice A et al. Ganciclovir-resistant cytomegalovirus clinical isolates: mode of resistance to ganciclovir. *Antimicrob Agents Chemother* 1991;35:2191–7.

51. Smee DF, Campbell NL, Matthews TR. Comparative anti-herpes-virus activities of 9-(1,3-dihydroxy-2-propoxymethyl)guanine, acyclovir, and two 2'-fluoropyrimidine nucleosides. *Antiviral Res* 1987;5:259–67.

52. Ho HT, Woods KL, Bronson JJ et al. Intracellular metabolism of the antiherpes agent (S)-1-(3-hydroxy-2-phosphonylmethoxypropyl)cytosine. *Mol Pharmacol* 1992;41:197–202.

53. Purves FC, Roizman B. UL13 gene of herpes simplex virus 1 encodes the functions for posttranslational processing associated with phosphorylation of the regulatory protein α22. *Proc Natl Acad Sci USA* 1992;89:7310–14.

54. Purves FC, Ogle WO, Roizman B. Processing of the herpes simplex virus regulatory protein α22 mediated by the UL13 protein kinase determines the accumulation of a subset of α and γ mRNAs and proteins in infected cells. *Proc Natl Acad Sci USA* 1993;90:6701–5.

55. Overton H, McMillan D, Hope L, Wong-Kai-In P. Production of host shutoff-defective mutants of herpes simplex virus type 1 by inactivation of the UL13 gene. *Virology* 1994;202:97–106.

56. Overton HA, McMillan DJ, Klavinskis LS et al. Herpes simplex virus type 1 gene UL13 encodes a phosphoprotein that is a component of the virion. *Virology* 1992;190:184–92.

57. Ng TI, Keenan L, Kinchington PR, Grose C. Phosphorylation of varicella-zoster virus open reading frame (ORF) 62 regulatory product by viral ORF 47-associated protein kinase. *J Virol* 1994;68:1350–9.

58. Talarico CL, Biron KK, Stanat SC *et al.* Analysis of the UL97 gene of ganciclovir-resistant cytomegalovirus isolated from AIDS patients. XVIII International Herpesvirus Workshop. Pittsburgh, Pennsylvania, 1993.

59. Chou S, Erice A, Jordan MC *et al.* Analysis of the UL97 phosphotransferase coding sequence in clinical cytomegalovirus isolates and identification of mutations conferring ganciclovir resistance. *J Infect Dis* 1995;171:576–83.

60. Wolf DG, Smith IL, Lee DJ *et al.* Mutations in human cytomegalovirus UL97 gene confer clinical resistance to ganciclovir and can be detected directly in patient plasma. *J Clin Invest* 1995;95:257–63.

61. Baldanti F, Silini E, Sarasini A *et al.* A three nucleotide deletion in the UL97 ORF is responsible for the ganciclovir resistance of a human cytomegalovirus clinical isolate. *J Virol* 1995;69:796–800.

62. Hanson MN, Preheim LC, Chou S *et al.* Novel mutation in the UL97 gene of a clinical cytomegalovirus strain conferring resistance to ganciclovir. *Antimicrob Agents Chemother* 1995;39:1204–5.

63. Sullivan V, Biron KK, Talarico C *et al.* A point mutation in the human cytomegalovirus DNA polymerase gene confers resistance to ganciclovir and phosphonylmethoxyalkyl derivatives. *Antimicrob Agents Chemother* 1993;37:19–25.

64. Erice A, Chou S, Gil-Roda C *et al.* Ganciclovir-resistant cytomegalovirus strains from AIDS patients with mutations in the DNA polymerase (*pol*) gene. 35th Interscience Conference on Antimicrobial Agents and Chemotherapy, 1995.

65. Chou S, Guentzel S, Michels KR, Miner RC, Drew WL. Frequency of UL97 phosphotransferase mutations related to ganciclovir resistance in clinical cytomegalovirus isolates. *J Infect Dis* 1995;172:239–42.

66. Taylor SS, Knighton DR, Zheng J, Ten Eyck LF, Sowadski JM. Structural framework for the protein kinase family. *Annu Rev Cell Biol* 1992;8:429–62.

67. Knighton DR, Zheng J, Eyck LFT *et al.* Structure of a peptide inhibitor bound to the catalytic subunit of cyclic adenosine monophosphate-dependent protein kinase. *Science* 1991;253:414–20.

68. Field AK, Biron KK. 'The end of innocence' revisited: resistance of herpesviruses to antiviral drugs. *Clin Microbiol Rev* 1994;7:1–13.

69. Kouzarides T, Bankier AT, Satchwell SC *et al.* Sequence and transcription analysis of the human cytomegalovirus DNA polymerase gene. *J Virol* 1987;61:125–33.

70. Teo IA, Griffin BE, Jones MD. Characterization of the DNA polymerase gene of human herpesvirus 6. *J Virol* 1991;65:4670–80.

71. Larder BA, Kemp SD, Darby G. Related functional domains in virus DNA polymerases. *EMBO J* 1987;6:169–75.

72. Lurain NS, Thompson KD, Holmes EW, Read GS. Point mutations in the DNA polymerase gene of human cytomegalovirus that result in resistance to antiviral agents. *J Virol* 1992;66:7146–52.

73. Gaillard R, Short S, Gaillard M, Stanat S, Biron K. Sequence alterations in the DNA polymerase genes of VZV strains selected for *in vitro* resistance to acyclovir or phosphonoacetic acid. 15th International Herpesvirus Workshop, Georgetown University, Washington DC, August 1990;154.

74. Haffey ML, Novotny J, Bruccoleri RE *et al.* Structure–function studies of the herpes simplex virus type I DNA polymerase. *J Virol* 1990;64:5008–18.

75. Stanat SC, Talarico CL, Safrin S, Biron KK. Sequential varicella zoster virus isolates from an AIDS patient: phenotype and genetic evidence for evolution of drug resistance at the thymidine kinase and DNA polymerase loci. *Antiviral Res* 1992;17(Suppl 1):51.
76. Bernad A, Blanco L, Lazaro JM, Martin G, Salas M. A conserved 3'→5' exonuclease active site in prokaryotic and eukaryotic DNA polymerases. *Cell* 1989;59:219–28.
77. Tatarowicz WA, Lurain NS, Thompson KD. A ganciclovir-resistant clinical isolate of human cytomegalovirus exhibiting cross-resistance to other DNA polymerase inhibitors. *J Infect Dis* 1992;166:904–7.
78. Lurain NS, Penland LK, Thompson KD. Ganciclovir-resistant DNA polymerase mutants isolated from an HCMV clinical specimen. 19th International Herpesvirus Workshop 1994; Abstract 211.
79. Sullivan V, Coen DM. Isolation of foscarnet-resistant human cytomegalovirus: patterns of resistance and sensitivity to other antiviral drugs. *J Infect Dis* 1991;164:781–4.
80. Sarasini A, Baldanti F, Furione M *et al*. Double resistance to ganciclovir and foscarnet of four human cytomegalovirus strains recovered from AIDS patients. *J Med Virol* 1995;47:237–44.
81. Baldanti F, Sarasini A, Silini E *et al*. Four dually-resistant human cytomegalovirus strains from AIDS patients: single mutations in UL97 and UL54 open reading frames are responsible for ganciclovir- and foscarnet-specific resistance, respectively. *Scand J Infect Dis* Suppl 1995; in press.
82. Morinet, personal communication.

8

Nucleosides and Foscarnet—Clinical Aspects

W. LAWRENCE DREW AND WILLIAM C. BUHLES

GANCICLOVIR

Clinical use of intravenous (i.v.) ganciclovir began in 1984 for the treatment of life-threatening and sight-threatening cytomegalovirus (CMV) infections in immunocompromised patients. Over the next four years thousands of patients received treatment with i.v. ganciclovir. However, by 1988 strains of CMV manifesting resistance to ganciclovir *in vitro* had been identified[1,2]. Emergence of CMV strains resistant to ganciclovir following i.v. ganciclovir treatment are now well documented. A number of methods have been used to determine *in vitro* susceptibility of CMV to ganciclovir, the plaque-reduction method being the most common. For the purposes of this chapter, the definitions, based upon susceptibility data described below and shown in Table 8.1, were used to classify strains.

Susceptibility of CMV clinical isolates prior to treatment

The initial reports of the anti-CMV activity of ganciclovir *in vitro* primarily utilized strains of CMV that had been maintained in the laboratory and passaged numerous times[3,4]. These studies indicated that most laboratory strains of CMV were inhibited *in vitro* by concentrations of ganciclovir of 0.25–1.50 μg/ml. In 1985 Plotkin *et al.*[5] reported the results of *in vitro* susceptibility testing of 54 clinical isolates of CMV collected in three different US cities, Boston, Philadelphia and San Francisco. Isolates were collected from 26 renal transplant allograft

Antiviral Drug Resistance. Edited by Douglas D. Richman © 1996 John Wiley & Sons Ltd

Table 8.1 Definitions to classify susceptibility of a CMV isolate based on the in vitro IC_{50} and IC_{90} values

IC_{50} (μg/ml)	IC_{90} (μg/ml)	*In vitro* susceptibility classification
<1.6	<3.1	Sensitive
<1.6	3.1–7.4	Sensitive
<1.6	>7.4	Intermediate
1.6–2.9	<3.1	Sensitive
1.6–2.9	3.1–7.4	Intermediate
1.6–2.9	>7.4	Resistant
>2.9	<3.1	Intermediate
>2.9	3.1–7.4	Resistant
>2.9	>7.4	Resistant

recipients, from six subjects with CMV mononucleosis, from one child with congenital CMV infection, and from 21 homosexual men who were shedding CMV. The method used to quantify susceptibility to ganciclovir *in vitro* was a plaque-reduction method using human embryo lung (HEL) cells. The methodology differed somewhat in the Boston laboratory, but was quite similar in the Philadelphia and San Francisco laboratories (Figure 8.1).

The mean IC_{50} of clinical isolates tested in Boston, most of which were from patients with CMV mononucleosis, was 1.48 μg/ml (5.9 μM), somewhat higher than the mean IC_{50} obtained in Philadelphia (0.83 μg/ml) or San Francisco (0.75 μg/ml). These differences were most probably due to differences in laboratory technique. Among all three locations, 47 out of 54 isolates (87%) had IC_{50} values of <1.5 μg/ml (<6 μM). In Philadelphia and San Francisco, 42 of the 45 clinical isolates tested (93%) had IC_{50} values of <1.5 μg/ml (<6 μM). The IC_{90} values were also calculated for the isolates tested in Philadelphia: typical IC_{90} concentrations were 0.15–4.0 μg/ml, with a mean IC_{90} of 2.0 μg/ml.

Drew *et al.*[6] evaluated the *in vitro* susceptibility of 31 CMV isolates cultured from subjects with AIDS and CMV retinitis prior to therapy with i.v. ganciclovir. Sensitivity was defined in this study as an $IC_{50} \leqslant 1.5$ μg/ml (6.0 μM) and an $IC_{90} \leqslant 3.0$ μg/ml (12 μM). Resistance was defined as an $IC_{50} > 3.0$ μg/ml (12 μM) or an $IC_{90} \geqslant 7.5$ μg/ml (30 μM). Isolates of CMV with IC values between these values were considered 'intermediate' in susceptibility. Thirty of the 31 isolates (97%) were designated sensitive, with a mean IC_{50} of 0.75 μg/ml (3 μM) and a mean IC_{90} of 1.43 μg/ml (5.72 μM). One isolate had intermediate susceptibility.

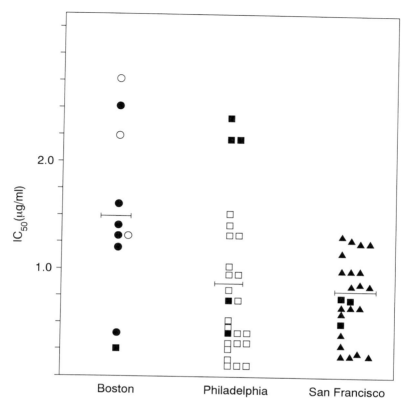

Figure 8.1 *Concentrations of DHPG giving 50% inhibition for strains of CMV as tested in three laboratories. The strains were derived from multiple sources: laboratory strain (■), renal transplant patient (▫), CMV mononucleosis (●), congenital CMV (○) and homosexual men (▲). Bars indicate mean ID_{50} for the respective laboratories. From reference 5, reproduced with permission*

The IC_{50} of all but one of the 31 isolates was less than 1.25 μg/ml (6 μM) prior to treatment.

Tseng[7] reported the results of ganciclovir susceptibility testing of CMV clinical isolates using a rapid shell vial culture assay. CMV isolates from two of 73 subjects (3%) who had not received treatment with ganciclovir showed *in vitro* resistance, and the remaining 71 isolates (97%) were designated sensitive.

Pepin *et al.*[8] reported on the *in vitro* susceptibility of CMV to ganciclovir among 10 subjects who were culture positive for CMV, either before ganciclovir treatment (eight subjects) or after only six days of i.v. ganciclovir treatment (two subjects). IC_{50} and IC_{90} values were higher than those reported by the investigators referred to above. However, all

10 isolates fell into either the sensitive or the intermediate susceptibility range defined above.

A recent evaluation was made of patients with newly diagnosed CMV retinitis and AIDS entering a randomized clinical trial of i.v. versus oral ganciclovir[9]. As shown in Table 8.2, 130 of 159 subjects were cultured for CMV prior to the start of any therapy, and 90 of these 130 were CMV culture positive (69%). Sixty-four of these were assayed for *in vitro* susceptibility, and only one (1.6%) was resistant, with an IC_{50} of 3.48 μg/ml. The mean IC_{50} was 0.59 μg/ml (2.36 μM).

Table 8.3 summarizes the findings from the above mentioned investigations. Care must be taken in interpretation across reports, as different methodologies were used in each laboratory and no standardization was involved. The results from the Boston site[5] and the results from Pepin in Paris[8] produced IC_{50} values clearly higher than those reported from the other laboratories, probably as a result of methodology rather than decreased susceptibility of these isolates. Excluding these results, the overall prevalence of isolates with an IC_{50} of >1.5 μg/ml was 4% from patients without significant prior ganciclovir treatment.

CMV drug resistance in subjects treated with intravenous ganciclovir

The potential for viral resistance to ganciclovir in subjects receiving intravenous treatment with ganciclovir was first studied by Fraser-Smith *et al.*[1], in work done at Syntex Research. They studied 19 subjects with

Table 8.2 *CMV culture and* in vitro *susceptibility results from subjects with a new diagnosis of CMV retinitis prior to any anti-CMV treatment*

No. subjects		159
No. subjects cultured		130
No. subjects culture pos. (%)		90 (69)
No. subjects tested		64
No. sensitive *in vitro* (%)		63 (98.4)
No. resistant *in vitro* (%)		1 (1.6)
IC_{50}	Mean (μg/ml)	0.59
	Median	0.53
	Range	0.02–3.48
IC_{90}	Mean (μg/ml)	2.15
	Median	1.75
	Range	0.28–12.5
IC_{99}	Mean (μg/ml)	4.49
	Median	4.25
	Range	1.23–12.5

Table 8.3   *Summary of all studies reporting in vitro susceptibility testing of CMV isolates either before or with very short duration anti-CMV treatment*

Reference	No. resistant/ no. tested	Percentage resistant	Mean IC_{50} (μg/ml)
[5] all locations	7/54	13	Not calculated
Boston	4/9	44	1.48
Philadelphia	3/24	13	0.83
San Francisco	0/21	0	0.75
[6]	1/31	3	0.75
[7]	2/73	3	Not calcutaled
[8]	4/10	40	1.28
[9]	1/64	1.6	0.59

CMV disease and an underlying immunocompromise who had received treatment with i.v. ganciclovir for varying periods of time under a compassionate use protocol. All 19 subjects were experiencing some degree of clinical treatment failure. Isolates were available from seven of the subjects prior to or during the first week of treatment, and all seven isolates were sensitive to ganciclovir *in vitro*. Eight subjects treated with i.v. ganciclovir had sequential cultures followed for up to eight months: isolates from four of these eight patients showed no increase in *in vitro* susceptibility. However, the other four subjects were found to be shedding CMV isolates that had significantly higher susceptibilities than the other isolates (Table 8.4). One subject had a blood culture isolate with an IC_{50} of 6.25 μg/ml following approximately four months of treatment with i.v. ganciclovir. One subject had an isolate from a liver biopsy with an IC_{50} of 3.75 μg/ml and an $IC_{90} > 6.25$ μg/ml following 10 months of treatment. One subject had a blood culture isolate of CMV with an IC_{50} of 4.25 μg/ml and an IC_{90} of 5.0 μg/ml following treatment with i.v. ganciclovir for an unspecified duration. One subject had an isolate cultured from the urine with an IC_{50} of 5.5 μg/ml after treatment with i.v. ganciclovir, also of unknown duration. The IC_{50} values of all four of

Table 8.4   *Identification of resistant CMV isolates from four patients treated with i.v. ganciclovir*

Patient number	Months on ganciclovir	Culture source	IC_{50} (μg/ml)
192	4	Blood	>6.25
827	10	Liver biopsy	3.75
1495	Not stated	Blood	4.25
2452	Not stated	Urine	5.50

these isolates fall into the resistant category (see Table 8.1). Unfortunately, none of these subjects had a baseline culture tested for susceptibility, thereby precluding the definitive determination of whether the resistance developed during ganciclovir treatment.

In 1989 Erice *et al.*[2] reported the recovery of CMV isolates resistant to ganciclovir from three subjects receiving treatment with ganciclovir. One subject had CMV retinitis and chronic lymphocytic leukemia, and was treated with ganciclovir for three courses of two to three weeks each. The CMV cultured from the urine at baseline had an IC_{50} of 3.6 $\mu g/ml$. At day 79 an isolate from a blood culture had an $IC_{50} = 7.63$ $\mu g/ml$. Shedding of CMV persisted in spite of treatment in this subject, and the retinitis responded only partially to the i.v. ganciclovir treatment. The second subject had a diagnosis of AIDS and CMV hepatitis followed by CMV retinitis that was treated with i.v. ganciclovir for more than three months. The IC_{50} of a blood isolate at day three of treatment was 0.53 $\mu g/ml$. After 131 days of intermittent courses of treatment the IC_{50} of a blood isolate was 4.43 $\mu g/ml$. This subject continued to shed CMV from the urine and oropharynx and the clinical condition eventually deteriorated, with a terminal diagnosis of CMV pneumonia. The third subject had AIDS and a history of CMV colitis treated with i.v. ganciclovir for 10 days. He then shed CMV in the lung and received additional therapy with i.v. ganciclovir. At the start of this treatment course the CMV isolate from the blood had an $IC_{50} = 0.35$ $\mu g/l$. After 60 days of treatment, during which time CMV cultures were frequently positive, the IC_{50} was found to be 4.1 $\mu g/ml$.

Among the three subjects described by Erice *et al.* the first had an isolate resistant to ganciclovir prior to treatment. It is interesting that this subject had received several courses of acyclovir treatment prior to the development of CMV retinitis. Restriction endonuclease analysis of the early and late isolates from this subject revealed that the two isolates were indistinguishable. In the second subject the susceptibility of the CMV isolated from serial cultures increased significantly. Restriction fragment analysis showed that the isolates were of the same strain. In the third subject resistance appeared to be the result of the emergence of a different strain of CMV during i.v. ganciclovir treatment, based on restriction fragment analysis. Thus, this report presented three possible scenarios for the clinical development of ganciclovir resistance.

In the report by Drew *et al.* in 1991[6], CMV was isolated from the urine of 18 subjects with AIDS and CMV retinitis during the first three months of treatment with i.v. ganciclovir, and from 27 subjects after more than three months of therapy. Among seven randomly selected isolates from subjects treated for less than three months, none was resistant. However, among 13 randomly selected isolates from those subjects treated for more than three months, five of the 13 (38%) were resistant and an additional two had intermediate susceptibility. The risk of developing resistance with i.v. ganciclovir treatment could thus be calculated. These authors documented that approximately 20% of subjects receiving treatment with i.v. ganciclovir will shed CMV at some time during therapy. If 38% of those shedding CMV were shedding a resistant strain, then the estimated prevalence of resistance in patients treated with i.v. ganciclovir for more than three months is 7.6% (20% times 38%). Although the study looked at prevalence, it is probable that resistance emerges gradually as drug pressure selects out a less susceptible viral subpopulation. These authors also noted that those subjects shedding resistent virus isolates often had progression of CMV retinitis, but progression was also seen in subjects shedding CMV sensitive to ganciclovir. Thus, resistance cannot be the sole cause of progression of CMV disease during treatment with i.v. ganciclovir.

Boivin et al.[9] reported on the *in vitro* susceptibility of clinical isolates of CMV from solid organ transplant recipients enrolled in a randomized trial of acyclovir versus ganciclovir prophylaxis. Forty-nine isolates were available from 42 subjects. About half of the subjects had received ganciclovir treatment for an average of 18–26 days, and all subjects had received prophylactic acyclovir or ganciclovir prior to CMV isolation. All 49 isolates of CMV were sensitive to ganciclovir, with a mean IC_{50} of 0.43 $\mu g/ml$ (range of $IC_{50} = 0.05$–1.33 $\mu g/ml$) and a mean IC_{90} of 0.7 $\mu g/ml$ (range of $IC_{90} = 0.33$–2.1 $\mu g/ml$). Presumably the absence of resistance in this series reflects the shorter duration of i.v. ganciclovir therapy given to these organ allograft recipients, compared to the series reported by Drew[6] in patients with CMV disease and AIDS. Also, patients with AIDS may have chronic replication of CMV at higher levels than allograft recipients.

Slavin et al.[10] evaluated the *in vitro* ganciclovir susceptibility of CMV isolates from bone marrow transplant recipients who had persistent isolation of CMV from bronchoalveolar lavage or lung tissue at autopsy following treatment with i.v. ganciclovir. Virus resistant to ganciclovir was isolated from one of 12 subjects after 17 days of treatment. This individual had received prior courses of ganciclovir. Among the other 11 subjects all isolates remained sensitive to ganciclovir after 9–32 days of treatment with ganciclovir and CMV immunoglobulin. The authors concluded that viral resistance could not account for the persistence of positive cultures in the lungs of these individuals. As in the report by Boivin[9], these patients received treatment for relatively shorter durations than would a person with AIDS.

Two trials studying oral ganciclovir treatment have added additional data concerning the prevalence of culture positivity and resistance following treatment with i.v. drug[11,12]. These two studies enrolled subjects with AIDS and stable CMV retinitis who had received treatment with i.v. ganciclovir for a minimum of four weeks. A total of 275 subjects with CMV retinitis and AIDS were enrolled, and cultures for CMV were performed at study entry in 253 of these individuals (92%). As shown in Table 8.5, 17 of the 253 subject cultures were positive for CMV (6.7%). Seven of these 17 isolates were tested by plaque reduction for *in vitro* susceptibility, and one was resistant. Using the same method for calculating the prevalence of resistant strains as used by Drew *et al.*[6], if 14% of those shedding CMV were shedding a resistant strain after more than one month of treatment with i.v. ganciclovir, and 6.7% were shedding CMV, then the estimated prevalence of resistance in this patient group treated with i.v. ganciclovir for an average of one to four months was 0.9% (14% times 6.7%).

Table 8.5 *Prevalence of isolation of CMV and in vitro susceptibility in subjects with CMV retinitis and AIDS after treatment for at least one month with i.v. ganciclovir*

No. subjects	275
No. with culture at baseline (%)	253 (92)
No. CMV positive at baseline (%)	17 (6.7)
No. tested for resistance	7
No. resistant *in vitro* (%)	1 (14)

Prevalence of resistance after treatment with oral ganciclovir

Oral ganciclovir has been in clinical development since 1987, and large-scale trials were initiated in 1991. The drug was approved in the USA for the maintenance treatment of CMV retinitis in 1994. The potential benefits of oral ganciclovir include convenience, improved tolerance and reduced cost. Oral ganciclovir is also potentially efficacious for the prevention of CMV disease in severely immunocompromised people. The pharmaco-kinetic characteristics of oral ganciclovir, however, are such that viral resistance might theoretically be more likely to emerge with oral treatment than with intravenous treatment. Intravenous ganciclovir given as a one-hour infusion results in a high peak concentration (about 6–12 μg/ml), a short half-life of two and a half to three hours, and rapid clearance via renal excretion. By eight to 12 hours after dosing serum concentrations are below those levels typically required to inhibit the replication of CMV *in vitro*. Oral ganciclovir, on the other hand, has low relative bioavailability but prolonged absorption from the gastrointestinal tract. A dose of oral ganciclovir results in relatively lower peak serum concentrations

(0.75–1.5 μg/ml) than an i.v. dose. With prolonged gastrointestinal absorption and multiple dosing during the day, however, measurable serum concentrations are maintained for 24 hours a day[11].

Buhles *et al.*[12] studied the prevalence of resistance of CMV isolates to ganciclovir from three clinical trials of oral ganciclovir. One of the studies was an open-label single-arm dose-rising study[11] (Syntex study 1505, ACTG 127). Two of the studies were randomized parallel comparisons of oral and i.v. ganciclovir maintenance treatment for CMV retinitis (Syntex studies ICM 1653 and 1774). Time to progression of CMV retinitis was measured by dilated indirect ophthalmoscopy and by masked assessment of fundus photographs. Subjects had cultures of urine, blood and semen for CMV performed at intervals prespecified in the protocols. A subset of those from whom CMV was isolated were tested for *in vitro* susceptibility to ganciclovir using a quantitative plaque-reduction method. *In vitro* susceptibility testing was performed prior to initiation of oral ganciclovir treatment, and for up to 270 days after treatment was initiated. The definition used to classify resistance was that shown in Table 8.1.

Resistance developed during therapy with oral ganciclovir, but was infrequent (Table 8.6). Culture and *in vitro* susceptibility results for subjects with CMV retinitis and AIDS randomized to maintenance treatment with either i.v. ganciclovir (5 mg/kg daily) or oral ganciclovir (3000 mg daily) are summarized from two studies. In neither was there a significant difference in the rate of CMV shedding in the rate of isolation of strains with a reduced *in vitro* susceptibility. These data are limited, however, by the fact that follow-up for most patients in these trials was for 100–120 days after randomization. It is not known if the rates of shedding or resistance might have increased if cultures had been performed later in the course of treatment. The absence of a higher prevalence of resistant virus in patients receiving oral drug may reflect the greater importance of intracellular versus serum drug levels, as the former may be similar in patients treated with oral or i.v. ganciclovir.

The susceptibility of CMV to ganciclovir is currently measured by

Table 8.6 *Culture and* in vitro *susceptibility results for patients with CMV retinitis and AIDS randomized to maintenance treatment with i.v. or oral ganciclovir*

Study no.	Prior treatment	Maint. i.v. No. pos./ no. cultured	Maint. i.v. No. resist./ no. tested	Maint. oral No. pos./ no. cultured	Maint. oral No. resist./ no. tested
1774	1–4 months i.v.	1/45	0/1	7/99	2/4
1653	None	3/48	1/2	4/44	0/2

tissue culture assay of a clinical isolate. *In vitro* testing may not reflect the spectrum of susceptibility of CMV strains in the infected host, since strains shed from one tissue may not necessarily be identical to CMV in other locations of the body. In addition, the estimates of the prevalence of resistance have been predicated upon the assumption that if a patient is infected with resistant CMV the individual will be culture positive, i.e. *in vitro* susceptibility testing can only be done after an isolate is obtained. Further evaluation of changes in susceptibility *in situ*, including strains that may be difficult to culture, will have to await utilization of nucleic acid assays to detect resistant genotypes.

Clinical relevance of CMV resistance

Anecdotal or single case reports or series suggest that if a patient has a strain of CMV resistant to ganciclovir *in vitro*, then clinical progression is more likely [1,2,6]. This fits a general model of microbial resistance, and the data presented here are not inconsistent with this observation. Many clinicians tend to assume that when a patient with CMV retinitis has progression of disease on therapy, viral resistance has developed. Data from the two randomized trials of i.v. versus oral ganciclovir, which utilized masked grading of retinal photographs to determine time to progression of CMV retinitis, show that this is not the case [12]. Only six of 117 patients (5%) were CMV culture positive at the time of progression of retinitis. Further, only one of nine patients (11%) who had *in vitro* susceptibility testing done at or after the diagnosis of progression of retinitis had a resistant CMV isolate [12]. Progression of CMV retinitis on therapy is probably the result of many factors, only one of which is the susceptibility of the CMV strain to the drug. Blood and tissue concentrations of ganciclovir, penetration of ganciclovir into the retinal tissue, and the host immune response probably play important roles in determining when clinical progression of CMV disease occurs.

Susceptibility testing of CMV to foscarnet

As with ganciclovir there is no standardized plaque-reduction susceptibility test for measuring the *in vivo* activity of foscarnet against CMV, although several laboratories are collaborating in an effort to develop the procedure. In a recent paper 58 isolates from patients who had never received foscarnet were tested by plaque reduction and the susceptibility results are shown in Figure 8.2 [13]. The distribution of IC_{50} is a typical population distribution, with a mean and median between 201 and 250 μM. Only five of 58 isolates had an $IC_{50} > 300$ μM and two isolates had an $IC_{50} > 400$ μM.

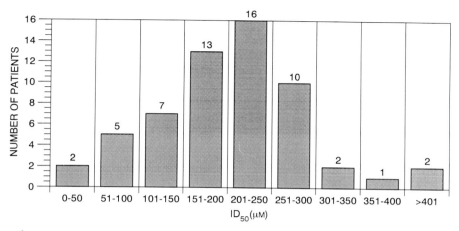

Figure 8.2 *Foscarnet new untreated patients. From reference 13, with permission*

On the basis of these results isolates tested by plaque-reduction assay using the method described (or a very similar method) were categorized as sensitive if their foscarnet IC_{50} is <400 μM. Isolates with higher IC_{50} are outside the range of pretherapy isolates and can be considered to exhibit varying degrees of resistance.

Foscarnet-resistant CMV

Sullivan and Coen[14] performed experiments which may account at least in part for the paucity of reports of foscarnet-resistant CMV isolated from patients. Pre-existing mutants of HSV, resistant to the foscarnet congener phosphonoacetic acid (PAA) occur at a frequency of $1:10^4$–$1:10^3$. In contrast, pre-existing foscarnet-resistant mutants of CMV could not be detected in the AD-169 strain, with a sensitivity of detection of a frequency of 1/70 000. The authors, however, were able to select foscarnet-resistant mutants of CMV by serial passage in increasing drug concentrations.

Resistant viruses derived by passage in foscarnet remained as susceptible to HPMPC as the parent AD–169; however, at least two clinical isolates of CMV were resistant to both foscarnet and HPMPC. One of these was recovered from blood after three months of foscarnet treatment (foscarnet IC_{50} = 870 μM; HPMPC IC_{50} 24 μM); previously the patient had also received long courses of ganciclovir, both prophylactically and therapeutically, which led to a mutation in the viral polymerase gene in addition to one in the UL97 region. The other isolate resistant to foscarnet and HPMPC was obtained from a patient prior to treatment with ganciclovir, and represented a minor (<1%) subpopulation of the patient's pretreatment isolate[15]. It was also resistant to ganciclovir, and was thought to be resistant to all three drugs on the basis of a mutation or mutations in viral DNA polymerase.

In contrast to numerous reports of ganciclovir-resistant CMV, there have been only a few scattered papers reporting foscarnet-resistant CMV. The clinical and virologic characteristics of these patients are summarized.

In 1991 Knox *et al.*[16] described the first clinical CMV isolate resistant to foscarnet from a bone marrow transplant recipient who had been treated with ganciclovir for CMV pneumonia. After 12 weeks of therapy an isolate from bronchoalveolar lavage was resistant to ganciclovir ($IC_{50} = 22$ μM) but sensitive to foscarnet ($IC_{50} = 312$ μM; control strain of CMV = 276 μM). The patient received foscarnet (105 mg/kg/day) for three weeks, followed by 38 mg/kg/day for one year. After approximately 12 months of maintenance treatment, CMV was isolated from her throat with an IC_{50} to foscarnet of 811 μM. Two months later a throat culture again yielded a foscarnet-resistant CMV ($IC_{50} > 1250$ μM). Despite recovery of these viruses the patient was continued on maintenance foscarnet, with no symptoms attributable to CMV and a well-functioning graft. The maintenance dosage was quite low in contrast to the 90–120 mg/day recommended for maintenance treatment of AIDS patients with CMV retinitis. This low dosage may have fostered the development of resistance and the authors do not state whether the maintenance dosage was increased following detection of the foscarnet-resistant CMV. It seems likely that since the graft was functioning well the degree of immunosuppression could be reduced, thus allowing host factors to suppress CMV replication.

The clinical significance of foscarnet resistance is more apparent in later reports. In 1993 Leport *et al.* reported an HIV-infected patient with multiple relapses of CMV retinitis despite maintenance treatment with i.v. foscarnet (115–127 mg/kg day)[17]. A CMV isolate from blood after three months of foscarnet therapy and just before a second relapse had an IC_{50} of 338 μM, with a mean of 147 μM for 11 control strains. The authors regarded the susceptibility of this isolate to foscarnet as intermediate, but it appeared to be sufficiently resistant to result in clinical failure of foscarnet therapy. Flores-Aguilar *et al.*[18] reported an AIDS patient with CMV viremia and clinically resistant retinitis despite foscarnet treatment. Isolates were obtained at weeks 58 and 88 after induction of foscarnet treatment, and the IC_{50} was >500 μM and >1000 μM respectively. Clinical failure occurred despite treatment with induction doses of foscarnet, resulting in peak and trough concentrations of 909 μM and 33 μM respectively[18].

Smith *et al.* reported three patients with blood or autopsy cultures positive for resistant isolates ($IC_{50} < 717$ 810 and >1000 μM), respectively, with four sensitive control viruses having a mean IC_{50} of 130 μM after two to four and a half months of foscarnet treatment[19]. Each patient demonstrated clinical signs of antiviral drug resistance.

Although there have been relatively few papers reporting clinical and laboratory resistance of CMV to foscarnet, as with ganciclovir most progression of retinitis in patients receiving foscarnet appears to be due to inadequate drug treatment rather than true viral resistance. Inadequate drug treatment may, in turn, be due to inadequate dosage attributable to poor patient compliance or drug toxicity. In addition, the concentration of drug in tissues such as the retina, central nervous system or gastrointestinal tract, may be inadequate to treat the virus in some patients. Thus the relative contributions to treatment failure of limited drug activity, altered pharmacokinetics or relative reductions in antiviral drug susceptibility are difficult to dissect.

REFERENCES

1. Fraser-Smith EB. Test for resistance of human cytomegalovirus to ganciclovir. Palo Alto (CA) Syntex Research, Institution of Agriscience, Department of Antimicrobial Research; 1988 October, Document No: RS-21592 CL 4617.
2. Erice A, Chou S, Biron KK *et al.* Progressive disease due to ganciclovir-resistant cytomegalovirus in immunocompromised patients. *New Engl J Med* 1989;320:289–93.
3. Tocci MJ, Livelli TJ, Perry HC, Crumpacker CS, Field AK. Effects of the nucleoside analog 2'-*nor*-2'-deoxyguanosine on human cytomegalovirus replication. *Antimicrob Agents Chemother* 1984;25:247–52.
4. Mar E, Cheng Y, Huang E. Effect of 9-(1,3-dihydroxy-2-propoxymethyl)guanine on human cytomegalovirus replication *in vitro*. *Antimicrob Agents Chemother* 1983;24:518–21.
5. Plotkin SA, Drew WL, Felsenstein D, Hirsch MS. Sensitivity of clinical isolates of human cytomegalovirus to 9-(dihydroxy-2-propoxymethyl)-guanine. *J Infect Dis* 1985;152:833–4.
6. Drew WL, Miner RC, Busch DF *et al.* Prevalence of resistance in patients receiving ganciclovir for serious cytomegalovirus infection. *J Infect Dis* 1991;163:716–9.
7. Tseng LF. Rapid and simple antiviral sensitivity testing of cytomegalovirus (CMV) (abstract). In: *Abstract Book of the 92nd General Meeting of the American Society for Microbiology*. New Orleans, USA, 1992:458.
8. Pepin J, Simon F, Dussault A *et al.* Rapid determination of human cytomegalovirus susceptibility to ganciclovir directly from clinical specimen primocultures. *J Clin Microbiol* 1992;30:2917.
9. Boivin G, Erice A, Crane DD, Dunn DL, Balfour HH Jr. Ganciclovir susceptibilities of cytomegalovirus (CMV) isolates from solid organ

transplant recipients with CMV viremia after antiviral prophylaxis. *J Infect Dis* 1993;168:332–5.

10. Slavin MA, Bindra RR, Gleaves CA, Pettinger MB, Bowden RA. Ganciclovir sensitivity of cytomegalovirus at diagnosis and during treatment of cytomegalovirus pneumonia in marrow transplant recipients. *Antimicrob Agents Chemother* 1993;37:1360–3.

11. Spector S, Busch D, Follansbee S *et al*. Pharmacokinetics, safety, and antiviral profiles of oral ganciclovir in persons infected with human immunodeficiency virus: a phase I/II study. *J Infect Dis* 1995;171:1431–7.

12. Buhles W, Drew WL, Miner RC for the Syntex Cooperative Oral Ganciclovir Study Group. Cytomegalovirus (CMV) resistance rates following treatment with IV and oral ganciclovir (GCV). Interscience Conference on Antimicrobial Agents and Chemotherapy. October 4–7 1994, Orlando, Florida.

13. Drew WL, Miner RC, Saleh E. Antiviral susceptibility testing of cytomegalovirus: criteria for detecting resistance to antivirals. *Clin Diagn Virol* 1993;1:179–85.

14. Sullivan V, Coen DM. Isolation of foscarnet-resistant human cytomegalovirus patterns of resistance and sensitivity to other antiviral drugs. *J Infect Dis* 1991;164:781–4.

15. Tatarowicz WA, Lurain NS, Thompson KD. A ganciclovir-resistant clinical isolate of human cytomegalovirus exhibiting cross-resistance to other DNA polymerase inhibitors. *J Infect Dis* 1992;166:904–7.

16. Knox KK, Drobyski WR, Carrigan DR. Cytomegalovirus isolate resistant to ganciclovir and foscarnet from a marrow transplant patient. *Lancet* 1991;337:1292–3.

17. Leport C, Puget S, Pepin JM *et al*. Meningoradiculoneuritis due to acyclovir-resistant varicella-zoster virus in a patient with AIDS. *J Infect Dis* 1993;168:1330–1.

18. Flores-Aguilar M, Kupperman BD, Quiceno JI *et al*. Pathophysiology and treatment of clinically resistant cytomegalovirus retinitis. *Ophthalmology* 1993;100:1022–30.

19. Smith RL, Jiles RE, Benbatoul KD *et al*. Molecular characterization of foscarnet resistant phenotypes of viral isolates from HCMV retinitis patients. Abstract presented at the 19th International Herpesvirus Workshop, Vancouver, BC, August 1994 (Abstract #213).

HUMAN IMMUNODEFICIENCY VIRUS

9
Nucleosides and Foscarnet—Mechanisms

BRENDAN A. LARDER

INTRODUCTION

Nucleoside analogues have proved to be the most fruitful source of human immunodeficiency virus (HIV) drugs to date, as numerous members of this class are potent inhibitors of HIV replication *in vitro*[1]. At present, five of these have been licensed for the treatment of HIV disease, namely 3'-azido-3'-deoxythymidine (AZT)[2], 2',3'-dideoxyinosine (ddI)[3], 2',3'-dideoxycytidine (ddC)[4], 2',3'-didehydro-2',3'-dideoxythymidine (d4T)[5] and (-)2'-deoxy-3'-thiacytidine (3TC)[9]. No HIV inhibitor of any other structural class received a treatment licence prior to these inhibitors. This is undoubtedly because many nucleoside analogues had already been synthesized before HIV infection became a recognized problem. When it became apparent that HIV-1 was a retrovirus, the unique viral-encoded reverse transcriptase (RT) (an essential enzyme for viral replication) became an obvious target for chemotherapeutic intervention. Since then many hundreds of nucleoside analogues have been tested for antiretroviral activity.

Although the RT has been successfully exploited as a chemotherapeutic target, it has also demonstrated a remarkable ability to evade the inhibitory activity of nucleoside analogues[6,7]. Not surprisingly, the emergence of HIV drug resistance was first seen with nucleoside analogues, specifically AZT[8]. Many of the lessons we learned from these early studies are now taken for granted when studying new HIV inhibitors, particularly the concept that resistance is due to the presence of specific, predictable mutations in the target enzyme. Much of our

Antiviral Drug Resistance. Edited by Douglas D. Richman © 1996 John Wiley & Sons Ltd

efforts to date in the study of HIV drug resistance have focused on the phenotypic and genotypic characterization of drug-resistant variants. Curiously, however, most of the knowledge obtained regarding AZT resistance and resistance to other nucleoside analogues has come from the study of HIV isolates during the clinical use of these drugs. Subsequent *in vitro* studies have proved invaluable in predicting the likelihood of resistance developing to a particular nucleoside analogue, and in allowing us to unravel the genetic basis of the observed resistance. Recent experiments involving 3TC resistance have also shown that *in vitro* studies may be very useful to establish a rationale to circumvent resistance development by exploiting mutational interactions in the RT[9].

In this chapter the mechanism of action of nucleoside analogues and foscarnet will be reviewed briefly. The following discussion of drug resistance will then be divided into the selection of drug-resistant variants, the genotypic characterisation of resistant strains, cross-resistance profiles and mutational interactions. Finally, structural and functional aspects of nucleoside analogue and foscarnet resistance will be discussed, in order to understand the mechanistic basis of resistance to these inhibitors and the potential effects the mutations have on replication of the virus.

MECHANISM OF ACTION OF NUCLEOSIDE ANALOGUES AND FOSCARNET

All nucleoside analogue inhibitors of HIV can be broadly classified as 2', 3'-dideoxynucleosides. Therefore it is not surprising that they all share a similar or common mode of action, culminating in chain termination of HIV DNA synthesis owing to the lack of a 3'-hydroxyl group. These inhibitors are only significantly active following conversion to the 5'-triphosphate form, which is mediated by a variety of cellular nucleoside and nucleotide kinases, since HIV does not encode such enzymes (for review, see[1]). The nucleotide analogues then behave as substrate mimics, binding to HIV RT in place of the natural triphosphates and leading to chain termination.

Obviously, the precise mechanism of action of each nucleoside analogue may differ, for example with respect to the relative phosphorylation rates of the unphosphorylated and various phosphorylated forms and the specific affinity of RT for the triphosphates. Taking AZT as an example, the 5'-triphosphate (AZT-TP) is a competitive inhibitor of HIV RT and an alternative substrate for thymidine triphosphate (TTP)[10-15]. The relative binding affinities observed for AZT-TP (K_i values between 2 and 120 nM[10-15]) suggest that this nucleotide analogue might bind more strongly to HIV RT than the natural substrate, TTP (K_m values of around 1–3 μM have been reported[12-15]). The actual K_m value of about 3–10 μM for incorporation of AZT-TP into newly synthesized viral DNA[13-15] is significantly higher than the K_i value for RT inhibition. This suggests that binding alone of AZT-TP to RT might in itself impede viral DNA synthesis by preventing TTP binding and incorporation. When AZT monophosphate becomes incorporated into the growing DNA chain, a dead-end complex of RT plus primer-template with inhibitor is formed. It has also been shown that primer-template chain terminated with AZT monophosphate is a strong RT inhibitor[12]. The reason why AZT-TP selectively inhibits HIV RT probably relates to the relatively weak interaction of this nucleotide analogue with cellular DNA polymerases. Thus, DNA polymerases α, β and γ appear to bind AZT-TP more weakly than HIV RT: in some cases K_i values are around 100 times higher than those determined for the viral enzyme[10,11].

One of the most structurally simple non-nucleoside inhibitors of HIV-1 RT is the pyrophosphate analogue foscarnet, or phosphonoformate[16]. This is a non-competitive inhibitor of TTP incorporation into viral DNA by HIV-1 RT, with a reported IC_{50} value of around 0.5 μM[16]. In addition, foscarnet is a non-competitive inhibitor when assessed with respect to primer-template. These data suggest that foscarnet does not bind to the same site on the RT as dNTPs (although it would be expected to interact at a putative pyrophosphate-binding site adjacent to the dNTP site). Furthermore, these kinetic data also suggest that the binding of foscarnet to RT does not itself affect binding of the primer-template to the enzyme.

SELECTION OF NUCLEOSIDE ANALOGUE RESISTANCE, ASSOCIATED GENOTYPIC CHANGES AND CROSS-RESISTANCE

AZT

Previous experience, particularly with herpesviruses and influenza viruses, has demonstrated the value of performing *in vitro* selection experiments to gain insights into the likely nature of resistance occurring during clinical use of antivirals. However, early selection studies with AZT failed to isolate HIV-1 mutants resistant to the drug[17]. Paradoxically, it was only when isolates from treated individuals were analysed that the mechanism of AZT resistance was discovered. Initially these isolates were found to have different levels of *in vitro* resistance, ranging from a few-fold change in IC_{50} value to a change of several hundredfold[8]. Inspection of ratios of IC_{50} to IC_{95} values for these isolates strongly suggested that mixed populations of wild type and mutant were common. Subsequent genotypic analysis confirmed that some of these isolates were indeed mixtures of viruses with different degrees of resistance[18]. In this analysis, full-length M13 RT clones were constructed following polymerase chain reaction (PCR) amplification of RT coding regions from infected cell DNA. Subsequently, comparative DNA sequence analysis of RT clones obtained from paired AZT-sensitive and -resistant isolates, led to identification of five specific amino acid substitutions: M41L, D67N, K70R, T215Y or F and K219Q[18,19]. Evidence of mixed populations of wild-type and mutant residues was apparent from this clonal analysis. In addition, it was clear that many different combinations of these mutations may exist in any one virus genome. Critical questions were posed by these observations, for example, what contribution did the respective mutations make to resistance and did these mutations appear in a specific order?

Absolute proof that the five identified amino acid substitutions were responsible for the observed phenotypes came from a series of site-directed mutagenesis studies. Molecularly cloned wild-type RT sequences were specifically altered *in vitro* to produce a series of mutant clones containing a large variety of combinations of the five mutations. These were then transferred into infectious HIV-1 proviral DNA, and the AZT sensitivity of virus recovered following transfection of T cells was assessed. When tested alone the codon 67 and 219 mutations did not alter AZT susceptibility. The codon 41 and 70 mutations alone increased the virus IC_{50} less than 10-fold[18-20]. The mutation of Thr215Tyr (caused by a double nucleotide change) conferred the most significant change of 15–20-fold in the wild-type HXB2-D background. Successive accumulation of these mutations in general caused an increase in resistance, although there are some important exceptions which will be discussed below. Combinations of four mutations (codons 41/67/70/215Tyr or 67/70/215Phe/219) or all five (codons 41/67/70/215Tyr/219) gave the most resistant viruses, with IC_{50} values increasing by more than 100-fold[18,19] (see Table 9.1 for a summary of these mutations).

Once it was clear that the above five mutations played a key role in AZT resistance it was of obvious interest to study the appearance of these during AZT therapy. Initial work focused on a cohort of asymptomatic individuals from whom sequential HIV-1 isolates were obtained for more than two years after initiation of AZT[21]. A common pattern was seen whereby the codon 70 mutation appeared first but was fairly quickly replaced by a population of viruses containing either the codon 41 or 215 mutations, or 70 linked with 215Tyr. Subsequently, viruses with linked 41 + 215Tyr mutations were frequently observed[22]. These findings could be rationalized by the site-directed mutagenesis data

Table 9.1 *Mutations in HIV-1 RT that confer nucleoside analogue resistance*

RT codon	Amino acid change	Most common inhibitor to select mutation	Approx fold increase in IC_{50}	Cross-resistance observed	Resistance suppression	Commonly associated mutations	Selected in vitro?	Selected in vivo?
41	Met-Leu	AZT	4x	3'-azido-nucleosides		67, 70, 215, 219	no	yes
62	Ala-Val	AZT + ddN	?			75, 77, 116, 151	no	yes
65	Lys-Arg	ddN	4–10x	ddN, 3TC		—	yes	yes
67	Asp-Asn	AZT	none	3'-azido-nucleosides		41, 70, 215, 219	yes	yes
69	Thr-Asp	ddC	5x			—	no	yes
70	Lys-Arg	AZT	8x	3'-azido-nucleosides		41, 67, 215, 219	yes	yes
74	Leu-Val	ddI	5–10x	ddC	AZT (not when 41Leu present)	—	yes	yes
75	Val-Thr	d4T	~5x	ddNs	AZT (partial)	—	yes	yes
75	Val-Ile	AZT + ddN	?			62, 77, 116, 151	no	yes
77	Phe-Leu	AZT + ddN	?			62, 77, 116, 151	no	yes
115	Tyr-Phe	1592U89	marginal			74, 184	yes	no
116	Phe-Tyr	AZT + ddN	?			62, 75, 77, 151	no	yes
151	Gln-Met	AZT + ddN	10x (AZT) ~5x (ddN)			62, 75, 77, 116	no	yes
184	Met-Val	3TC	>500x	ddNs	AZT	—	yes	yes
184	Met-Ile	3TC	~125x	ddNs	AZT	—	yes	yes
210	Leu-Trp	AZT	none	?		41, 215,	no	yes
215	Thr-Tyr	AZT	15–20x	3'-azido-nucleosides		41, 67, 70, 219	yes	yes
215	Thr-Phe	AZT	~10x	3'-azido-nucleosides		41, 67, 70, 219	no	yes
219	Lys-Gln	AZT	none	3'-azido-nucleosides		41, 67, 70, 215	no	yes
219	Lys-Glu	AZT	none	?		41, 67, 70, 215	yes	?

which demonstrated that genetic linkage of the codon 41 + 215Tyr mutations resulted in a virus with substantial AZT resistance (around 60–70-fold increase in IC_{50} value compared to wild-type virus). By contrast, the combination of the codon 70 + 215Tyr mutations led to a virus that was more AZT sensitive than anticipated (with an IC_{50} value around 0.06 μM) and significantly less resistant than the 41 + 215Tyr mutant strain[22]. Therefore, it seems that the appearance of particular combinations of AZT resistance mutations is largely dictated by the absolute change in sensitivity conferred by the mutations. The reason why the codon 70 mutation appears first is not clear, although it is possible that this strain pre-exists at a low but significant level in the wild-type population. Thus, in the presence of AZT selection pressure, virus with the codon 70 mutation would rapidly outgrow wild-type virus and persist until the much more resistant 41 + 215Tyr strain developed. If this is the case, it seems unlikely that highly AZT-resistant virus pre-exists in a wild-type population, especially as virus with four or five of the mutations only appears late in therapy after progression to AIDS.

During the time AZT-resistant clinical isolates were being analysed, attempts were being made to select variants in cell culture by passaging HIV in the presence of AZT[17]. Different laboratories reported similar results in that resistant strains were finally isolated by such passage procedures[23,24]. It was gratifying that these viruses had acquired the same RT mutations as observed in clinical isolates. Furthermore, in one passage series there was evidence that the order of appearance of these mutations was similar to that previously seen with clinical isolates[23]. Specifically, passage of wild-type virus resulted initially in the development of the codon 70 mutation followed by 215Tyr. At this time there was evidence that virus with the codon 70 mutation had diminished in the population. These data were the first to confirm the potential value of such *in vitro* selection experiments in predicting the likely ease of antiretroviral resistance development in the clinic, and the nature of mutations conferring resistance.

There has been continued interest in attempting to uncover additional RT mutations that might also decrease AZT susceptibility, besides the five amino acid substitutions described above in RT that collectively confer AZT resistance. One such suggestion is that amino acid variation at codon 210 (Leu to Trp) might play a role in AZT resistance[25]. However, the significance of this variation for resistance remains unclear, as conflicting data have been obtained in different laboratories. The consensus of opinion is that 210Trp alone in a wild-type background has no effect on AZT susceptibility[25-27]. However, opinions differ as to the relative effect of this change on AZT resistance in the background of pre-existing AZT resistance mutations[25,27]. This is especially the case with the 41Leu plus 215Tyr background (with which the codon 210 change is often associated), where 210Trp has been reported to have only a modest or quite significant effect on AZT resistance[25,27].

Dideoxynucleoside analogues

Initial indications that HIV-1 could acquire ddI and ddC resistance again came from the study of isolates obtained from treated individuals. The first such study was of a group of patients who switched therapy from AZT to ddI[28]. Virus isolates were obtained prior to and after therapy was switched, and were assessed for AZT and ddI susceptibility. IC_{50} values for ddI increased about 10-fold after six to 12 months of ddI treatment, and these isolates were also similarly cross-resistant to ddC. Curiously, those isolates with a pre-existing 215Tyr mutation in RT retained this mutation but regained AZT sensitivity[28]. The nature of this phenotypic 'reversion' will be discussed in more detail below. DNA sequence analysis of the ddI-resistant isolates revealed a novel RT mutation at codon 74 (Leu to Val). Virus reconstruction experiments, in which the codon 74 change was introduced into a wild-type background by site-directed mutagenesis, confirmed that this change was responsible for the observed resistance[28]. Subsequent studies have also identified 74Val as a mutation associated with ddI therapy[29,30].

A number of additional mutations have been identified through the study of clinical isolates, or by *in vitro* selection experiments, that confer reduced susceptibility to ddI[31–33], ddC[31–34] or d4T[35] (see Table 9.1 for a summary of these mutations). Isolates from a small number of patients receiving long-term ddC therapy were reported to contain a mutation at codon 69 of RT (Thr to Asp) that confers modest resistance to ddC but not cross-resistance to ddI[34]. More recently, a mutation of Lys to Arg at codon 65 has been shown to confer a degree of both ddI and ddC resistance[32,33]. This was identified by *in vitro* selection with ddC and also by sequence analysis of isolates from individuals treated with either ddI or ddC. An additional mutation at codon 184 (Met to Val) can also be selected both *in vitro* and *in vivo* by ddC[31]. This mutation also confers cross-resistance (albeit low level) to ddI[31]. Finally, only limited data relating to d4T resistance are available. These are mainly from a single *in vitro* study where a virus was selected with an RT mutation at codon 75 (Val to Thr). Site-directed mutagenesis experiments confirmed that this mutation caused about a sevenfold decrease in IC_{50} to d4T, in addition to cross-resistance to ddI and ddC[35]. A subsequent study focusing on the analysis of HIV isolates from d4T-treated individuals failed to sub-stantiate completely the earlier *in vitro* results, in that d4T therapy did not appear to result consistently in the appearance of 75Thr in RT[36]. Surprisingly, analysis of similar mutant virus strains created by site-directed mutagenesis did not confirm the phenotypic effect of 75Thr reported in the first study[36].

Drug resistance data have also been obtained for a carbocyclic nucleoside analogue, 1592U89 [(1S,4R)-4-(2-amino-6-cyclopropylamino)-9H-purin-9-yl)-2-cyclopentene-1-methanol], which is currently in clinical trials[37]. This nucleoside is converted during intercellular phosphorylation to the triphosphate form of carbovir[37]. *In vitro* passage experiments showed that resistance develops relatively slowly to 1592U89, and multiple mutations are required to give significant levels of resistance (>10-fold)[38]. Passage of wild-type virus resulted initially in the RT mutation Met184 to Val. This was followed by Leu74 to Val and Lys65 to Arg (or Tyr115 to Phe in place of the codon 65 mutation). Analysis of virus variants constructed with single, double and triple combinations of these mutations confirmed their significance for 1592U89 resistance[38]. As expected from this pattern of RT mutations, these variants were also cross-resistant to ddI, ddC and 3TC.

It is apparent from the above discussion that there are common patterns of resistance to dideoxynucleosides. First, all of the above mutations (except Asp69) confer resistance to both ddI and ddC. This suggests that a common mechanism of 'ddN' resistance may exist via mutation at a number of residues in RT. Furthermore, the magnitude of resistance conferred by each mutation to ddI and ddC is similarly modest (i.e. around a five- to 20-fold increase in IC_{50} compared to parental virus). This might be because large changes in sensitivity to these nucleosides are not necessary to allow the virus to evade the activity of these inhibitors *in vivo*.

3TC

Resistance to 3TC, and the closely related inhibitor (-)-2'-deoxy-5-fluoro-3'-thiacytidine (FTC), was observed by a number of groups after *in vitro* passage experiments with wild-type HIV-1[39-42]. Unlike such selection studies with other nucleoside analogues, resistance to 3TC or FTC occurs extremely rapidly within two to three passages in cell culture. The magnitude of this resistance is even more remarkable, in that virus variants are selected with IC_{50} values 500–1000 times higher than wild-type virus. DNA sequencing of resistant strains and site-directed mutagenesis studies identified two mutations at RT codon 184, Met to Val or Ile, that are responsible for the observed phenotype[39-42]. As anticipated from the discussion in the previous section, variants with these codon 184 mutations showed a low level of cross-resistance to ddC and ddI[40,42]. Interestingly, it has also been noted that HIV-1 variants with the Lys65 to Arg mutation also exhibit low-level cross-resistance to 3TC[32].

As both the 184Val and 184Ile mutations can be selected with either 3TC or FTC, starting with viruses having different genetic backgrounds, it was initially thought that these mutations were equivalent. However, further investigation of viruses containing each mutation has revealed some subtle differences. For example, it appears that 184Val confers a higher degree of resistance to both 3TC and FTC than the 184Ile mutation[43]. In addition, growth competition experiments with mixtures of virus variants containing 184Val or Ile demonstrated that the 184Val variant is able to compete out the 184Ile mutant[9]. This occurred both in the absence and presence of either 3TC or FTC[9]. These *in vitro* data suggest that during treatment of individuals with 3TC the inhibitor selection pressure will allow both variants to appear, although 184Val is likely to be dominant. In fact, this phenomenon has been seen during the study of 3TC-resistant isolates in a 3TC monotherapy clinical trial[44]. This raises the question as to why the 'less fit' 184Ile mutant emerges at all both *in vitro* and *in vivo*. It has been suggested that this might be related to the relatively high mutation frequency observed for G to A transitions (i.e. AT$\underline{G}$ [Met] to AT$\underline{A}$ [Ile]), creating an Ile substitution, compared to A to G transitions (i.e. $\underline{A}$TG [Met] to $\underline{G}$TG [Val]) which causes a Val substitution[9].

SELECTION OF FOSCARNET-RESISTANT VARIANTS AND ASSOCIATED GENOTYPIC CHANGES

The first indication that HIV-1 could acquire resistance to foscarnet came from early RT site-directed mutagenesis studies[45]. A cloned RT fragment was mutated at codons corresponding to conserved regions in the enzyme. A number of these mutations allowed viable viral replication when they were introduced into an infectious molecular clone[46]. In particular, Asp113 to Glu and Ala114 to Ser conferred resistance to foscarnet in cell culture, although surprisingly these mutant viruses were both hypersensitive to AZT[46]. Another mutant virus, with a change in RT of Glu89 to Gly, was isolated by screening RT clones *in vitro* for resistance to ddGTP[47]. This was also found to be foscarnet resistant, but not resistant to nucleoside analogues.

Recent information has been reported on the selection of foscarnet-resistant HIV-1 strains by selection with the inhibitor in cell culture. In one study, virus with about 10-fold decreased susceptibility to foscarnet was isolated after multiple passages in cell culture[48]. This virus also

Table 9.2   Mutations in HIV-1 RT that confer foscarnet resistance

RT codon	Amino acid change	Approx. fold increase in IC_{50}	Hypersusceptibility	Commonly associated mutations	Selected in vitro?	Selected in vivo?
88	Trp–Ser	$3-4\times$	none	161,208	no	yes
89	Glu–Gly	$13-14\times$	none	—	yes	no
89	Glu–Lys	$5\times$ with 92	AZT, NNRTIs	92	yes	no
92	Leu–Ile	$5\times$ with 89	AZT, NNRTIs	89	yes	no
113	Asp–Glu	$5\times$	AZT	—	SDM	no
114	Ala–Ser	$5\times$	AZT	—	SDM	no
161	Gln–Leu	$10\times$	AZT, NNRTIs	88, 208	yes	yes
208	His–Tyr	marginal	AZT, NNRTIs (with 161Leu)	88, 161	yes	yes

displayed increased susceptibility to AZT (90-fold) and to non-nucleo-side RT inhibitors such as nevirapine. Genetic analysis of this isolate revealed two mutations in RT: Gln161 to Leu and His208 to Tyr[48]. In addition, the same mutations plus Trp88 to Ser were found in the RT of HIV-1 isolates from individuals receiving foscarnet. Site-directed mutagenesis studies demonstrated that the codon 161 mutation alone conferred about a 10-fold reduction in foscarnet susceptibility[48]. The other mutations appeared to confer marginal resistance to the inhibitor. However, since the codon 88 mutation did not alter AZT susceptibility it was reasoned that this might appear more frequently in virus isolated from individuals receiving simultaneous AZT and foscarnet therapy. In a separate study[49], strains showing about fivefold foscarnet resistance were selected by in vitro passage that had different mutations in RT from those described above. One such variant had a Glu89 to Lys mutation and another had a change of Leu92 to Ile. Both of these mutations also rendered the virus hypersusceptible to AZT and non-nucleoside RT inhibitors[49] (see Table 9.2 for a summary of these mutations).

MUTATIONAL INTERACTIONS: MULTIDRUG RESISTANCE AND RESISTANCE SUPPRESSION

The first indication that specific interactions between various nucleoside analogue resistance mutations can occur came from a close examination of HIV-1 strains containing different combinations of AZT resistance mutations[22]. Although it appeared initially that there was a broad increase in AZT resistance with increasing numbers of mutations in one genome, this was not always the case. The combination of 70Arg and 215Tyr gives a less resistant virus than anticipated (an IC_{50} value of 0.06 μM, compared with 0.08 μM for 70Arg alone, or 0.16 μM for 215Tyr alone in viruses derived from molecular clones)[22]. As described above, virus with 41Leu and 215Tyr in contrast has a considerably higher IC_{50} value than these mutations singly. Thus, it appears that the codon 70 mutation has a suppressive effect on 215Tyr. It is perhaps not too surprising that virus with 41Leu and 215Tyr becomes dominant in a population during AZT therapy[22].

In view of the above, the possibility of suppression of phenotypic resistance to one nucleoside inhibitor by generation of simultaneous resistance to a second was of considerable interest. Indeed, a number of such examples of suppression of AZT resistance have been documented, through both *in vitro* and *in vivo* observations. The first demonstration of this came from a study of HIV-1 isolates obtained from ddI-treated individuals who had already received AZT[28]. As described above, resistance to ddI occurred within 12 months owing to the 74Val mutation in RT. However, it appeared that although these isolates retained AZT-resistance mutations (notably 215Tyr), they became phenotypically more AZT sensitive when 74Val was induced[28]. Subsequent analysis of virus variants derived by site-directed mutagenesis and containing 74Val with 215Tyr confirmed that 74Val can reverse the effect of 215Tyr. In this initial study other AZT-resistance mutations seen when therapy was switched (41Leu and 70Arg) did not persist after the 74Val mutation emerged[28].

Suppression of AZT resistance has also been documented to occur owing to induction of resistance to non-nucleoside RT inhibitors (NNRTIs). During *in vitro* passage experiments where pre-existing AZT-resistant virus was exposed to various NNRTIs, resistance to these inhibitors occurred rapidly as a result of a mutation in RT of Tyr181 to Cys[50]. Concurrently this virus regained susceptibility to AZT, even though AZT-resistance mutations such as 41Leu and 215Tyr persisted in RT[50]. Similar observations were made during clinical trials with the NNRTI nevirapine. Thus, when individuals harbouring pre-existing AZT-resistant virus were treated with nevirapine alone, the virus rapidly became NNRTI resistant, acquiring the 181Cys mutation[51]. However, the pattern of resistance was different when nevirapine was given in combination with AZT. In this case a number of different RT mutations appeared rather than the AZT resistance 'suppression' mutation 181Cys[51]. As these mutations do not suppress AZT resistance, the simultaneous presence of AZT-resistance mutations resulted in a dual resistant phenotype. This is a clear example of alternative resistance 'pathways' that can occur depending on the specific inhibitor selection pressure.

In view of the above observations there has been considerable interest in determining whether HIV-1 can tolerate multiple mutations in RT in order to develop co-resistance to multiple RT inhibitors. A report that initially created considerable excitement claimed to demonstrate that specific mutational constraints existed in RT which prevented the development of such multidrug resistance[52]. Specifically, it was reported that simultaneous co-resistance to AZT, ddI and nevirapine could not occur, since the combinations of mutations required to confer such resistance were detrimental to the replication of the virus[52]. Unfortunately, it turned out that owing to technical flaws in one of the critical mutagenesis experiments[53] the supposed replication-'defective' virus was in fact perfectly viable[54,55]. In addition, virus variants with the relatively simple RT genotype 41Leu, 74Val, 106Ala and 215Tyr were co-resistant to these inhibitors[54]. Such virus was selected by passage of a 41Leu/74Val/215Tyr mutant in all three drugs[54].

A more recent example of AZT-resistance suppression has been seen with the codon 184 mutations in RT that confer high-level resistance to 3TC and other thionucleoside analogues[9,39,42]. The suppressive effect of this mutation on AZT resistance was discovered in two ways. First, pre-existing AZT-resistant mutant viruses had 184Ile or Val incorporated into RT by site-directed mutagenesis[9,39,42]. The resulting virus strains (based on the HXB2-D parent) were highly resistant to 3TC but had regained AZT susceptibility. Both the Ile and Val substitutions at codon 184 had a similar suppressive effect on AZT resistance[9,39,42]. For example, virus with 41Leu + 215Tyr became completely AZT sensitive when 184Met was changed to either Ile or Val. *In vitro* selection experiments starting with AZT-resistant strains based on HXB2-D confirmed the suppressive effect of codon 184 mutations on AZT resistance. For example, when AZT-resistant virus with 41Leu + 215Tyr was passaged in the presence of 3TC, this virus became rapidly 3TC resistant and simultaneously AZT susceptible, owing to codon 184 mutations[9]. Passage of the same virus in both AZT and 3TC gave essentially the same result, although it took about 10 passages rather than three before 184Val was detected[9]. Nevertheless, this virus was ultimately 3TC resistant and AZT susceptible[9]. These *in vitro* selection experiments demonstrated that there was no obvious alternative 3TC-resistance pathway that could evolve in order to allow co-resistance between AZT and 3TC to occur.

Clinical studies in which the combination of AZT and 3TC was assessed have largely confirmed these *in vitro* observations. In AZT-naive individuals, the rate of AZT resistance development was significantly slower with the combination than with AZT monotherapy, even though 3TC resistance rapidly appeared[9]. This early induction of the 184Val mutation might have caused the subsequent slow appearance of AZT-resistance mutations owing to the suppressive effect of this mutation on AZT resistance. The picture in previously AZT-treated individuals was more complex, since the virus from many of these individuals already contained AZT-resistance mutations before combination therapy commenced. However, the 184Val mutation again appeared very rapidly in this population, and the pattern of AZT-resistance mutations seemed to be unaffected[56]. Thus it is possible that a number of these strains had regained AZT susceptibility as a result of the 184Val mutation, although there is now some evidence that dual resistant isolates can occur[57]. These studies again confirmed that the dominant pathway to high-level 3TC resistance was via induction of the 184Val mutation in RT.

The first documentation of AZT/3TC dual resistance came from *in vitro* passage experiments using a pre-existing AZT-resistant clinical isolate of HIV-1[58]. In addition to the recognized AZT-resistance mutations at RT codons 41, 67, 70 and 215, this strain also had over 20 other amino acid differences in RT with respect to HXB2-D[59]. Passage of the virus in the presence of both AZT and 3TC eventually resulted in virus that was 3TC resistant and still retained a fairly high level of resistance to AZT[58,59]. Genotypic analysis revealed that exposure to 3TC once again resulted in the appearance of 184Val, thus accounting for the observed increase in 3TC resistance[59]. However, it was not immediately obvious why the codon 184 mutation in this strain did not suppress AZT resistance, as had been observed with other strains. A series of marker transfer genetic mapping and site-directed mutagenesis experiments eventually led to the conclusion that pre-existing amino acid variation in this mutant strain was responsible. Surprisingly, a change of Gly333Glu appeared sufficient to prevent the AZT-resistance suppressive activity of the 184Val mutation[59]. Thus, when 333Glu was reverted by mutagenesis to 333Gly the dual-resistant virus regained AZT susceptibility[59]. Preliminary analysis of HIV-1 strains from individuals with pre-existing AZT-resistant virus undergoing AZT and 3TC combination therapy revealed little variation at RT codon 333[56]. It is therefore not clear at present whether variation at this codon will play a significant role in the development of AZT/3TC co-resistance.

There have been a number of recent reports claiming that HIV-1 can become resistant to multiple dideoxynucleosides owing to selection of novel mutations in RT[60,61]. These strains were identified by the analysis of HIV-1 variants that emerged during combination therapy with AZT and ddI or ddC. Although these strains appeared at a relatively low frequency, their initial description caused some interest and raised a number of questions that have yet to be answered. During combination therapy it was found that the virus could gradually accumulate five novel mutations in RT (Ala62Val, Val75Ile, Phe77Leu, Phe116Tyr and Gln151Met)[60,61]. It appeared that the Gln151Met mutation was pivotal in this 'alternative' resistance pathway, since it was the first to be detected (and alone could confer co-resistance to AZT, ddI, ddC and d4T)[60,61]. It is not clear why these mutations should occasionally emerge in response to the simultaneous pressure of AZT combined with a ddN, since the accumulation of 'conventional' resistance mutations in RT can also confer similar co-resistance. In addition, it is also not obvious why the codon 151 mutation alone is not selected with single ddN therapy, as this mutation can itself confer fairly broad co-resistance. It is possible that the specific amino acid background in RT is important in 'dictating' the resistance pathway HIV-1 can take as a result of drug pressure. Large-scale comprehensive sequence analysis of RT before and after ddN combination therapy might be required to resolve this issue.

STRUCTURAL AND FUNCTIONAL ASPECTS OF NUCLEOSIDE ANALOGUE AND FOSCARNET RESISTANCE

In contrast to the large amount of data that has accumulated during the last few years on the genotypic nature of nucleoside analogue and foscarnet resistance, relatively little information has been obtained regarding the enzymatic mechanisms of such resistance. This is despite the fact that good-quality RT crystallographic data have been available for some time. The first clue that the biochemical nature of nucleoside analogue resistance was not straightforward came from early studies of AZT-resistant mutants. It was anticipated that simple RT inhibition experiments with enzyme derived from AZT-resistant virus would reveal that there was *in vitro* resistance to AZT triphosphate (AZT-TP). Surprisingly, this did not appear to be the case[8]. Numerous attempts to demonstrate a difference in binding of AZT-TP to mutant RT relative to wild-type enzyme have been unsuccessful. Detailed comparisons of the kinetic properties of RT derived from virions or purified recombinant enzyme only revealed small differences between enzymes from sensitive or AZT-resistant viruses (up to a threefold change in sensitivity)[8,62]. A variety of other parameters have been investigated in order to elucidate the biochemical mechanism of AZT resistance; these include the susceptibility of the RT endogenous activity to AZT-TP; comparison of the fidelity of mutant and wild-type enzymes; and the relative modulating activity of AZT monophosphate on the inhibitory activity of AZT-TP[62]. Unfortunately, none of these studies have so far been able to explain how RT from AZT-resistant virus can escape inhibition by AZT-TP. It might be that the small but reproducible kinetic changes seen between RT from sensitive and resistant viruses are somehow sufficient to confer a high degree of resistance on the virus. Perhaps a small perturbation of the chain terminating activity of AZT-TP could translate into significant levels of virus resistance. However, until we are able to demonstrate convincingly that this is the case, the central dichotomy of AZT resistance will remain a mystery.

In contrast to the inconclusive biochemical data obtained with 'conventional' AZT-resistance mutations, kinetic data with mutant RTs from ddN-resistant viruses has been less perplexing. For example, RT with 74Val shows 'biochemical resistance' to ddATP with the magnitude of change similar to that seen with the mutant virus to ddI[63]. Similarly, it has been demonstrated that mutant enzyme with 184Val is significantly resistant *in vitro* to 3TC triphosphate (3TC-TP)[41]. Another study with RT containing the ddN resistance mutation 65Arg showed that there was decreased chain termination by ddCTP, ddATP, 3TC-TP and AZT-TP in a cell-free assay system compared to wild-type enzyme[64]. These data are consistent with those obtained in whole virus cell culture assays using ddI, ddC and 3TC, but not with AZT since 65Arg confers no AZT resistance. Curiously, RT studied from one of the rare multiple ddN-resistant isolates (containing mutations at residues 62, 75, 77, 116 and 151) was considerably insensitive to AZT-TP relative to RT from the paired pretherapy isolate[60]. This suggests that the particular mechanism of resistance conferred by the 'conventional' AZT-resistance mutations might be different from the multiple resistant variants.

It was anticipated that the recently available RT crystal structure data[65-70] would shed some light on the specific underlying mechanisms by which the observed mutations in RT confer nucleoside analogue resistance. However, unlike the NNRTI-resistance mutations which all cluster around the NNRTI-binding pocket in the enzyme[65,68,70], the situation with nucleoside analogue resistance mutations is still far from clear[65,68]. It was assumed before the structure of HIV-1 RT was known that the nucleoside resistance mutations would also be found in a cluster. Surprisingly few of the numerous residues that mutate to confer nucleoside resistance appear to lie very close to the polymerase active site, comprising the catalytic Asp residues 110, 185 and 186 in the p66 'palm' domain of RT (see Plate 1)[65,68,69]. In fact, most of these residues are located in both the 'fingers' and 'palm' domains of the p66 subunit of RT[65,68]. Thus, it seems that rather than interacting directly with nucleotide substrates or inhibitors, mutation at these residues could alter the interaction of the enzyme with the primer-template, resulting in a subtle 'repositioning' in the active site. Direct evidence that this might indeed be the case, at least for dideoxynucleosides, came from a recently reported biochemical study of RT containing the ddN-resistance mutation 74Val[71]. Using primer-templates that could be extended different lengths, it was shown that wild-type enzyme is only sensitive to the active form of ddI (ddATP) when the template extends more than three or four nucleotides beyond the end of the primer strand (and beyond the catalytic site). In contrast, the mutant enzyme is resistant to ddATP whatever the length of the template extension[71]. These data suggest that 'long-distance' mutations, in this case 74Val, may cause primer-template repositioning in the RT active site and specifically change the ability of the enzyme to accept or reject an incoming nucleotide (i.e. ddATP). From a mechanistic perspective, the mutation at residue 184 in RT which confers high-level resistance to 3TC appears to be an exception to the other nucleoside analogue resistance mutations, owing to its position in the RT structure. This is located directly in the active site of the enzyme, close to the catalytic Asp residues (see Plate 1). It seems probable that mutation of this residue (to Val or Ile) results in direct blocking of 3TC-TP binding in the active site. This seems especially likely as the 184Val mutant shows marked 'resistance' to 3TC-TP in cell-free RT assays.

When considering foscarnet resistance mutations, the probable enzymatic mechanisms of resistance might be similar to those discussed above for nucleosides. As foscarnet is a pyrophosphate analogue, it is assumed that it binds to the RT active site in the region of the catalytic Asp residues. Mutation of residue 161, which is located close to this site, might therefore have a direct effect on foscarnet binding by altering the confirmation of the putative dNTP-binding site[48]. However, this is probably not the case with the mutations that cluster from residue 88 to 92, as these lie in a region of the p66 subunit that is involved in primer-template binding[68]. Thus, it has been suggested that the foscarnet resistance mutations in this region could also alter the positioning of the primer-template in the active site, similar to the situation with the 74Val ddI-resistance mutation[48,49]. As the location of residue 208 in the RT structure is neither close to the active site, nor appears to contact the primer-template, it is not clear how this mutation alters foscarnet susceptibility.

SUMMARY

An enormous wealth of nucleoside analogue- and foscarnet-resistance data has accumulated since the first description of AZT resistance. This has been derived both from *in vitro* selection studies and by the analysis of HIV-1 isolates during clinical use of these inhibitors. In general, the *in vitro* studies have been surprisingly predictive of the nature and patterns of resistance seen in the clinic. However, in a number of cases, notably AZT, initial resistance data were derived from clinical isolates and not from cell culture selection experiments. The advances in molecular technology enabling the analysis and verification of HIV-1 drug resistance have resulted in a detailed understanding and cataloguing of genotypic resistance. This has a number of important benefits. First, we now have the ability to rapidly detect the emergence of drug-resistant strains using highly sensitive molecular tools. It seems only a matter of time before such assays become common in the overall management strategies of infected individuals in order to optimize therapy. Secondly, the intriguing interactions between resistance mutations that have been documented will hopefully be 'harnessed' to improve future combination therapy. Perhaps the increased potency seen with the AZT + 3TC combination is the first example of utilizing the 'resistance reversal' phenomenon.

One of the more perplexing aspects of HIV-1 resistance to nucleoside analogues and foscarnet has been unravelling the precise way in which the mutations structurally cause loss of inhibitor susceptibility. This is perhaps now becoming a little clearer in some cases, for example with the 74Val ddI-resistance mutation. However, a number of mysteries still surround the biochemical mechanism of AZT resistance, despite the fact that high-resolution RT structural data are available and the locations of the mutations are known. To gain further insight into the mechanisms of resistance it will probably be important to solve the crystal structure of RT enzymes that have defined drug-resistance mutations (both alone and in various combinations). It might also be necessary to solve mutant RT structures that are complexed with primer-template and dNTP in order to deduce the effects of multiple resistance mutations. Resolving this puzzle will not only be of clear scientific interest, but could lead to a better understanding of how to use drug combinations in a more rational way, perhaps allowing resistance to drugs such as AZT to be avoided.

REFERENCES

1. De Clercq E. HIV inhibitors targeted at the reverse transcriptase. *AIDS Res Hum Retroviruses* 1992;8:119–34.
2. Wilde MI, Langtry HD. Zidovudine. An update of its pharmacodynamic and pharmacokinetic properties, and therapeutic efficacy. *Drugs* 1993;46:515–78.
3. Yarchoan R, Mitsuya H, Thomas RV et al. *In vivo* activity against HIV and favourable toxicity profile of 2'-,3'-dideoxyinosine. *Science* 1989;245:412–15.
4. Broder S, Yarchoan R. Dideoxycytidine: current clinical experience and future prospects. A summary. *Am J Med* 1990;88:1S–33S.

5. Balzarini J, Kang GJ, Dalal M *et al.* The anti-HTLV-III (anti-HIV) and cytotoxic activity of 2',3'-didehydro-2',3'-dideoxyribonucleosides: a comparison with their parental 2',3'-dideoxyribonucleosides. *Mol Pharmacol* 1987;32:162–7.

6. Larder BA. Reverse transcriptase inhibitors and drug resistance. In: Skalka AM, Goff SP, eds. *Reverse Transcriptase.* New York: Cold Spring Harbor Laboratory Press, 1993:205–22.

7. Richman DD. Resistance of clinical isolates of human immunodeficiency virus to antiretroviral agents. *Antimicrob Agents Chemother* 1993;37:1207–13.

8. Larder BA, Darby G, Richman DD. HIV with reduced sensitivity to zidovudine (AZT) isolated during prolonged therapy. *Science* 1989;243:1731–4.

9. Larder BA, Kemp SD, Harrigan PR. Potential mechanism for sustained antiretroviral efficacy of AZT-3TC combination therapy. *Science* 1995;269:696–9.

10. Cheng Y-C, Dutschman GE, Bastow KF, Sarngadharan MG, Ting RYC. Human immunodeficiency virus reverse transcriptase. General properties and its interactions with nucleoside triphosphate analogs. *J Biol Chem* 1987;262:2187–9.

11. St. Clair MH, Richards CA, Spector T *et al.* 3'-azido-3'-deoxythymidine triphosphate as an inhibitor and substrate of purified human immunodeficiency virus reverse transcriptase. *Antimicrob Agents Chemother* 1987;31:1972–7.

12. Heidenreich O, Kruhoffer M, Grosse F, Eckstein F. Inhibition of human immunodeficiency virus 1 reverse transcriptase by 3'-azidothymidine triphosphate. *Eur J Biochem* 1990;192:621–5.

13. Kedar PS, Abbotts J, Kovacs T *et al.* Mechanism of HIV reverse transcriptase: enzyme–primer interaction as revealed through studies of a dNTP analogue, 3'-azido-dTTP. *Biochemistry* 1990;29:3603–11.

14. Reardon JE, Miller WH. Human immunodeficiency virus reverse transcriptase: substrate and inhibitor kinetics with thymidine 5'-triphosphate and 3'-azido-3'-deoxythymidine 5'-triphosphate. *J Biol Chem* 1990;265:20302–7.

15. Parker WB, White EL, Shaddix SC *et al.* Mechanism of inhibition of human immunodeficiency virus type 1 reverse transcriptase and human DNA polymerases α, β and γ by the 5'-triphosphates of Carbovir, 3'-azido-3'-deoxythymidine, 2',3'-dideoxyguanosine, and 3'-deoxythymidine. A novel template for the evaluation of antiretroviral drugs. *J Biol Chem* 1991;266:1754–62.

16. Vrang L, Oberg B. PPi analogs as inhibitors of human T-lymphotropic virus type III reverse transcriptase. *Antimicrob Agents Chemother* 1986;29:867–72.

17. Smith MS, Brian EL, Pagano JS. Resumption of virus production after human immunodeficiency virus infection of T-lymphocytes in the presence of azidothymidine. *J Virol* 1987;61:3769–73.

18. Larder BA, Kemp SD. Multiple mutations in HIV-1 reverse transcriptase confer high-level resistance to zidovudine (AZT). *Science* 1989;246:1155–8.

19. Kellam P, Boucher CA, Larder BA. Fifth mutation in human immunodeficiency virus type 1 reverse transcriptase contributes to the development of high-level resistance to zidovudine. *Proc Natl Acad Sci USA* 1992:89:1934–8.

20. Larder BA, Kellam P, Kemp SD. Zidovudine resistance predicted by direct detection of mutations in DNA from HIV-infected lymphocytes. *AIDS* 1991;5:137–44.

21. Boucher CA, O'Sullivan E, Mulder JW *et al.* Ordered appearance of zidovudine resistance mutations during treatment of 18 human immunodeficiency virus-positive subjects. *J Infect Dis* 1992;165:105–10.

22. Kellam P, Boucher CA, Tijnagel JM, Larder BA. Zidovudine treatment results in the selection of human immunodeficiency virus type 1 variants whose genotypes confer increasing levels of drug resistance. *J Gen Virol* 1994;75:341–51.

23. Larder BA, Coates KE, Kemp SD. Zidovudine-resistant human immunodeficiency virus selected by passage in cell culture. *J Virol* 1991;65:5232–6.

24. Gao Q, Gu ZX, Parniak MA, Li XG, Wainberg MA. *In vitro* selection of variants of human immunodeficiency virus type 1 resistant to 3'-azido-3'-deoxythymidine and 2',3'-dideoxyinosine. *J Virol* 1992;66:12–19.

25. Hooker DJ, Tachedjian G, Solomon AE *et al.* An *in vivo* mutation from leucine to tryptophan at position 210 in human immunodeficiency virus type 1 reverse transcriptase contributes to high-level resistance to 3'-azido-3'-deoxythymidine (AZT). (submitted for publication).

26. Harrigan PR, Kinghorn I, Bloor S *et al.* Significance of amino acid variation at HIV-1 reverse transcriptase residue 210 for 3'-azido-3'deoxythymidine (AZT) susceptibility. *J Virol*, in press.

27. Fitzgibbon JE, Farnham AE, Sperber SJ, Kim H, Dubin DT. Human immunodeficiency virus type 1 *pol* gene mutations in an AIDS patient treated with multiple antiretroviral drugs. *J Virol* 1993;67:7271–5.

28. St Clair MH, Martin JL, Tudor-Williams G *et al.* Resistance to ddI and sensitivity to AZT induced by a mutation in HIV-1 reverse transcriptase. *Science* 1991;253:1557–9.

29. Shafer RW, Kozal MJ, Winters MA *et al.* Combination therapy with zidovudine and didanosine selects for drug-resistant human immunodeficiency virus type 1 strains with unique patterns of *pol* gene mutations. *J Infect Dis* 1994;169:722–9.

30. Kozal MJ, Kroodsma K, Winters MA *et al.* Didanosine resistance in HIV-infected patients switched from zidovudine to didanosine monotherapy. *Ann Intern Med* 1994;121:263–8.

31. Gu Z, Gao Q, Li X, Parniak MA, Wainberg MA. Novel mutation in the human immunodeficiency virus type 1 reverse transcriptase gene that encodes cross-resistance to 2',3'-dideoxyinosine and 2',3'-dideoxycytidine. *J Virol* 1992;66:7128–35.

32. Gu Z, Gao Q, Fang H *et al.* Identification of a mutation at codon 65 in the IKKK motif of reverse transcriptase that encodes human immunodeficiency virus resistance to 2',3'-dideoxycytidine and 2',3'-dideoxy-3'-thiacytidine. *Antimicrob Agents Chemother* 1994;38:275–81.

33. Zhang D, Caliendo AM, Eron JJ *et al.* Resistance to 2',3'-dideoxycytidine conferred by a mutation in codon 65 of the human immunodeficiency virus type 1 reverse transcriptase. *Antimicrob Agents Chemother* 1994;38:282–7.

34. Fitzgibbon JE, Howell RM, Haberzettl CA *et al.* Human immunodeficiency virus type 1 *pol* gene mutations which cause decreased susceptibility to 2',3'-dideoxycytidine. *Antimicrob Agents Chemother* 1992;36:153–7.

35. Lacey SF, Larder BA. Novel mutation (V75T) in human immunodeficiency virus type 1 reverse transcriptase confers resistance to 2',3'-didehydro-2',3'-dideoxythymidine in cell culture. *Antimicrob Agents Chemother* 1994;38:1428–32.

36. Lin PF, Samanta H, Rose RE *et al*. Genotypic and phenotypic analysis of human immunodeficiency virus type 1 isolates from patients on prolonged stavudine therapy. *J Infect Dis* 1994;170:1157–64.

37. Deluge SM, Good SS, Martin MT *et al*. 1592U89 succinate—a novel carbocyclic nucleoside analog with potent, selective anti-HIV activity. Abstracts of the 34th Interscience Conference on Antimicrobial Agents and Chemotherapy, 1994, Orlando, FL, USA, p.7.

38. Tisdale M, Parry NR, Cousens D, St. Clair MH, Boone LR. Anti-HIV activity of (1S,4R)-4-(2-amino-6-cyclopropylamino)-9H-purin-9-yl)-2-cyclopentene-1-methanol (1592U89). Abstracts of the 34th Interscience Conference on Antimicrobial Agents and Chemotherapy, 1994, Orlando, FL, USA, p.92.

39. Boucher CA, Cammack N, Schipper P *et al*. High-level resistance to (-)enantiomeric 2'-deoxy-3'-thiacytidine *in vitro* is due to one amino acid substitution in the catalytic site of human immunodeficiency virus type 1 reverse transcriptase. *Antimicrob Agents Chemother* 1993;37:2231–4.

40. Gao Q, Gu Z, Parniak MA *et al*. The same mutation that encodes low-level human immunodeficiency virus type 1 resistance to 2',3'-dideoxyinosine and 2',3'-dideoxycytidine confers high-level resistance to the (-)enantiomer of 2',3'-dideoxy-3'-thiacytidine. *Antimicrob Agents Chemother* 1993;37:1390–2.

41. Schinazi RF, Lloyd RM Jr, Nguyen MH *et al*. Characterization of human immunodeficiency viruses resistant to oxathiolane-cytosine nucleosides. *Antimicrob Agents Chemother* 1993;37:875–81.

42. Tisdale M, Kemp SD, Parry NR, Larder BA. Rapid *in vitro* selection of human immunodeficiency virus type 1 resistant to 3'-thiacytidine inhibitors due to a mutation in the YMDD region of reverse transcriptase. *Proc Natl Acad Sci USA* 1993;90:5653–6.

43. Kemp SD, Larder BA. *In vitro* studies with 3TC-resistant HIV-1: growth properties and cross-resistance profile. Abstracts of the 3rd International HIV Drug Resistance Workshop, 1994, Kauai, Hawaii, p.33.

44. Schuurman R, Nijhuis M, van Leeuwen R *et al*. Rapid changes in human immunodeficiency virus type 1 (HIV-1) RNA load and appearance of drug-resistant virus populations in persons treated with lamivudine (3TC). *J Infect Dis* 1995;171:1411–19.

45. Larder BA, Purifoy DJM, Powell KL, Darby G. Site-specific mutagenesis of AIDS virus reverse transcriptase. *Nature* 1987;327:716–17.

46. Larder BA, Kemp SD, Purifoy DJM. Infectious potential of human immunodeficiency virus type 1 reverse transcriptase mutants with altered inhibitor sensitivity. *Proc Natl Acad Sci USA* 1989;86:4803–7.

47. Prasad VR, Lowy I, de-los-Santos T, Chiang L, Goff SP. Isolation and characterization of a dideoxyguanosine triphosphate-resistant mutant of human immunodeficiency virus reverse transcriptase. *Proc Natl Acad Sci USA* 1991;88:11363–7.

48. Mellors JW, Bazmi HZ, Schinazi RF *et al*. Novel mutations in reverse transcriptase of human immunodeficiency virus type 1 reduce susceptibility to foscarnet in laboratory and clinical isolates. *Antimicrob Agents Chemother* 1995;39:1087–92.

49. Tachedjian G, Hooker D, Gurusinghe A *et al*. Characterisation of foscarnet-resistant strains of human immunodeficiency virus type 1. *Virology* 1995;212:58–68.

50. Larder BA. 3'-Azido-3'-deoxythymidine resistance suppressed by a mutation

conferring human immunodeficiency virus type 1 resistance to nonnucleoside reverse transcriptase inhibitors. *Antimicrob Agents Chemother* 1992;36:2664–9.

51. Richman DD, Havlir D, Corbeil J *et al.* Nevirapine resistance mutations of human immunodeficiency virus type 1 selected during therapy. *J Virol* 1994;68:1660–6.
52. Chow YK, Hirsch MS, Merrill DP *et al.* Use of evolutionary limitations of HIV-1 multidrug resistance to optimize therapy. *Nature* 1993;361:650–4.
53. Chow YK, Hirsch MS, Kaplan JC, D'Aquila RT. HIV-1 error revealed. *Nature* 1993;364:679.
54. Larder BA, Kellam P, Kemp SD. Convergent combination therapy can select viable multidrug-resistant HIV-1 *in vitro. Nature* 1993;365:451–3.
55. Emini EA, Graham DJ, Gotlib L *et al.* HIV and multidrug resistance. *Nature* 1993;364:679.
56. Harrigan PR, Bloor S, Kinghorn I, the Lamivudine European HIV Working Group, Larder BA. Virological response to AZT/3TC combination therapy in AZT experienced patients (trial NUCB3002). Abstracts of the 4th International HIV Drug Resistance Workshop, 1995, Sardinia, Italy, p.54.
57. Johnson VA, Wagner SF, Overbay CB *et al.* Drug resistance and viral load in NUCA3002: a comparative trial of lamivudine (3TC) (high or low dose)/zidovudine (ZDV) combination therapy vs. ZDV/dideoxycytidine (ddC) combination therapy in ZDV-experienced ($\geq$24 weeks) patients (CD4 cells 100–300/mm^3). Abstracts of the 4th International HIV Drug Resistance Workshop, 1995, Sardinia, Italy, p.55.
58. Goulden MG, Cammack N, Hopewell PL, Penn CR, Cameron JM. Selection *in vitro* of an HIV-1 variant resistant to both 3TC and AZT. *AIDS* (in press).
59. Kemp SD, Kohli A, Larder BA. Genotypic characterisation of an HIV-1 mutant co-resistant to AZT and 3TC. Abstracts of the 4th International HIV Drug Resistance Workshop, 1995, Sardinia, Italy, p.51.
60. Shirasaka T, Kavlick MF, Ueno T *et al.* Emergence of human immunodeficiency virus type 1 variants with resistance to multiple dideoxynucleosides in patients receiving therapy with dideoxynucleosides. *Proc Natl Acad Sci USA* 1995;92:2398–402.
61. Iversen AKN, Wehrly K, Shafer RW *et al.* Multidrug-resistant or partially replication incompetent HIV resulting from combination antiviral therapy. Abstracts of the 2nd National Conference on Human Retroviruses, 1995, Washington, USA, p.138.
62. Lacey SF, Reardon JE, Furfine ES *et al.* Biochemical studies on the reverse transcriptase and RNase H activities from human immunodeficiency virus strains resistant to 3'-azido-3'-deoxythymidine. *J Biol Chem* 1992;267:15789–94.
63. Martin JL, Wilson JE, Haynes RL, Furman PA. Mechanism of resistance of human immunodeficiency virus type 1 to 2',3'-dideoxyinosine. *Proc Natl Acad Sci USA* 1993;90:6135–9.
64. Gu Z, Arts EJ, Parniak MA, Wainberg MA. Mutated K65R recombinant reverse transcriptase of human immunodeficiency virus type 1 shows diminished chain termination in the presence of 2',3'-dideoxycytidine 5'-triphosphate and other drugs. *Proc Natl Acad Sci USA* 1995;92:2760–4.
65. Kohlstaedt LA, Wang J, Friedman JM, Rice PA, Steitz TA. Crystal structure at 3.5 Å resolution of HIV-1 reverse transcriptase complexed with an inhibitor. *Science* 1992;256:1783–90.
66. Jacobo-Molina A, Clark AD Jr, Williams RL *et al.* Crystals of a ternary complex of human immunodeficiency virus type 1 reverse transcriptase with

a monoclonal antibody Fab fragment and double-stranded DNA diffract X-rays to 3.5-Å resolution. *Proc Natl Acad Sci USA* 1991;88:10895–9.

67. Jacobo-Molina A, Ding J, Nanni RG *et al.* Crystal structure of human immunodeficiency virus type 1 reverse transcriptase complexed with double-stranded DNA at 3.0 Å resolution shows bent DNA. *Proc Natl Acad Sci USA* 1993;90:6320–4.

68. Tantillo C, Ding J, Jacobo-Molina A *et al.* Locations of anti-AIDS drug binding sites and resistance mutations in the three-dimensional structure of HIV-1 reverse transcriptase. Implications for mechanisms of drug inhibition and resistance. *J Mol Biol* 1994;243:369–87.

69. Ren J, Esnouf R, Garman E *et al.* High resolution structures of HIV-1 RT from four RT-inhibitor complexes. *Nature Struct Biol* 1995;2:293–302.

70. Esnouf R, Ren J, Ross C *et al.* Mechanism of inhibition of HIV-1 reverse transcriptase by non-nucleoside inhibitors. *Nature Struct Biol* 1995;2:303–8.

71. Boyer PL, Tantillo C, Jacobo-Molina A *et al.* Sensitivity of wild-type human immunodeficiency virus type 1 reverse transcriptase to dideoxynucleotides depends on template length; the sensitivity of drug-resistant mutants does not. *Proc Natl Acad Sci USA* 1994;91:4882–6.

10

Nucleosides and Foscarnet—Clinical Aspects

RICHARD T. D'AQUILA

INTRODUCTION

Replication of drug-resistant HIV-1 during antiretroviral therapy has been hypothesized to cause treatment failure because the dynamism of HIV-1 replication within infected individuals has been linked to CD4+ T-lymphocyte turnover and the pathogenetic spiral to fatal immune system collapse[1-3]. Studies of nucleosides and foscarnet relevant to this hypothesis are reviewed in this chapter. These agents are considered together because nucleosides and foscarnet have similar mechanisms of inhibition of the HIV-1 reverse transcriptase (RT). Nucleosides, including zidovudine (ZDV), didanosine (ddI), zalcitabine (ddC), stavudine (d4T) and lamivudine (3TC) require intracellular phosphorylation to the active nucleotide triphosphate inhibitor. Cellular mechanisms for nucleoside resistance therefore also may be relevant to understanding drug failure, but remain less well defined and will not be detailed in this chapter. In contrast, foscarnet is a pyrophosphate analog and does not require intracellular activation. The genetic and biochemical mechanisms of HIV-1 resistance to these agents are described by Larder in Chapter 9. Following a summary of laboratory methods for identifying HIV-1 isolates which are resistant to RT inhibitors, the biologic effects of these viruses and their impact on the virologic and clinical aspects of HIV-1 disease and its therapy will be described. The available data indicate that resistance to some of these agents accounts for at least some of the loss of their antiviral effect. However, drug resistance is not the only factor determining pathogenesis, and its contribution may differ for each of these agents.

Antiviral Drug Resistance. Edited by Douglas D. Richman © 1996 John Wiley & Sons Ltd

LABORATORY MONITORING FOR VIRUSES RESISTANT TO NUCLEOSIDES OR FOSCARNET

Susceptibility of HIV-1 to RT inhibitors can theoretically be quantified based on laboratory assays of the phenotype of either virus replication or RT enzyme activity. If all mutations that confer resistance to these drugs were known and all possible interactive effects of the different mutations catalogued, characterization of viral genotype at all relevant positions would theoretically also suffice to characterize the nature and magnitude of resistance phenotype. In practice, complexities of virus and RT biology mean that these different methods are complementary.

Phenotypic assays

Based on virus replication in cell culture

Assaying the susceptibility of HIV-1 isolates to drugs permits assessment of the interactive effects of different resistance mutations on ZDV resistance[4] (see also Chapter 9) and of the overall phenotype of the diverse assortment of viral genetic variants that comprises an isolate. ZDV susceptibility phenotyping is restricted to assays based on virus replication because such resistance cannot currently be completely assessed using cell-free assays of RT enzymatic activity. ZDV-selected RT T215Y and K219E in RT p66, which cause only a minimal degree of virus ZDV resistance, do decrease binding of ZDV triphosphate (ZDV-TP) to the RT in studies of recombinant-expressed enzymes[5,6]. Multiply mutant viruses, including RT D67N, K70R, T215Y and K219Q, have high-level resistance to ZDV defined as more than a 100-fold increase in 50% inhibitory concentration (IC_{50}) of ZDV for viral replication in cell culture. However, the RTs from such viruses have only a minimal difference from wild-type enzyme in AZT-TP inhibition in cell-free assays of recombinant-expressed enzymes[5-7]. Thus, measurement of the ZDV susceptibility phenotype of virus replication is currently the preferred method for the assessment of ZDV resistance, despite the need for cumbersome assays.

In contrast to the simplicity of plaque-reduction assays for many lytic viruses that grow in adherent cells in culture, quantification of the amount of HIV-1 replicating at different drug concentrations is more difficult because its host cells only grow in suspension and may not show detectable cytopathic effects. A plaque reduction-like assay was developed for HIV-1 using certain HeLa cell lines which grow in an adherent monolayer and express the cell-surface CD4 molecule, the receptor for HIV-1 virion gp120[8-10]. Within a few days after infection expression of HIV-1 proteins, including gp120, leads to fusion of the initially infected CD4+ HeLa cell with neighboring cells. These foci of HIV-1-infected multinucleated giant cells, loosely called 'plaques' even though the cells are not lysed, can be visualized microscopically in different ways[8,10,11]. IC_{50} can be determined from plots of percentage reduction in the number of foci of multinucleated giant cells versus drug concentration. This assay is relatively inexpensive, rapid and reproducible. It was used to great advantage in the first published studies that described ZDV resistance[9]. However, a large proportion of clinical isolates do not yield visible foci of multinucleated giant cells in CD4+ HeLa cell cultures, limiting evaluation to only a subset of patient isolates and raising concern that epidemiologic conclusions may be affected by a selection bias for only those viruses which can 'plaque'.

This problem can be circumvented by employing phytohemagglutinin (PHA)-stimulated peripheral blood mononuclear cells (PBMC) as the host for characterization of drug susceptibility in cell culture. HIV-1 can be isolated from nearly all patients using such cells[12,13]. Measurements of virus replication in such primary cells have included quantification of HIV-1 core (p24) antigen[14-18] or RT enzyme activity[19,20] in culture supernatant fluid, as well as quantification of the amount of HIV-1 RNA[21] or DNA[22] in the infected cells. A standardized method for ZDV susceptibility testing of clinical HIV-1 isolates has been validated and gained fairly widespread acceptance[17]. The IC_{50}s for clinical isolates from patients who have never received ZDV were <0.16 μM ZDV and, as in the CD4+ HeLa cell assay, the most highly ZDV-resistant multiply mutant isolates have IC_{50}s > 1 μM ZDV. This is a wide enough range of IC_{50}s to reliably discriminate among isolates and minimize concern that assay variability will confound results. Cordblood lymphocytes have been reported to perform similarly to PBMC in such assays[23].

There are some limitations to such assays on primary cells, however. Under optimum conditions it requires a lengthy process which makes timely characterization nearly impossible: initial isolation of a virus (two to three weeks), infectivity titration of the isolate (one week), and then susceptibility testing itself (one week). If modified to serve as a qualitative screening assay for high-level ZDV resistance, rather than an accurate determination of an IC_{50}, the assay can be done more rapidly. There have been concerns that the drug susceptibility phenotype of an isolate may be modified by either initial culture or repeated passage in PBMCs before susceptibility testing is undertaken[15,24].

This methodology has only been standardized for ZDV susceptibility testing, but data have also been published which indicate that it performs relatively well for testing the susceptibility of clinical isolates to a number of other agents, including the other nucleoside analogs and foscarnet[25-29]. One study using the ACTG/DoD PBMC-based assay to test genetically uncharacterized clinical isolates from ZDV-experienced patients who denied using other nucleosides found about a twofold increase in ddI and ddC IC_{50}s for every 10-fold increase in AZT IC_{50}[25]. The correlation between ZDV and dideoxynucleoside IC_{50}s of isolates from ZDV-experienced patients may be less apparent with other methodologies[22]. Two alternative explanations seem possible, given that the characterized ZDV resistance mutations do not confer dideoxynucleoside cross-resistance[10]: ZDV therapy may select for as yet unidentified RT mutations which confer dideoxynucleoside cross-resistance, or some isolates may have growth characteristics *in vitro* attributable to genetic changes in genes other than the RT, which result in a decrease in dideoxynucleoside susceptibility in the ACTG/DoD PBMC-based assay. Some recent data support the latter possibility[26].

Genetically characterized mutants resistant to ddI, ddC, d4T and foscarnet have only a slightly higher IC_{50} (two to 10 times higher) than wild-type susceptible virus in a number of different phenotypic assays[6,19,22,27,30-35]. The higher magnitude of resistance observed for the inhibitors with non-physiologic sugars (ZDV and 3TC) suggests that their triphosphate derivatives can be more readily differentiated by the viral enzyme from physiologic nucleotide triphosphates than can those of the inhibitors with more physiologic sugar residues (ddI, ddC, d4T).

A different approach to phenotypic testing avoids any potential for culture to introduce biased sampling, and can evaluate all molecular species present *in vivo*, including those which are replication-incompetent. Such methods involve the regeneration of an infectious virus by recombination of RT polymerase chain reaction (PCR) products into an HIV-1 DNA plasmid clone with a deleted RT coding region[36]. The recombinant virus produced by co-transfection of these DNAs into a T-cell line can then undergo rapid susceptibility testing in the CD4+ HeLa cell assay.

Direct cultivation of HIV-1 from a patient sample in the presence of the drug of interest has been attempted to speed identification of resistant isolates[37,38]. There are, however, a number of potential technical problems that may lead to the mischaracterization of a susceptible virus as resistant in such assays. A patient sample with a higher inoculum will replicate better, and appear more resistant, than a sample with a lower inoculum, even if the viruses have identical IC_{50}s in the more standardized multistep assay systems described above. Attempts to control this by simultaneous titration and drug testing of multiple dilutions of each patient sample have been presented[38], but this approach has not been validated by a rigorous comparison to a more standardized assay.

Based on RT enzymatic activity

Resistance to ddI, ddC, 3TC and foscarnet differs from that to ZDV: there is a parallel between enzyme-based and virus replication-based measurements of resistance to each of the drugs other than ZDV[5,6,34,39–41]. Assays of polymerase enzymatic activity in the presence of the nucleotide triphosphates of these inhibitors can involve the use of native virion RT in solution, generally following polyethylene glycol precipitation to concentrate virions from a clinical isolate. Either incorporation of a radiolabeled deoxynucleotide triphosphate (dNTP) into an extending primer or methodologies that do not involve radioactivity[6,34] can be used. PCR can also be used to construct molecular clones of recombinant HIV-1 RT DNA in expression vectors, which can be assayed either in solution or by *in situ* RT assays[42]. With *in situ* RT assays, bacterial colonies containing recombinant-expression plasmids are transferred to a membrane filter and the expressed RTs are renatured on the membrane to test for incorporation of dNTPs in the presence of the inhibitor. Such enzyme activity assays do not necessitate virus isolation in cell culture and can theoretically be performed from virtually all patient samples. The *in situ* assays also allow assessment of the proportion of a viral population which has a functional, enzymatically active RT.

RT enzymatic activity, and perhaps its resistance to ZDV-TP, ddCTP and other inhibitors, may be able to be assessed by the ability of the HIV-1 RT to complement the growth of certain polymerase-mutant *Escherichia coli* strains[43,44]. The HIV-1 RT can substitute for *E. coli* DNA polymerase I function, enabling an *E. coli* mutant with a temperature-sensitive phenotype due to mutations in two *E. coli* genes (*polA* and *recA*) to grow at the non-permissive temperature. ZDV was able to inhibit growth of bacteria expressing a wild-type HIV-1 RT at a non-permissive temperature, but did not inhibit growth of bacteria expressing a T215Y mutant HIV-1 RT[43]. If such work can be confirmed and extended, this may prove to be a relatively simple and rapid methodology for evaluating susceptibility to ZDV and perhaps other HIV-1 RT inhibitors.

Genotypic assays

DNA sequencing is the current 'gold standard' for determining the genotype relevant to HIV-1 inhibitor resistance[45,46]. Advances in PCR amplification of RT gene sequences from clinical samples and in systems for non-radioactive electrophoretic detection of sequence, automated base calling, sequence analysis and data storage (i.e. automated sequencers) have begun to allow commercial availability of this service, as well as expanded capacity for research laboratories. However, sequencing remains relatively expensive and laborious. It is not practical to use it to monitor for resistance mutations longitudinally in all patients undergoing therapy. With continuing technical advances, however, it may become more practical and reproducible to detect multiple specific point mutations than small changes in virus or RT susceptibility phenotype for agents such as ddI, ddC, d4T and foscarnet.

More rapid assays to detect specific point mutations have also been developed, notably selective PCR assays[47-49] which have been widely used by many investigators[31-33,50-54]. They are based on the requirement that the 3' terminal base in an amplification primer must be matched to its template in order to prime synthesis efficiently and yield a PCR product of a specific size. The use of two different amplification primer pairs, with either a wild-type or a mutant base at the 3' terminus of one of the primers, allows for scoring of a sample as either wild-type, mutant or mixed. Because of the extreme sensitivity of PCR, the assay cannot reliably quantify proportions of wild-type and mutant genomes if a mixture is seen. It is important to maintain specificity of amplification as a stringent control in such assays: at high enough input template copy numbers some PCR product may be generated from a mismatched primer. The ZDV resistance T215Y or F substitutions each require two adjacent base pair changes, which allows the use of primers with both the penultimate and terminal bases matched to either wild-type or mutant sequence. This helps maintain sequence specificity for detection of these particular mutations in codon 215, although this approach has also been successfully applied to specific detection of many single base point mutations.

A different rapid assay, called the point mutation assay, allows quantification of the proportion of each of the four different bases at a particular position in the viral RT coding sequence by allowing each of the four possible radioactively-labeled chain-terminating dideoxynucleotide triphosphates to be added on to the 3' end of a primer annealed to an amplification product template just 5' to the base being interrogated[55]. This has allowed study of the evolution of resistance mutations at a number of specific positions in RT during different therapies[56-58].

Other techniques have also been used to rapidly assess RT genotype. ZDV resistance mutations have been detected by oligonucleotide-specific hybridization of DNA amplified from RT genes[24,59,60]. The mutant versus wild-type sequence at codon 215 has been identified using RNase A digestion patterns[61]. The ddI-resistance conferring L74V has been detected semi-quantitatively using a novel assay relying on ligation of two pairs of matched oligonucleotides (either wild type or mutant at the 3' end of one of the oligonucleotides) annealed to a PCR-amplified template[62]. All the rapid genotyping assays, including the selective PCR and point mutation assays, tend to lose any practical advantage over DNA sequencing if many different mutation sites must be assessed, as is necessary for comprehensive evaluation of viruses from patients receiving either sequential monotherapies or simultaneous combination therapy.

There are a number of techniques under development to speed and simplify DNA sequencing. This seems necessary for comprehensive evaluation of viral selection during sequential monotherapies and combination therapies. One of the most promising new methods involves sequencing by hybridization to an array of thousands of different oligonucleotides immobilized on small silica chips[63]. It is being developed for 'resequencing' of patient-derived HIV-1 polymerase amplicons, including both protease and RT coding regions.

If methods for HIV-1 phenotyping and genotyping become more practical for routine use in clinical virology laboratories, assessment of both phenotype and genotype may be optimal in the future as sequential and combination therapies become more common. Non-nucleoside RT inhibitor-, ddI- and 3TC-selected mutations can suppress effects of at least some ZDV resistance mutations[4,6,19,64,65]. Such a resistance-suppressing interactive effect of a resistance mutation not previously known to cause this effect can only be seen using phenotypic assays. However, only genotypic assays provide information about what pre-existing genotypes might have the potential to rapidly dominate the virus population when a new therapy is started.

Should circulating cells or plasma be assayed?

A selective PCR assay detected the codon 215 mutation in cell-free serum virions (following *in vitro* reverse transcription) as early as two months after starting therapy, and months before it was identified in PBMC DNA[51,56]. (The initial report identifying the codon 215 mutation in plasma RNA before it was detectable in PBMC DNA may have been flawed by use of a primer for reverse transcription which was the same sense as the RNA template and must have hybridized non-specifically in order to yield product[51]. However, this methodologic problem has been addressed[66,67] and the results have also been independently confirmed[56].) Other evidence suggests that different ZDV resistance genotypes[3,68] and envelope genotypic variants[69] are present in plasma HIV-1 RNA compared to PBMC HIV-1 DNA. The HIV-1 DNA sequences found in circulating PBMC from infected patients are those that were present in plasma virus populations at an earlier point in time[69,70]. Most of the replication of HIV-1 occurs in lymph nodes, particularly during the earlier stages of the disease[71,72]. There is recent evidence that a decrease in plasma HIV-1 RNA levels during antiretroviral therapy indeed reflects down regulation of replication in lymph nodes[73]. The current working hypothesis is that a drug-resistant mutant emerges first in virus replicating in lymphoid tissue, and it can also be found in plasma virus RNA or infectious HIV-1 which can be isolated from PBMC circulating at that time. However, the dominant circulating virus at that time may only be detectable in HIV-1 DNA sequences in PBMC at a later time, perhaps one to eight months later.

CLINICAL SIGNIFICANCE OF VIRUSES RESISTANT TO NUCLEOSIDES OR FOSCARNET

The question of whether resistance causes therapeutic failure must be broken down into a number of separate questions, in order to attempt to explicate HIV-1 pathogenesis. It is instructive to consider recent lessons about how drug-resistant viruses are selected from the pre-existing population of replicating HIV-1 before dividing the discussion of the clinical significance of viruses resistant to nucleosides or foscarnet into whether they are transmissible, associated with increased virus load *in vivo*, predictive of more rapid disease progression during therapy, or a potential laboratory marker useful for clinical management. A number of different factors can independently contribute to failure of HIV-1 therapy. Patients clearly progress with drug-susceptible virus whether they receive antiretroviral therapy or not. Insufficient inhibition of virus replication, syncytium-inducing virus phenotype, other viral factors and host immunologic factors may all contribute to increasing virus load during treatment and accelerating progression of immunodeficiency, singly or in combination with each other or with drug resistance. Moreover, the earliest studies of ZDV resistance established a fact confirmed by subsequent work: that some clinically stable patients may harbor ZDV-resistant virus.

HIV-1 population dynamics *in vivo* and in cell culture

The emergence of drug-resistant HIV-1 during therapy *in vivo* indicates that the drug in question suppressed replication of some of the genetic variants in the complex HIV-1 population present *in vivo* (i.e. it exerted a selective pressure)[74] and that viruses that were more 'fit' in the presence of the drug continued to replicate. The latter fact becomes more understandable in light of the less than two-day half-life for free plasma HIV-1 virions, indicating that at least 30% of the enormous pool of HIV-1 in plasma ($>10^{10}$ virions) is replaced every day[2,3,58]. The degree of inhibition of HIV-1 replication achieved *in vivo* to date may be many orders of magnitude less than needed to stop all ongoing HIV-1 replication.

It is much easier to block the spread of a relatively small number of infectious viruses in PBMC cultures using some combinations of RT inhibitors[75-77] than it is to limit spread in a human harboring orders of magnitude more HIV-1. Control cultures where virus replication resumed following a period of suppression have taught us a valuable lesson: in at least some cases, prevention of the development of resistance is not the mechanism for the better effectiveness of some regimens, compared to others, in cell culture[77]. The viruses which 'break through' drug inhibition in cultures treated with simultaneous regimens of three or four drugs are not resistant to all the drugs[77]; this was a confirmation of an earlier observation in cell cultures treated with ZDV monotherapy[78]. The mechanism of prevention of spread in cell culture probably involves achieving a magnitude of antiviral inhibition that is greater than the rate of increase in progeny viruses[77]. Incomplete inhibition of replication is a more likely explanation for virus 'breakthrough' in such cell culture systems than is drug resistance.

However, drug-resistant virus can be selected under some cell culture conditions, depending on the level of genetic diversity in the virus population used as initial inoculum in the *in vitro* experiment. The major reason why some resistant viruses have only been noted *in vivo* and have been harder to select for *in vitro* probably relates to the fact that the size of the replicating virus population in any cell culture experiment is many orders of magnitude smaller than that in the infected person. If the steady-state frequency of a pre-existing mutant resistant to the given drug is lower than the amount of diversity in the cell culture inoculum, a degree of drug inhibition that allows ongoing replication and generation of diversity in the infected culture over many replication cycles may be necessary to select a drug-resistant mutant. The frequency of the mutant, relative to the wild type, in any HIV-1 population prior to drug pressure has been hypothesized to depend on the degree to which mutant virus replicates less well than wild-type virus in the absence of the drug[1]. Indeed, wild-type genomes generally predominate in the HIV-1 populations in infected individuals, and mutations in the RT that confer resistance to ZDV, ddC, 3TC, d4T and other RT inhibitors have only been identified at a low frequency in untreated individuals[79,80]. This supports the concept that therapy selectively amplifies pre-existing, drug-resistant variants of HIV-1 from the diverse virus population *in vivo*.

Transmissibility of drug-resistant viruses

ZDV-resistant HIV-1 has been isolated from semen and vaginal washings of ZDV-treated individuals[81], as well as blood. However, it might be questioned whether ZDV-resistant HIV-1 replicates well enough to be transmissible *in vivo*, given that drug-resistant HIV-1 may be present at a low frequency in infected individuals without dominating the population in the absence of drug selection pressure. Person-to-person transmission of ZDV-resistant virus has now been documented by inoculation parenterally[82,83], via sexual intercourse[38,84–87], and to a fetus from an infected mother who had treatment with ZDV for a prolonged period prior to her pregnancy[88]. There are shortcomings in some of these reports. The drug susceptibility phenotyping methodology in one can be criticized[38]. Some reports did not characterize the virus present in the donor to confirm that the mutant indeed originated in the donor's viral population[82,84], but others confirmed the relatedness of viruses from the donor and recipient by sequencing[83,85–87]. In one case, the route of transmission was not proved, although it appeared likely to involve unrecognized, probably percutaneous, exposure of the recipient to the donor's blood[83]. Taken as a whole, these data establish that transmission of ZDV-resistant HIV-1 occurs, although further investigation is needed to evaluate if wild-type HIV-1, rather than a ZDV-resistant mutant, may be preferentially transmitted from a mixed population[86]. In any case, preliminary data suggest that the prevalence of ZDV-resistant codon 215 mutant HIV-1 as the initially infecting virus is increasing among adults who are recent seroconverters[89].

It has not yet been conclusively documented that initial infection with a ZDV-resistant mutant is associated with a different rate of virologic, immunologic or clinical progression, compared to initial infection with wild-type HIV-1. In cell culture a wild-type virus may often be selected following passage of a genetically heterogeneous ZDV-resistant clinical isolate in the absence of drug[15,79], probably owing to preferential outgrowth of a minority wild-type species rather than genetic reversion[79]. In two recipients of ZDV-resistant viruses via sexual intercourse, however, ZDV-resistant mutants persisted and the patients' CD4 cell counts were low for early disease[84,85]. Only one of these two patients received ZDV treatment for a prolonged illness associated with seroconversion[84]. Other preliminary data suggest that the ZDV-resistance substitution at codon 215 may not persist following seroconversion with a codon 215 mutant[87,90]. Long-term prospective studies of newly infected patients are needed to compare the persistence of ZDV-resistant virus and the relative disease progression rates of patients harboring either wild-type or ZDV-resistant viruses in the presence and absence of therapy.

There are no published data confirming person-to-person transmission of HIV-1 resistant to any other drug. There seems to be no reason why viruses resistant to other nucleosides or foscarnet should differ in this regard from ZDV-resistant viruses.

Associations between resistance and escape from suppression of HIV-1 replication

Zidovudine monotherapy

Until recently it had been difficult to demonstrate an association between the emergence of a ZDV-resistant virus and escape from suppression of HIV-1 replication during ZDV monotherapy, unlike the experience with non-nucleoside RT inhibitor (NNRTI)-resistant virus. Individual patients treated with NNRTIs had increases in plasma RNA levels within days to weeks after starting therapy, at the same time as highly NNRTI-resistant virus with single point mutations could be detected[91,92]; this temporal correlation was apparent in virtually every patient studied. In contrast, ZDV-resistant viruses are selected more slowly as mutants in up to five or six different codons of the RT progressively accumulate as the dominant viruses in the population in a fairly ordered sequence; the codon 215 mutations are selected relatively early in this process[93]. The K70R mutation often appears transiently and is quickly followed by codon 215. The codon 70 mutation may confer some disadvantage until other compensating mutations are added; K70R can often be found later linked to other mutations as M41L and D67N are added to T215Y or F[93]. Highly ZDV-resistant isolates with multiple mutations and ⩾100-fold increases in ZDV IC_{50}, relative to fully wild-type virus, are identified only after many months to years of therapy, and only in some patients[94,95]. In the initial characterization of highly resistant isolates from ZDV-treated patients, increases in p24 antigenemia levels were not temporally associated with the emergence of highly resistant isolates[9]. It has been speculated that p24 antigenemia is a poor measure of circulating virus load, and that any changes in virus load may be gradual over the long process of selection.

One study found that patients treated with zidovudine for two years or more who had the codon 215 RT mutation detected by selective PCR in their PBMC had a ninefold higher amount of HIV-1 DNA in their PBMC, as detected by quantitative PCR, than did those with a wild-type codon 215[51]. Others have also reported increased virus load associated with the presence of the codon 215 mutations[53]. Codon 215 mutant isolates can have a wide range of ZDV IC_{50}s, however, depending on whether other mutations are also present[10,54]. Another study of advanced patients who had received prolonged ZDV therapy also found that patients with codon 215 mutant HIV-1 isolated from patient PBMC had a higher level of plasma HIV-1 RNA than those with codon 215 wild-type isolates[96]. High-level phenotypic resistance to ZDV ($IC_{50} ⩾ 1$ μM ZDV) did not correlate with higher plasma RNA levels in that same group of patients, however[96].

Studies examining serum HIV-1 RNA levels at frequent time points starting soon after initiation of ZDV therapy have begun to illuminate this issue[56,97]. The most marked antiviral effect of ZDV, in terms of suppression of circulating cell-free HIV-1 RNA, may last only a few weeks in some patients (phase 1 in Figure 10.1), and the rapid partial increase in serum virus RNA level toward its pretherapy baseline seen in many of the patients in this study (phase 2 in Figure 10.1) was due to resurgence of predominantly ZDV-susceptible wild-type virus. In two patients in one study, the virus populations in serum did not have any detectable drug resistance mutations, and in five other patients' sera the proportion of resistant mutant virus genotypes was insufficient to account for the observed increase in serum HIV-1 RNA[56]. Another group has also presented preliminary data suggesting that the increase in plasma RNA levels during the first three months after starting ZDV

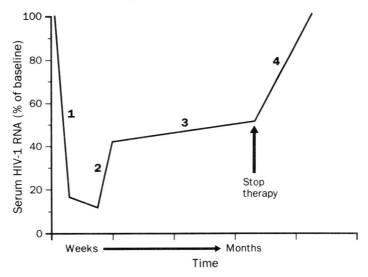

Figure 10.1 *Phases of patients' virologic responses to zidovudine (ZDV). Phase 1: early prompt fall in circulating HIV-1 RNA load over days to a few weeks. Phase 2: a prompt return toward baseline (which does not reach the pretreatment level) over several weeks. This is not completely explained by the appearance of known ZDV resistance mutations and appears to be due, at least in part, to increased replication of wild-type ZDV-susceptible virus. Phase 3: a prolonged period of many months where circulating virus load continues to return toward baseline, although much more slowly than during phase 2. The gradual increase in virus load appears to correlate with an increasing proportion of the virus population containing a progressive accumulation of multiple mutations conferring increasing ZDV resistance. Phase 4: in some patients who stopped antiretroviral therapy, continuing suppression by ZDV became apparent because of the rebound to baseline level of virus load seen after ZDV withdrawal. Adapted from reference 56 with permission*

therapy was independent of detection of resistance mutations in plasma RNA[97]. This differs from the early escape from NNRTI inhibition, which can apparently be entirely explained by increasing amounts of resistant mutant virus RNA in the plasma[91,92]. The mechanism that allows resurgent wild-type virus replication *in vivo* within weeks after starting ZDV therapy is still undefined. Mathematical modeling suggests that the increase in host CD4+ cells drives increased virus replication; such 'predator–prey' models suggest that virus RNA rebounds because of the greater availability of the 'prey' CD4+ host cells[97,98]. Changes in cellular enzymes that phosphorylate ZDV have also been hypothesized as a possible explanation for the early rebound[56].

Most patients have a gradual return of serum RNA toward pretreatment levels over months, in temporal association with an increasing proportion of serum HIV-1 RNA containing ZDV resistance mutations (phase 3 in Figure 10.1). In one study the return toward pretherapy baseline levels of plasma HIV-1 RNA between three and six months after starting therapy was associated with outgrowth of K70R, singly mutant virus variants and selection for additional mutations causing increasing levels of ZDV resistance continued after the six-month time point[97]. In five of six patients who stopped ZDV therapy in another study there was a further rebound increase of virus load toward baseline, suggesting at least some continuing suppression of resistant virus by ZDV (phase 4 in Figure 10.1). In summary, these data suggest that ZDV resistance may not be the only factor causing viral escape from ZDV inhibition *in vivo* (phase 2 in Figure 10.1), that some suppression of virus replication by ZDV is gradually lost owing to ZDV resistance as resistance mutations accumulate (phase 3 in Figure 10.1), and that ZDV may continue to partially suppress replication of at least some ZDV-resistant viruses (phase 4 in Figure 10.1).

Other monotherapies

Didanosine-resistant clinical isolates have also been identified after months of ddI therapy in patients who switched from ZDV to ddI monotherapy, and in patients who started therapy with ddI[6,16,18,19,99]. In the absence of the ZDV-resistance mutation in codon 41, development of the L74V ddI-resistance mutation suppressed the phenotypic effects of other pre-existing ZDV resistance mutations[6,19,65]; this would be expected to be relevant to mutant selection during combination therapy with ZDV and ddI in the subset of patients lacking the codon 41 ZDV-resistance mutation. A different interactive effect of ZDV and ddI-resistance mutations is relevant to ddI monotherapy: the presence of some ZDV-resistance mutations in the same genome with the codon 74 ddI-resistance mutation conferred a greater degree of ddI resistance than did the codon 74 mutation alone[6]. Indeed, isolates with mutations in both codons 74 and 215 have been detected commonly in patients switched from ZDV to ddI monotherapy, consistent with the hypothesized selective advantage of that combination in that situation[66,100]. Patients with circulating cell-free ddI-resistant mutant virions have a slightly statistically significantly greater circulating HIV-1 RNA burden after months of ddI monotherapy than patients with circulating virions that remained wild type at codon 74[66]. It is important to recall that ddI IC_{50} of an L74V mutant virus is increased only ≤10-fold, compared to wild type.

Although V75T HIV-1 with about a fivefold decrease in susceptibility to d4T has been selected by *in vitro* passage[35], phenotypic analyses identified only two of 13 patients treated for 18–22 months with isolates having similar low levels of d4T resistance in a PBMC-based assay[26]. A mutation in the RT could not be implicated in causing d4T resistance in these isolates, however; the codon 75 mutation was not observed[26]. A pair of chimeric viruses constructed by inserting RT sequences from isolates with different d4T susceptibilities into a standard laboratory HIV-1 strain genetic background did not have substantially different IC_{50}s for d4T, suggesting that growth differences attributable to other HIV-1 genes may have accounted for the isolates' different susceptibilities to d4T in the PBMC-based assay[26]. Correlations between d4T resistance and virus load *in vivo* have not been presented. Studies of the impact of ddC or foscarnet resistance on plasma virus load have not been reported either.

Codon 184 mutant viruses which have a 500- to 1000-fold increased 3TC IC_{50} emerge in every patient studied during 3TC monotherapy[101]. This selection occurs more rapidly *in vivo* than does selection for either ZDV- or ddI-resistant viruses during monotherapy. Selection for 3TC-resistant mutants is at a similar pace to selection of NNRTI-resistant viruses. An initial isoleucine (ATA) mutant is favored over the wild-type methionine (ATG) at codon 184, but this is followed rapidly by emergence of valine (GTG) mutants; the latter completely dominate the circulating population within 12 weeks[101]. The isoleucine (ATA) genotype may occur more frequently in pre-existing virus populations, perhaps because of the HIV-1 RT's preference for G-to-A transitions. The eventual outgrowth of the valine (GTG) genotype could be consistent with relative differences between the two mutants in level of 3TC resistance, viral replicative fitness and/or host immune control. The initial rapid decline in circulating virus load due to 3TC inhibition of wild-type virus was rapidly reversed, and in some patients the resurgence could be completely explained by increasing amounts of the drug-resistant mutant RNA[101]. However, sustained suppression of plasma

RNA below the pre-therapy baseline was seen in some patients despite evolution of a 100% mutant codon 184 (valine) population. Median plasma RNA levels for this and other groups of patients treated with the highest doses of 3TC monotherapy in phase I/II trials remained below baseline over a few months[101-103]. Although data remain limited, they do not suggest that a gradual return toward baseline circulating virus load may be associated with increasing 3TC resistance, such as occurs during ZDV monotherapy (phase 3 in Figure 10.1). It is clear that high-level 3TC resistance is not invariably associated with complete loss of inhibition of mutant virus replication[101]. This suggests the hypothesis that codon 184 mutant, 3TC-resistant virus replication is impaired by the M184V substitution in RT which may compromise virus fitness[39,104-106], still inhibited by 3TC, or better controlled by the immune system than wild-type virus. In conjunction with the circulating virus load response pattern during ZDV therapy (Figure 10.1), these data on 3TC resistance suggest the general hypothesis that high-level HIV-1 nucleoside resistance indicates at least partial, but not necessarily complete, escape from antiviral suppression.

Combination regimens

A temporal correlation between the development of co-resistance to all agents in any combination regimen and escape from inhibition of virus replication has not yet been presented. Phenotypic and genotypic resistance was more common among patients with only transient suppression of plasma HIV-1 RNA levels during two years of ZDV + ddI combination therapy, compared to those with either no suppression or sustained suppression[107]. However, such data do not yet permit any conclusions about whether resistance caused escape or vice versa.

Indirect support for the hypothesis that resistance causes escape from antiviral inhibition might be gleaned from comparisons of virus load and resistance during combination regimens to those seen during monotherapy, based on the assumption that the greater magnitude of antiviral suppression observed during combination therapy[108-111] would slow selection for resistant mutants compared to the pace seen during monotherapy. However, the two-drug combination regimens including ZDV which have been studied to date do not markedly slow development of ZDV resistance[109,112-115], except that preliminary data suggest that ZDV resistance may develop more slowly among previously untreated patients during ZDV + 3TC combination therapy than during ZDV monotherapy[57,116]. ZDV-containing two-drug combination therapies do seem to limit resistance to the second agent. Resistance to ddI as the second agent has clearly been documented to be less frequent than seen with monotherapy[109,113,115]. It is more difficult to compare ddC monotherapy with AZT + ddC combination therapy because only limited data are available to assess resistance frequency during ddC monotherapy[33,34]. However, ddC resistance was also very uncommon during ZDV + ddC therapy[112,115,117]. Again, the regimen of ZDV + 3TC represents an apparent exception. Preliminary data suggest that 3TC resistance develops in virtually all patients treated with ZDV + 3TC, although its emergence is minimally slowed in previously untreated patients receiving ZDV + 3TC compared to those receiving 3TC monotherapy[57].

Different RT mutations may emerge during combination regimens from those that emerge during monotherapy with the same agents. For example, some degree of NNRTI resistance was found in virtually all patients during NNRTI + ZDV combination therapy, but it was mediated by a different spectrum of substitutions from those seen during NNRTI monotherapy[92,118]. However, only one alternative genotype has been noted in ZDV + dideoxynucleoside-treated patients to date that has not been seen during monotherapy with either agent. Two groups have reported a few isolates from patients treated with ZDV + dideoxynucleoside that have a multiply mutant RT genotype (A62V, V75I, F77L, F116Y, Q151M) and resistance to all nucleosides tested, including ZDV, ddI, ddC, d4T and perhaps 3TC[18,107,113].

The alternative routes to resistance during combination therapy may be explained in part by some constraints on the virus' mutational options: suppression of the phenotypic effects of ZDV-resistance mutations. The ddI-resistance mutation L74V[19] can suppress the effects of some ZDV-resistance mutations and both the NNRTI-resistance mutation Y181C[65] and the 3TC-resistance mutation M184V[64] can suppress effects of all ZDV-resistance mutations. Perhaps some foscarnet-resistance mutations can also suppress ZDV resistance[27,119]. Since the ddC resistance mutations K65R and T69D have not been reported to suppress the ZDV-resistance phenotype, and the frequently occurring L41M-containing ZDV-resistant mutants do not have their ZDV resistance suppressed by L74V, suppression of ZDV resistance may not be the only mechanistic explanation for infrequent detection of isolates resistant to dideoxynucleosides during combination therapy. It seems unlikely that lack of selective pressure of the dideoxynucleoside is an explanation, because the addition of ddI or ddC to ZDV enhances antiviral activity *in vivo*.

Resistance to the second agent in two-drug combinations including ZDV has generally emerged by selection of an alternative route to resistance to the dideoxynucleoside or NNRTI, so pre-existing ZDV resistance is not suppressed under continuing ZDV selection pressure. However, an alternative route to 3TC resistance other than the codon 184

3TC-resistance mutation has not yet been noted *in vitro* or *in vivo*. Preliminary data indicate that the strong ZDV-suppressive effect of M184V consistently occurred during a number of ZDV + 3TC-resistance selections *in vitro*, but that eventually another RT mutation which reversed the M184V-mediated suppression of the persistent pre-existing ZDV-resistance mutations was also selected in the same genome[120,121]. Preliminary data also suggest that M184V is virtually always selected as the only mutation by ZDV + 3TC combination therapy *in vivo*[28,29,116,122], although ZDV-resistance suppression may not be evident in all isolates obtained from ZDV-experienced patients treated with ZDV + 3TC[28].

Another intriguing phenomenon that merits further investigation has been noted during attempts to correlate changes in circulating virus load with the development of resistance during combination therapy. Plasma HIV-1 RNA containing a ZDV-resistance mutation in RT codon 215 was less well suppressed than codon 215 wild-type plasma HIV-1 RNA in patients switched from prolonged ZDV monotherapy to combination therapy with ZDV + ddI; all of the effect of the combination on plasma RNA was attributable to suppression of codon 215 wild-type RNA[60]. The suggestion that codon 215 mutant plasma RNA may also not be suppressed in patients switched from ZDV monotherapy to ZDV + nevirapine combination therapy[60] raises the possibility that a mechanism other than potential cross-resistance to ddI explains the apparently better replication of the codon 215 mutant virus compared to codon 215 wild-type virus[25].

Is drug resistance independently predictive of more rapid disease progression?

Progression of immunodeficiency during antiretroviral therapy, as assessed by decreases in circulating CD4 cell counts or the occurrence of new clinical endpoints (i.e. opportunistic infections or malignancies), is an imperfect indicator of loss of therapeutic effectiveness. CD4 cell count is only a partial surrogate for therapeutic effect: an antiretroviral-related improvement in CD4 cell count does not necessarily predict more prolonged survival. And, as Richman has pointed out, 'the connection between clinical endpoints and the failure of antiretroviral therapy is not precise and direct'[123]. Opportunistic infections occur because of random events such as pathogen exposure, as well as the declining level of immune function. Other viral and host pathogenetic factors may also contribute to advancing immunodeficiency, and can be intertwined with the emergence of drug resistance.

One of the major pathogenetic factors linked with the development of resistance is the level of immune function. The prevalence of ZDV resistance in a group of patients is related to duration of therapy, and resistance emerges more rapidly in patient groups with more advanced disease, i.e. lower baseline CD4 cell count[94]. The emergence of high levels of resistance associated with multiply mutant isolates is not necessary for clinical disease progression, and the development of resistance need not be temporally correlated with disease progression[93]. However, among a group of 38 ZDV-treated patients who were matched at a relatively high CD4 cell count at the start of therapy (about 400 cells/mm^3), those who had a ZDV-resistance mutation in codon 215 detected in the proviral DNA of circulating cells during the subsequent two years of therapy had a greater decrease in CD4 cell count than did those who remained wild type at codon 215[51]. This may be consistent with resistance as either a cause or an effect of decreased CD4 cell count. Others have also noted that detection of the codon 215 mutation was associated with decreases in CD4 cell count[52,124]. However, 26 patients in the study by Kozal et al.[51] had serial serum samples taken and the time point when the 215 mutations were first detectable in serum HIV-1 RNA could be determined. Although CD4 counts were similar at baseline, those who had the mutation detected in serum RNA had a drop in CD4 count over the next 12 months, whereas those whose serum persistently contained only wild-type codon 215 sequences had a minimal increase in CD4 cell count[51]. Thus, resistance often precedes a fall in the CD4 cell count, perhaps consistent with resistance causing the decline in CD4 cell count.

The first demonstration that ZDV resistance was associated with more rapid clinical progression during therapy was in a group of 19 children among whom higher ZDV IC_{50}s were associated with more clinical endpoints, higher levels of p24 antigenemia and lower CD4 cell counts over six months of therapy[125,126]. However, the children who had clinical progression had lower age-adjusted CD4 cell counts at baseline, and either their lower CD4 cell counts, higher levels of ZDV resistance or both may have caused more rapid clinical progression[125,126]. Another study of a small group of children also noted more frequent clinical progression and lower CD4 cell counts among those who had ZDV-resistant isolates[127]. In a study of 50 adults receiving ZDV monotherapy over two and a half years, 26 were found to have disease progression and 15 of these were patients who developed highly ZDV-resistant isolates ($\geq$50-fold increased IC_{50})[128]. The development of high-level ZDV resistance conferred a doubling of progression risk, which was significantly increased compared to the risk for patients with more susceptible virus, even after adjustment for the CD4/CD8 ratio which was itself a significant predictor of progression[128].

Another factor which may confound analysis of the association of resistance with progression is syncytium-inducing (SI) viral phenotype, which also accelerates the rate of CD4 depletion and clinical progression[129,130]. In one study, high-level ZDV resistance was associated with the SI phenotype encoded within the HIV-1 envelope gene[131]. In another small case-control study of ZDV-treated adults, there was a stronger association between SI phenotype and clinical progression than between ZDV resistance and clinical progression[132].

None of these studies of associations between either ZDV resistance or SI phenotype and disease progression controlled for all the factors identified as associated with progression, and the most commonly used definition of progression included diagnosis of a new opportunistic infection or malignancy. The practical impact on survival of some opportunistic events which can be promptly and effectively treated may be minimal. If there was an association between ZDV resistance and survival, the clinical relevance of detection of ZDV-resistant virus would be undeniable. A collaborative multicenter virologic study by the AIDS Clinical Trials Group (ACTG) Virology Committee Resistance Working Group sought to determine the relative contribution of ZDV resistance, baseline CD4 cell count, symptomatic disease stage, SI phenotype and other factors to the rate of clinical progression in a well characterized group of 170 adults who had been randomized to prolonged monotherapy with either ZDV or ddI after a median of 14 months of prior ZDV use[95]. The patients studied had participated in ACTG protocol 116B/117[113], a randomized comparison of a switch to ddI versus continued ZDV monotherapy in patients who had received ≥16 weeks of previous ZDV therapy and had advanced HIV-1 disease (median baseline CD4 cell count of 48 cells/mm^3 for virologically studied patients).

Compared with all the other patients studied virologically, the 15% (26 of 170) with baseline HIV-1 isolates showing high-level ZDV resistance ($IC_{50} \geq 1~\mu M$ ZDV) had 1.74 times the risk of progressing during the subsequent period of observation to a new AIDS-defining event or death (95% confidence interval (CI) 1.00–3.03) and 2.78 times the risk of death (95% CI 1.21–6.39) (Table 10.1)[95]. These risks were determined by proportional hazards regression analyses that controlled for baseline CD4 cell count, SI HIV-1 phenotype, disease stage and randomized treatment assignment[95]. Patients with baseline isolates having only moderate levels of resistance ($IC_{50} \geq 0.2~\mu M$, but <1.0 μM ZDV) did not differ significantly in disease progression risk from those with susceptible viruses at baseline. The increased risk for progression to either endpoint was not significantly decreased when adjusted for other factors that were also associated with progression (compare unadjusted relative hazard to adjusted relative hazard in Table 10.1). It is of practical importance to clinicians that the predictive ability of high-level ZDV resistance was not explained by the SI phenotype[95]. In this study, which

Table 10.1   Risk factors for rate of death among patients in ACTG 116B/117[*]

Factor	Unadjusted relative hazard (95% CI)[†]	Adjusted relative hazard (95% CI)[‡]
Zidovudine resistance of baseline HIV-1 isolates[§]		
High level	2.24 (1.08–4.65)	2.78 (1.21–6.39)
Moderate	1.33 (0.64–2.77)	1.48 (0.67–3.28)
Baseline CD4 + T-lymphocyte count[**]	0.71 (0.50–0.81)	0.85 (0.68–1.07)
Syncytium-inducing phenotype of baseline HIV-1 isolate	2.93 (1.23–6.95)	3.29 (1.06–10.26)
AIDS diagnosis at study entry	4.96 (2.89–8.69)	3.13 (1.55–6.35)
Random assignment to didanosine treatment	0.62 (0.36–1.08)	0.58 (0.30–1.15)

[*] ACTG, AIDS Clinical Trials Group
[†] Unadjusted relative hazard indicates the rate of death for patients with the listed factor, relative to patients who did not have that factor. This was determined from a proportional hazards regression model including only that single independent variable. A relative hazard greater than 1 indicates that patients with a specific factor died sooner than those who did not have that factor; a relative hazard less than 1 indicates that patients with a specific factor died later than those without the factor.
[‡] Adjusted relative hazard indicates adjustment to control for the effects of each of the other listed factors, as determined from a proportional hazards regression model including all the multiple listed factors as independent variables.
[§] Patients with baseline isolates with high ($IC_{50} \geq 1.0\ \mu M$ zidovudine) and moderate (50% inhibitory concentration $\geq 0.2\ \mu M$, but $<1.0\ \mu M$ zidovudine) levels of zidovudine resistance were each compared with patients having zidovudine-susceptible isolates ($IC_{50} < 0.2\ \mu M$ zidovudine).
[**] The unadjusted relative hazard for death of baseline CD4 + T-lymphocyte count of 0.71 indicates a 29% decrease in risk for each doubling in baseline CD4 + T-lymphocyte count. Reprinted from reference 95 with permission

is the largest reported to date, an increased risk for death was associated with both high-level ZDV resistance and the SI phenotype at baseline after adjustment for the alternate virologic factor and other relevant variables, including baseline CD4 cell count (Table 10.1)[95]. More rapid genotypic assays were also evaluated in this patient group[54]. The detection by selective PCR of ZDV-resistance mutations in codons 41 and 215 was independently associated with an increased risk for progression in analyses that controlled for other predictors[54].

Thus there is now strong evidence that ZDV resistance, as detected by either phenotypic or genotypic assays, can predict disease progression independently of other pathogenetic factors with which resistance development is intertwined. Studies need to be extended to less advanced patients and those with shorter durations of ZDV therapy to ascertain if the results from the advanced ACTG 116B/117 population can be generalized. There are minimal data yet on whether resistance to any other antiretroviral drug predicts clinical progression. The finding that moderate levels of ZDV resistance were not predictive of accelerated progression during therapy[95] may suggest that the predictive ability of resistance to some of the other single agents which have not yet been noted to select for highly resistant viruses may not be similar to that noted for high-level ZDV resistance. However, Kozal *et al.*[66] have reported that detection of the ddI-resistance mutation at RT codon 74 may predict decreases in CD4 cell counts during ddI therapy: patients who developed the RT codon 74 mutation in serum RNA had greater decreases in CD4 cell counts than did patients in whom the mutation was not present. The virologic data that circulating virus load may continue to be stably suppressed for some time following the development of 3TC resistance also suggest that additional complexities remain to be learned from further studies aimed at understanding whether there is any clinical impact of 3TC resistance during combination therapy with ZDV + 3TC[28,29,116,122]. The ability of resistance to different regimens to predict disease progression during therapy does seem as if it may differ.

Can laboratory monitoring for resistance guide antiretroviral treatment decisions?

The patient population studied by the ACTG Resistance Working Group was chosen for a thorough virologic analysis, partly in order to attempt to answer another question that emerged from the results of the clinical trial comparing continued ZDV to a switch to ddI[133]. The working hypothesis underlying the design of this clinical trial was that the efficacy of ZDV would diminish over time for a number of reasons, including resistance. It was anticipated that in a group of advanced patients treated for a prolonged time the frequency of resistant isolates would be quite high[94]. ZDV was felt to be a more potent inhibitor than ddI *in vitro*. (However, the complexity of comparing inhibitor potency *in vivo* was emphasized by a subsequent report. Effective intracellular levels of ZDV-TP were greater in mitogen-activated cells than in resting cells, but effective levels of the active triphosphate form of ddI (ddATP) were greater in resting cells than in activated cells[134].) Because the characterized ZDV resistance mutations were not reported to confer ddI cross-resistance[10], it was expected that an increasing frequency of ZDV resistance would lead to greater relative benefit of switching from ZDV to ddI among those with longer previous therapy. However, the primary analysis of the clinical trial showed that prior duration of ZDV therapy was clearly not associated with the benefit of switching to ddI[133]. This raised a question about whether the benefit of ddI therapy was limited to patients failing ZDV therapy because of high-level ZDV resistance, as many had hypothesized it would be.

Four results from the subsequent virologic analyses of the ACTG 116B/117 population were indeed not consistent with the hypothesis that benefit of ddI treatment was greater in patients with high-level ZDV-resistant baseline isolates. First, and most importantly, the number of patients with evidence of high-level ZDV resistance was too small to explain the observed approximately 40% lower risk of disease progression during ddI therapy, compared to continued ZDV. Only 15% of patients had highly ZDV-resistant baseline isolates in the phenotypic assay $(IC_{50} \geqslant 1.0\ \mu\text{M ZDV})$[95] and only 21% of baseline isolates had mutations in both codons 41 and 215 detected in the genotypic assays[54]. This is a much lower prevalence of resistance than had been anticipated for such heavily pretreated advanced disease patients, and suggests that most patients retain ZDV susceptibility longer than had been expected. Secondly, in an analysis limited to patients assigned to ddI, those with high-level phenotypic ZDV-resistant baseline isolates had a significantly increased risk of death during ddI therapy, compared to patients with baseline isolates that were more susceptible to ZDV[95]. Thirdly, the relative benefit of randomization to ddI therapy was essentially unchanged when the few patients with highly ZDV-resistant isolates were excluded from analysis[95]. Fourthly, randomization to ddI therapy was associated with a significantly reduced risk of progression after controlling for the presence at baseline of mutations at codons 41 and 215 (and in the absence of a significant interaction between treatment assignment and presence of the mutations)[54]. These results suggest that patients with advanced HIV-1 disease may benefit from a switch from ZDV to ddI monotherapy, regardless of whether high-level ZDV resistance is present. Although this was not expected, it is consistent with observations that viruses with known ZDV-resistance mutations are as susceptible to ddI *in vitro* as are wild-type viruses[6,10,19]. Subsequently, other clinical trials have confirmed the clinical superiority of ddI monotherapy to ZDV monotherapy[135].

The finding that baseline high-level ZDV resistance was associated with increased risk of progression during ddI therapy has suggested 'host failure' rather than ZDV failure to some[123]. The reasoning was that the infected person who allowed ZDV-resistant viruses to dominate and who did not respond to an agent (ddI) to which ZDV-resistant viruses are susceptible *in vitro* probably would not respond to any 'salvage' therapy. However, another interpretation of this finding is that ddI is somewhat less inhibitory *in vivo* for highly ZDV-resistant viruses than for more ZDV-susceptible viruses. Possible mechanisms include augmentation of ddI resistance due to ZDV-selected mutations[6,25]. There is also some support for the hypothesis that ZDV-resistant mutants may have a replication advantage over wild-type virus that is unrelated to cross-resistance. Increased replication of codon 215 mutant viruses, relative to codon 215 wild-type viruses, has been found *in vivo* during different alternate therapies[60]. Persistent accumulation of increasing proportions of codon 41 and 215 resistant mutant viruses in circulating viral RNA has been reported for months after ZDV therapy is withdrawn, consistent with a biologic advantage for such mutants over wild-type viruses in the absence of an antiretroviral[56]. *In vitro*, one genotype of highly ZDV-resistant mutant virus (D67N, K70R, T215Y, K219Q) had a replication advantage over wild-type virus in the absence of drug in PBMC infected when they were quiescent (unstimulated PBMC) and then subsequently activated many days later by a mitogen[136]. The two viruses replicated similarly in PBMC activated by a mitogen three days before they were infected, which is the standard methodology to maximize HIV-1 replication *in vitro*[136]. The fact that unstimulated PBMC contain less effective levels of AZT-TP than activated PBMC[134] may result in a selective advantage for viruses with improved replication efficiency in unstimulated cells during AZT therapy that was not present before initiation of AZT therapy because they could reverse transcribe their genome in the presence of lower effective levels of AZT-TP.

The virologic analyses of ACTG protocol 116B/117 suggested that assessment of ZDV resistance was not useful as a laboratory guide for when to switch from ZDV to ddI monotherapy. Although it remains to be proven, laboratory monitoring of resistance may be of greater practical utility for other treatment decisions, for example when to switch to a combination regimen. Indeed, preliminary data have been presented that median increases in CD4 cell count were greater for patients harboring HIV-1 isolates with $IC_{50}s \geq 1$ μM ZDV who switched to combination therapy with ZDV + ddI, than for those with high-level ZDV resistance who either switched to ddI monotherapy or continued ZDV monotherapy[137]. In that study patients with baseline isolates with intermediate ZDV susceptibility had greater CD4 cell increases following a switch to either ddI monotherapy or ZDV + ddI combination therapy, but did not benefit from continuing ZDV[137]. These results are consistent with the hypothesis that highly ZDV-resistant viruses may have a replication advantage over more ZDV-susceptible viruses present in patients after prolonged ZDV monotherapy, and also speak against high-level ZDV resistance as an indicator of 'host failure'. However, increasing use of the strategy of adding rather than switching anti-retrovirals and the availability of plasma RNA measurements may limit the utility of monitoring resistance as a guide to timing therapeutic changes. Increasing horizontal and vertical transmission of drug-resistant HIV-1, and the likelihood that there are pre-existing drug-resistant minority sub-populations in individuals with dominant drug-susceptible circulating virus genotypes, suggests that initial assessment of drug resistance may become increasingly important before starting antiretroviral therapy. This remains to be investigated.

CONCLUSION

Laboratory methods to monitor for nucleoside RT inhibitor- and foscarnet-resistant HIV-1 are becoming increasingly informative. However, assessment of resistance is not yet proved to aid in clinical decisions about specific therapeutic changes. Escape from antiviral suppression because of resistance or any other mechanism appears to be best detected by serial quantitative assays of circulating HIV-1 RNA.

Many observations indicate that resistance is not the only pathogenetic mechanism operative during antiretroviral therapy, and suggest that detection of resistant virus is not completely predictive of treatment failure. Some early escape from ZDV suppression appears due to resurgent replication of wild-type virus, suggesting a role for non-resistance mediated pathogenetic mechanisms. However, the clinical significance of resistance to these antiretroviral agents is supported by a number of lines of evidence. ZDV-resistant viruses are transmissible. All of the early escape from 3TC suppression, and a portion of the escape from ZDV suppression, can be attributable to replication of resistant virus. Virologic suppression is gradually lost during ZDV therapy, commensurate with the development of increasingly ZDV-resistant isolates. High-level ZDV resistance predicts more rapid progression during therapy even after controlling for other pathogenetic factors. There are some less conclusive data about the effects of ddI on virus load and CD4 cell counts. Virtually nothing is known about the impact of ddC, d4T or foscarnet resistance on virus load, CD4 cell counts or clinical progression. Antiviral suppression may persist even in the face of high-level 3TC resistance during ZDV + 3TC combination therapy; to a lesser extent even high-level ZDV resistance may not mean that all virologic effectiveness of ZDV is lost. Mechanisms for persistent antiviral effect despite high-level resistance require definition, and may include suppression of ZDV resistance, decreased replication capacity of some mutants, adequate drug levels to allow some continuing partial suppression of the resistant virus, or immune effects against the drug-selected viral population. Further understanding of the biology of resistance to nucleoside RT inhibitors appears likely to lead to major improvements in the magnitude and duration of chemotherapeutic suppression of HIV-1 replication.

REFERENCES

1. Coffin JM. HIV population dynamics *in vivo*: implications for genetic variation, pathogenesis, and therapy. *Science* 1995;267:483–9.
2. Ho DD, Neumann AU, Perelson AS *et al*. Rapid turnover of plasma virions and CD4 lymphocytes in HIV-1 infection. *Nature* 1995;373:123–6.
3. Wei X, Ghosh SK, Taylor ME *et al*. Viral dynamics in human immunodeficiency virus type 1 infection. *Nature* 1995;373:117–22.
4. Larder BA. Interactions between drug resistance mutations in human immunodeficiency virus type 1 reverse transcriptase. *J Gen Virol* 1994;75:951–7.
5. Martin JL, Wilson JE, Haynes RL, Furman PA. Mechanism of resistance of human immunodeficiency virus type 1 to 2',3'-dideoxyinosine. *Proc Natl Acad Sci USA* 1993;90:6135–9.
6. Eron JJ, Chow Y-K, Caliendo AM *et al*. *pol* mutations conferring zidovudine and didanosine resistance with different effects *in vitro* yield multiply resistant human immunodeficiency virus type 1 isolates *in vivo*. *Antimicrob Agents Chemother* 1993;37:1480–7.
7. Lacey SF, Reardon JE, Furfine ES *et al*. Biochemical studies of the reverse transcriptase and RNase H activities from human immunodeficiency virus strains resistant to 3'-azido-3'-deoxythymidine. *J Biol Chem* 1992;267:15789–94.
8. Chesebro B, Wehrly K. Development of a sensitive quantitative focal assay for human immunodeficiency virus infectivity. *J Virol* 1988;62:3779–88.
9. Larder BA, Darby G, Richman DD. HIV with reduced sensitivity to zidovudine (AZT) isolated during prolonged therapy. *Science* 1989;243:1731–4.
10. Larder B, Chesebro B, Richman D. Susceptibilities of zidovudine-susceptible and -resistant human immunodeficiency virus isolates to antiviral agents determined by using a quantitative plaque reduction assay. *Antimicrob Agents Chemother* 1990;34:436–41.
11. Kimpton J, Emerman M. Detection of replication competent and pseudotyped human immunodeficiency virus with a sensitive cell line on the basis of activation of an integrated beta-galactosidase gene. *J Virol* 1992;66:2232–9.
12. Hollinger F, Bremer J, Myers L, Gold J, McQuay L and the NIH/NIAID/DAIDS/ACTG Virology Laboratories. Standardization of sensitive human immunodeficiency virus coculture procedures and establishment of a multicenter quality assurance program for the AIDS Clinical Trials Group. *J Clin Microbiol* 1992;30: 1787–94.
13. Jackson JB, Coombs RW, Sannerud K, Rhame FS, Balfour HH. Rapid and sensitive viral culture method for human immunodeficiency virus type 1. *J Clin Microbiol* 1988;26:1416–18.
14. Johnson VA, Merrill DP, Videler JA *et al*. Two-drug combinations of zidovudine, didanosine, and recombinant interferon-alpha A inhibit replication of zidovudine-resistant human immunodeficiency virus type 1 synergistically *in vitro*. *J Infect Dis* 1991;164:646–55.
15. Mayers D, McCutchan FE, Sanders-Buell EE *et al*. Characterization of HIV-1 isolates arising after prolonged zidovudine therapy. *J AIDS* 1992;5:749–59.
16. McLeod GX, McGrath JM, Ladd EA, Hammer SM. Didanosine and zidovudine resistance patterns in clinical isolates of human immunodeficiency virus type 1 as determined by a replication endpoint concentration assay. *Antimicrob Agents Chemother* 1992;36:920–5.

17. Japour AJ, Mayers DL, Johnson VA *et al*. Standardized peripheral blood mononuclear cell culture assay for determination of drug susceptibilities of clinical human immunodeficiency virus type 1 isolates. The RV-43 Study Group, the AIDS Clinical Trials Group Virology Committee Resistance Working Group. *Antimicrob Agents Chemother* 1993;37:1095–101.

18. Shirasaka T, Yarcjoan R, O'Brien MC *et al*. Changes in drug sensitivity of human immunodeficiency virus type 1 during therapy with azidothymidine, dideoxycytidine, and dideoxyinosine: an *in vitro* comparative study. *Proc Natl Acad Sci USA* 1993;90:562–6.

19. St. Clair MH, Martin JL, Tudor-Williams G *et al*. Resistance to ddI and sensitivity to AZT induced by a mutation in HIV-1 reverse transcriptase. *Science* 1991;253:1557–9.

20. Brun-Vezinet F, Ingrand D, Deforges L *et al*. HIV-1 sensitivity to zidovudine: a consensus culture technique validated by genotypic analysis of the reverse transcriptase. *J Virol Meth* 1992;37:177–88.

21. Japour A, Chatis P, Eigenrauch H, Crumpacker C. Detection of human immunodeficiency virus type 1 clinical isolates with reduced sensitivity to zidovudine and dideoxyinosine by RNA-RNA hybridization. *Proc Natl Acad Sci USA* 1991;88:3092–6.

22. Eron JJ, Gorczyca P, Kaplan JC, D'Aquila RT. Susceptibility testing by polymerase chain reaction DNA quantitation: a method to measure drug resistance of human immunodeficiency virus type 1 isolates. *Proc Natl Acad Sci USA* 1992;89:3241–5.

23. Salomon H, Belmonte A, Nguyen K *et al*. Comparison of cord blood and peripheral blood mononuclear cells as targets for viral isolation and drug sensitivity studies involving human immunodeficiency virus type 1. *J Clin Microbiol* 1994;32:2000–2.

24. Richman DD, Guatelli JC, Grimes J, Tsiatis A, Gingeras T. Detection of mutations associated with zidovudine resistance in human immunodeficiency virus by use of the polymerase chain reaction. *J Infect Dis* 1991;164:1075–81.

25. Mayers DL, Japour AJ, Arduino JM *et al*. and the RV43 Study Group. Dideoxynucleoside resistance emerges with prolonged zidovudine monotherapy. *Antimicrob Agents Chemother* 1994;38:307–14.

26. Lin PF, Samanta H, Rose RE *et al*. Genotypic and phenotypic analysis of human immunodeficiency virus type 1 isolates from patients on prolonged stavudine therapy. *J Infect Dis* 1994;170:1157–64.

27. Mellors JW, Bazmi HZ, Schinazi RF *et al*. Novel mutations in reverse transcriptase of human immunodeficiency virus type 1 reduce susceptibility to foscarnet in laboratory and clinical isolates. *Antimicrob Agents Chemother* 1995;39:1087–92.

28. Johnson VA, Wagner SF, Overbay CB *et al*. Drug resistance and viral load in NUCA 3002: a comparative trial of lamivudine (3TC) (high or low dose)/zidovudine (ZDV) combination therapy vs. ZDV/dideoxycytidine combination therapy in ZDV-experienced (≥24 weeks) patients (CD4 cells 100–300/mm^3). Fourth International HIV Drug Resistance Workshop, Sardinia, Italy, 1995:55 and *J AIDS* (in press).

29. Kuritzkes DR, Bell S, Shugarts D *et al*. Development of resistance to lamivudine (3TC) in NUCA 3001, a phase II comparative trial of 3TC vs zidovudine (ZDV) plus 3TC. Second National Conference on Human Retroviruses, Washington DC, American Society for Microbiology, 1995: Abstract LB36.

30. Fitzgibbon JE, Howell RM, Haberzettl CA *et al.* Human immunodeficiency virus type 1 *pol* gene mutations which cause decreased susceptibility to 2',3'-dideoxycytidine. *Antimicrob Agents Chemother* 1992;36:153–7.

31. Gao Q, Gu Z, Parniak MA, Li X, Wainberg MA. *In vitro* selection of variants of human immunodeficiency virus type 1 resistant to 3'-azido-3'-deoxythymidine and 2',3'-dideoxyinosine. *J Virol* 1992;66:12–19.

32. Gao Q, Gu Z, Hiscott J, Dionne G, Parniak MA. Generation of drug-resistant variants of human immunodeficiency virus-type 1 by *in vitro* passage in increasing concentrations of 2',3'-dideoxycytidine and 2',3'-dideoxy-3'-thiacytidine. *Antimicrob Agents Chemother* 1993;37:130–3.

33. Gu Z, Gao Q, Fang H *et al.* Identification of a mutation at codon 65 in the IKKK motif of reverse transcriptase that encodes human immunodeficiency virus resistance to 2',3'-dideoxycytidine and 2',3'-deoxythiacytidine. *Antimicrob Agents Chemother* 1994;38:275–81.

34. Zhang D, Caliendo AM, Eron JJ *et al.* Resistance to 2',3'-dideoxycytidine conferred by a mutation in codon 65 of the human immunodeficiency virus type 1 reverse transcriptase. *Antimicrob Agents Chemother* 1994;38:282–7.

35. Lacey SF, Larder BA. Novel mutation (V75T) in human immunodeficiency virus type 1 reverse transcriptase confers resistance to 2',3'-didehydro-2',3'-dideoxythymidine in cell culture. *Antimicrob Agents Chemother* 1994;38:1428–32.

36. Kellam P, Larder BA. Recombinant virus assay: a rapid, phenotypic assay for assessment of drug susceptibility of human immunodeficiency virus type 1 isolates. *Antimicrob Agents Chemother* 1994;38:23–30.

37. Rooke R, Tremblay M, Soudeyns H. Isolation of drug-resistant variants of HIV-1 from patients on long-term zidovudine therapy. *AIDS* 1989;3:411–15.

38. Mohri H, Singh MK, Ching WT, Ho DD. Quantitation of zidovudine-resistant human immunodeficiency virus type 1 in the blood of treated and untreated patients. *Proc Natl Acad Sci USA* 1993;90:25–9.

39. Wakefield JK, Jablonski SA, Morrow CD. *In vitro* enzymatic activity of human immunodeficiency virus type 1 reverse transcriptase mutants in the highly conserved YMDD amino acid motif correlates with the infectious potential of the proviral genome. *J Virol* 1992;66:6806–12.

40. Prasad V, Lowy I, Santos TD, Chiang L, Goff SP. Isolation and characterization of a dideoxyguanosine triphosphate-resistant mutant of HIV-1 RT. *Proc Natl Acad Sci USA* 1991;88:11363–7.

41. Schinazi RF, Lloyd RM, Nguyen M-H *et al.* Characterization of human immunodeficiency viruses resistant to oxathiolane-cytosine nucleosides. *Antimicrob Agents Chemother* 1993;37:875–81.

42. Prasad VR, Goff SP. A novel in situ colony screening method to detect human immunodeficiency virus reverse transcriptase activity expressed in bacteria: isolation of pseudorevertants of reverse transcriptase mutants. *J Biol Chem* 1989;264:16689–93.

43. Kim B, Loeb LA. Human immunodeficiency virus reverse transcriptase substitutes for DNA polymerase I in *Escherichia coli. Proc Natl Acad Sci USA* 1995;92:684–8.

44. Kim B, Loeb L. A screen in *Escherichia coli* for nucleoside analogs that target human immunodeficiency virus reverse transcriptase and herpes simplex virus thymidine kinase. *J Virol* 1995;69:6563–6.

45. Wahlberg J, Albert J, Lundeberg J *et al.* Dynamic changes in HIV-1 quasispecies from azidothymidine (AZT)-treated patients. *FASEB J* 1992;6:2843–7.

46. Larder BA, Kohli A, Kellam P et al. Quantitative detection of HIV-1 drug resistance mutations by automated DNA sequencing. *Nature* 1993;365:671–3.
47. Boucher C, Tersmette M, Lange J et al. Zidovudine sensitivity of human immunodeficiency viruses from high-risk, symptom free individuals during therapy. *Lancet* 1990;336:585–90.
48. Larder BA, Kellam P, Kemp SD. Zidovudine resistance predicted by direct detection of mutations in DNA from HIV-infected lymphocytes. *AIDS* 1991;5:137–44.
49. Larder BA, Boucher CAB. Polymerase chain reaction detection of human immunodeficiency virus drug resistance mutations. In: Persing DH, Smith TF, Tenover FC, White TJ, eds. *Diagnostic Molecular Microbiology. Principles and Applications*. Washington DC: American Society for Microbiology, 1993:527–33.
50. Jung M, Agut H, Candotti D et al. Susceptibility of HIV-1 isolates to zidovudine: correlation between widely applicable culture test and PCR analysis. *J AIDS* 1992;5:359–64.
51. Kozal MJ, Shafer RW, Winters MA, Katzenstein DA, Merigan TC. A mutation in human immunodeficiency virus reverse transcriptase and decline in CD4 lymphocyte numbers in long-term zidovudine recipients. *J Infect Dis* 1993;167:526–32.
52. Principi N, Marchisio P, DePasquale MP et al. HIV-1 reverse transcriptase codon 215 mutation and clinical outcome in children treated with zidovudine. *AIDS Res Hum Retroviruses* 1994;10:721–6.
53. Luque F, Caruz A, Pineda JA et al. Provirus load changes in untreated and zidovudine-treated human immunodeficiency virus type 1-infected patients. *J Infect Dis* 1994;169:267–73.
54. Japour AJ, Welles S, D'Aquila RT et al. for the AIDS Clinical Trials Group 116B/117 Study Team and the Virology Committee Resistance Working Group. Prevalence and clinical significance of zidovudine resistance mutations in human immunodeficiency virus isolated from patients following long-term zidovudine treatment. *J Infect Dis* 1995;171:1172–9.
55. Kaye S, Loveday C, Tedder RS. A microtitre format point mutation assay: application to the detection of drug resistance in human immunodeficiency virus type-1 infected patients treated with zidovudine. *J Med Virol* 1992;37:241–6.
56. Loveday C, Kaye S, Tenant-Flowers M et al. HIV-1 RNA serum-load and resistant viral genotypes during early zidovudine therapy. *Lancet* 1995;345:820–4.
57. Loveday C, Kaye S, Comber E, Collis P, Tedder RS. Acquisition of genotypic resistance in drug naive patients receiving 3TC/ZDV combination therapy or ZDV monotherapy. Fourth International HIV Drug Resistance Workshop, Sardinia, Italy, 1995:58 and *J AIDS* (in press).
58. Nowak MA, Bonhoeffer S, Loveday C et al. HIV results in the frame. Results confirmed. *Nature* 1995;375:193.
59. Gingeras TR, Propandovich P, Latimer T et al. Use of self-sustained sequence replication amplification reaction to analyze and detect mutations in zidovudine resistant HIV. *J Infect Dis* 1991;164:1066–74.
60. Holodniy M, Mole L, Margolis D et al. Determination of human immunodeficiency virus RNA in plasma and cellular and viral RNA genotypic zidovudine resistance and viral load during zidovudine-didanosine combination therapy. *J Virol* 1995;69:3510–16.

61. Lopez-Galindez C, Rojas JM, Najera R, Richman DD, Perucho M. Characterization of genetic variation and AZT resistance mutations of HIV by RNase A mismatch method. *Proc Natl Acad Sci USA* 1991;88:4280–4.

62. Frenkel LM, Wagner LEN, Atwood SM, Cummins TJ, Dewhurst S. Specific, sensitive, and rapid assay for human immunodeficiency virus type 1 *pol* mutations associated with resistance to zidovudine and didanosine. *J Clin Microbiol* 1995;33:342–7.

63. Pease AC, Solas D, Sullivan EJ *et al.* Light-generated oligonucleotide arrays for rapid DNA sequence analysis. *Proc Natl Acad Sci USA* 1994;91:5022–6.

64. Larder BA, Kellam P, Kemp SD. Convergent combination therapy can select viable multi-drug resistant HIV-1 *in vitro*. *Nature* 1993;365:451–3.

65. Larder BA. 3'-Azido-3'-deoxythymidine resistance suppressed by a mutation conferring human immunodeficiency virus type 1 resistance to nonnucleoside reverse transcriptase inhibitors. *Antimicrob Agents Chemother* 1992;36:2664–9.

66. Kozal M, Kroodsma K, Winters MA *et al.* Didanosine resistance in HIV-infected patients switched from zidovudine to didanosine monotherapy. *Ann Intern Med* 1994;121:263–8.

67. Kozal MJ, Shafer RW, Winters MA, Katzenstein DA, Merigan TC. Clarification of a method to reverse transcribe human immunodeficiency virus RNA. *J Infect Dis* 1995;171:1072.

68. Smith MS, Koerber KL, Pagano JS. Zidovudine-resistant human immunodeficiency virus type 1 genomes detected in plasma distinct from viral genomes in peripheral blood mononuclear cells. *J Infect Dis* 1993;167:445–8.

69. Zhang Y-M, Dawson SC, Landsman D, Lane HC, Salzman NP. Persistence of four related human immunodeficiency virus subtypes during the course of zidovudine therapy: relationship between virion RNA and proviral DNA. *J Virol* 1994;68:425–32.

70. Simmonds P, Zhang LQ, McOmish F *et al.* Discontinuous sequence change of HIV-1 *env* sequences in plasma viral and lymphocyte associated proviral populations *in vivo*: implications for models of HIV pathogenesis. *J Virol* 1991;65:6266–76.

71. Pantaleo G, Graziosi C, Deunarest JF *et al.* HIV infection is active and progressive in lymphoid tissue during the clinically latent stage of disease. *Nature* 1993;362:355–8.

72. Embretson J, Zupanic M, Ribas JL *et al.* Massive covert infection of helper T lymphocytes and macrophages by HIV during the incubation period of AIDS. *Nature* 1993;362:359–62.

73. Cohen OJ, Pantaleo G, Holodniy M *et al.* Decreased human immunodeficiency virus type 1 plasma viremia during antiretroviral therapy reflects downregulation of viral replication in lymphoid tissue. *Proc Natl Acad Sci USA* 1995;92:6017–21.

74. Herrmann ECJ, Herrmann JA. A working hypothesis—virus resistance development as an indicator of specific antiviral activity. *Ann N Y Acad Sci* 1977;284:632–7.

75. Vasudevachari MB, Battista C, Lane HC *et al.* Prevention of the spread of HIV-1 infection with nonnucleoside reverse transcriptase inhibitors. *Virology* 1992;190:269–77.

76. Chow Y-K, Hirsch MS, Merrill DP *et al.* Use of evolutionary limitations of HIV-1 multi-drug resistance to optimize therapy. *Nature* 1993;361:650–4 (and correction 364:679).

77. Mazzulli T, Rusconi S, Merrill DP *et al.* Alternating versus continuous drug regimens in combination chemotherapy of HIV-1 infection *in vitro*. *Antimicrob Agents Chemother* 1994;38:656–61.

78. Smith MS, Brian EL, Pagano JS. Resumption of virus production after human immunodeficiency virus infection of T lymphocytes in the presence of azidothymidine. *J Virol* 1987;61:3769–73.

79. Najera I, Richman DD, Olivares I *et al.* Natural occurrence of drug resistance mutations in the reverse transcriptase of human immunodeficiency virus type 1 isolates. *AIDS Res Hum Retroviruses* 1994;10:1479–88.

80. Najera I, Holguin A, Quinones-Mateu ME *et al. Pol* gene quasispecies of human immunodeficiency virus: mutations associated with drug resistance in virus from patients undergoing no drug therapy. *J Virol* 1995;69:23–31.

81. Wainberg MA, Beaulieu R, Tsoukas C, Thomas R. Detection of zidovudine-resistant variants of HIV-1 in genital fluids. *AIDS* 1993;7:433–4.

82. Anonymous. HIV seroconversion after occupational exposure despite early prophylactic zidovudine therapy. *Lancet* 1993;341:1077–8.

83. Fitzgibbon JE, Gaur S, Frenkel LD *et al.* Transmission from one child to another of human immunodeficiency virus type 1 with a zidovudine-resistance mutation. *New Engl J Med* 1993;329:1835–41.

84. Erice A, Mayers DL, Strike DG *et al.* Brief report: primary infection with zidovudine-resistant human immunodeficiency virus type 1. *New Engl J Med* 1993;328:1163–5.

85. Conlon CP, Klenerman P, Edwards A, Larder BA, Phillips RE. Heterosexual transmission of human immunodeficiency virus type 1 variants associated with zidovudine resistance. *J Infect Dis* 1994;169:411–5.

86. Wahlberg J, Fiore J, Angarano G, Uhlen M, Albert J. Apparent selection against transmission of zidovudine-resistant human immunodeficiency virus type 1 variants. *J Infect Dis* 1994;169:611–4.

87. Cooper DA, Imrie A, the Sydney Primary HIV Infection Study Group. Sexual transmission of zidovudine resistant HIV-1. *AIDS* 1994;8 (Suppl 4): Abstract 5.3.

88. Siegrist CA, Yerly S, Kaiser L, Wyler CA, Perrin L. Mother to child transmission of zidovudine-resistant HIV-1. *Lancet* 1994;344:1771–2.

89. Mayers DL, Yerly S, Perrin L *et al.* Prevalence and clinical impact of seroconversion with AZT-resistant HIV-1 between 1988 and 1994. The Second National Conference on Human Retroviruses and Related Infections. Washington DC: American Society for Microbiology, 1995: Abstract 385.

90. Perrin L, Yerly S, Rakik A, Kinloch S, Hirschel B. Transmission of 215 mutants in primary HIV infection and analysis after 6 months of ZDV. Fourth International HIV Drug Resistance Workshop, Sardinia, Italy, 1995:21 and *J AIDS* (in press).

91. Saag MS, Emini EA, Laskin OL *et al.* A short-term clinical evaluation of L-697,661, a non-nucleoside inhibitor of HIV-1 reverse transcriptase. L-697,661 Working Group. *New Engl J Med* 1993;329:1065–72.

92. Richman DD, Havlir D, Corbeil J *et al.* Nevirapine resistance mutations of human immunodeficiency virus type 1 selected during therapy. *J Virol* 1994;68:1660–6.

93. Boucher CAB, O'Sullivan E, Mulder JW *et al.* Ordered appearance of zidovudine resistance mutations during treatment of 18 human immunodeficiency virus-positive subjects. *J Infect Dis* 1992;165:105–10.

94. Richman DD, Grimes JM, Lagakos SW. Effect of stage of disease and drug

dose on zidovudine susceptibilities of isolates of human immunodeficiency virus. *J AIDS* 1990;3:743–6.

95. D'Aquila RT, Johnson VA, Welles SL *et al.* for the AIDS Clinical Trials Group Protocol 116B/117 Team and the Virology Committee Resistance Working Group. Zidovudine resistance and human immunodeficiency virus type 1 disease progression during antiretroviral therapy. *Ann Intern Med* 1995;122:401–8.

96. Hooper C, Welles S, D'Aquila R *et al.* and the ACT6 Virology PCR Validation and Resistance Working Groups. HIV-1 RNA level in plasma and association with disease progression, zidovudine sensitivity phenotype and genotype, syncytium-inducing phenotype, CD4+ cell count and clinical diagnosis of AIDS. Third International HIV Drug Resistance Workshop. Kauai, Hawaii, 1994:67.

97. de Jong MD, Veenstra J, Stilianakis N *et al.* Host–parasite dynamics and outgrowth of virus containing a single k70R amino acid change in reverse transcriptase are responsible for the loss of human immunodeficiency virus type I RNA load suppression by zidovudine. *Proc Natl Acad Sci USA* 1996 (in press).

98. Frost SD, McLean AR. Quasispecies dynamics and the emergence of drug resistance during zidovudine therapy of HIV infection. *AIDS* 1994;8:323–32.

99. Reichman RC, Tejani N, Lambert JL *et al.* Didanosine (ddI) and zidovudine (ZDV) susceptibilities of human immunodeficiency virus (HIV) isolates from long-term recipients of ddI. *Antiviral Res* 1993;20:267–77.

100. Masquelier B, Pellegrin I, Ruffault A *et al.* Genotypic evolution of HIV-1 isolates from patients after a switch of therapy from zidovudine to didanosine. *J AIDS Retrovirol* 1995;8:330–4.

101. Schuurman R, Nijhuis M, van Leeuwen R *et al.* Rapid changes in human immunodeficiency virus type 1 RNA load and appearance of drug-resistant virus populations in persons treated with lamivudine (3TC). *J Infect Dis* 1995;171:1411–9.

102. Pluda JM, Cooley TP, Montaner JS *et al.* A phase I/II study of 2'-deoxy-3'-thiacytidine (lamivudine) in patients with advanced human immunodeficiency virus infection. *J Infect Dis* 1995;171:1438–47.

103. van Leeuwen R, Katlama C, Kitchen V *et al.* Evaluation of safety and efficacy of 3TC (lamivudine) in patients with asymptomatic or mildly symptomatic human immunodeficiency virus infection: a phase I/II study. *J Infect Dis* 1995;171:1166–71.

104. Boyer PL, Hughes SH. Analysis of mutations at position 184 in reverse transcriptase of human immunodeficiency virus type 1. *Antimicrob Agents Chemother* 1995;39:1624–8.

105. Back NKT, Nijhuis M, Boucher CAB *et al.* Reduced *in vitro* polymerase activity of 3TC-resistant reverse transcriptase enzymes. Third International HIV Drug Resistance Workshop. Kauai, Hawaii, 1994:32.

106. Wainberg MA, Quan Y, Gu Z, Li Z. Kinetics and chain termination studies performed with recombinant mutated M184V and K65R HIV reverse transcriptase. Fourth International HIV Drug Resistance Workshop, Sardinia, Italy, 1995:5 and *J AIDS* (in press).

107. Shafer RW, Iversen AKN, Winters MA *et al.* and the AIDS Clinical Trials Group 143 Virology Team. Drug resistance and heterogeneous long-term virologic responses of human immunodeficiency virus type 1-infected subjects to zidovudine and didanosine combination therapy. *J Infect Dis* 1995;172:70–8.

108. Collier AC, Coombs RW, Fischl MA *et al.* Combination therapy with zidovudine and didanosine compared with zidovudine alone in HIV-1 infection. *Ann Intern Med* 1993;119:786–93.

109. Kojima E, Shirasaka T, Anderson BD *et al.* Human immunodeficiency virus type 1 (HIV-1) viremia changes and development of drug-related mutations in patients with symptomatic HIV-1 infection receiving alternating or simultaneous zidovudine and didanosine therapy. *J Infect Dis* 1995;171:1152–8.

110. Yarchoan R, Lietzau JA, Nguyen B-Y *et al.* A randomized pilot study of alternating or simultaneous zidovudine and didanosine therapy in patients with symptomatic human immunodeficiency virus infection. *J Infect Dis* 1994;169:9–17.

111. Meng T-C, Fischl MA, Boota AM *et al.* Combination therapy with zidovudine and dideoxycytidine in patients with advanced human immunodeficiency virus infection: a phase I/II study. *Ann Intern Med* 1992;116:13–20.

112. Richman DD, Meng T-C, Spector SA *et al.* Resistance to AZT and ddC during long-term combination therapy in patients with advanced infection with human immunodeficiency virus. *J AIDS* 1994;7:135–8.

113. Shafer RW, Kozal MJ, Winters MA *et al.* Combination therapy with zidovudine and didanosine selects for drug-resistant human immunodeficiency virus type 1 strains with unique patterns of *pol* gene mutations. *J Infect Dis* 1994;169:722–9.

114. St. Clair MH, Pennington KN, Larder BA, the Protocol 34,225-02 Collaborative Group. A placebo controlled trial of AZT alone or in combination with ddI or ddC: *in vitro* AZT resistance analysis as determined by PBMC assay. Third International HIV Drug Resistance Workshop. Kauai, Hawaii, 1994:72.

115. Larder BA, Kemp SD, Kinghorn I *et al.* The Protocol 34-CG. A placebo controlled trial of AZT alone or in combination with ddI or ddC: genotypic and phenotypic resistance analysis. Third International HIV Drug Resistance Workshop. Kauai, Hawaii, 1994:73.

116. Larder BA, Kemp SD, Harrigan PR. Potential mechanism for sustained antiretroviral efficacy of AZT-3TC combination therapy. *Science* 1995;269:696–9.

117. Sylvester S, Caliendo A, An D *et al.* HIV-1 resistance mutations and plasma RNA during ZDV + ddC combination therapy. Fourth International HIV Drug Resistance Workshop, Sardinia, Italy, 1995:47 and *J AIDS* (in press).

118. Staszewski S, Massari FE, Kober A *et al.* Combination therapy with zidovudine prevents selection of human immunodeficiency virus type 1 variants expressing high-level resistance to L-697,661, a nonnucleoside reverse transcriptase inhibitor. *J Infect Dis* 1995;171:1159–65.

119. Tachedjian G, Birch C, Mills J. Failure to select HIV-1 with dual resistance to zidovudine (AZT) and foscarnet (PFA). Fourth International HIV Drug Resistance Workshop, Sardinia, Italy, 1995:17 and *J AIDS* (in press).

120. Kemp SD, Kohli A, Larder BA. Genotypic characterization of an HIV-1 mutant co-resistant to AZT and 3TC. Fourth International HIV Drug Resistance Workshop, Sardinia, Italy, 1995:51 and *J AIDS* (in press).

121. Goulden MG, Hopewell P, Viner KC *et al.* Selection of high level resistance to both 3TC™ and AZT. Fourth International HIV Drug Resistance Workshop, Sardinia, Italy, 1995:50 and *J AIDS* (in press).

122. Harrigan PR, Bloor S, Kinghorn I, Group TLEHW, Larder BA. Virologic response to AZT/3TC combination therapy in AZT experienced patients (Trial NUCB 3002). Fourth International HIV Drug Resistance Workshop. Sardinia, Italy, 1995:54 and *J AIDS* (in press).

123. Richman DD. Resistance, drug failure, and disease progression. *AIDS Res Hum Retroviruses* 1994;10:901–4.

124. Husson RN, Shirasaka T, Butler KM, Pizzo PA, Mitsuya H. High-level resistance to zidovudine but not to zalcitabine or didanosine in human immunodeficiency virus from children receiving antiretroviral therapy. *J Pediatr* 1993;123:9–16.

125. Tudor-Williams G, St Clair MH, McKinney RE *et al*. HIV-1 sensitivity to zidovudine and clinical outcome in children. *Lancet* 1992;339:15–19.

126. Tudor-Williams G, St Clair MH, McKinney RE *et al*. HIV-1 sensitivity to zidovudine and clinical outcome. *Lancet* 1992;339:627.

127. Ogino MTS Dankner WM, Spector SA. Development and significance of zidovudine resistance in children infected with human immunodeficiency virus. *J Pediatr* 1993;123:1–8.

128. Montaner JSG, Singer J, Schecter MT *et al*. Clinical correlates of *in vitro* HIV-1 resistance to zidovudine. Results of the Multicentre Canadian AZT Trial. *AIDS* 1993;7:189–96.

129. Koot M, Keet IPM, Vos HV *et al*. Prognostic value of HIV-1 syncytium-inducing phenotype for rate of CD4$^+$ cell depletion and progression to AIDS. *Ann Intern Med* 1993;118:681–8.

130. Bozzette SA, McCutchan JA, Spector SA, Wright B, Richman DD. A cross-sectional comparison of persons with syncytium- and non-syncytium-inducing human immunodeficiency virus. *J Infect Dis* 1993;168:1374–9.

131. Boucher CAB, Lange JMA, Miedema FF *et al*. HIV-1 biologic phenotype and the development of zidovudine resistance in relation to disease progression in asymptomatic individuals during treatment. *AIDS* 1992;6:1259–64.

132. St. Clair MH, Hartigan PM, Andres JC *et al*. Zidovudine resistance, syncytium-inducing phenotype, and HIV disease progression in a case-control study. *J AIDS* 1993;6:891–7.

133. Kahn JO, Lagakos SW, Richman DD *et al*. and the NIAID AIDS Clinical Trials Group. A controlled trial comparing continued zidovudine with didanosine in human immunodeficiency virus infection. *New Engl J Med* 1992;327:581–7.

134. Gao W-Y, Agbaria R, Driscoll JS, Mitsuya H. Divergent antihuman immunodeficiency virus activity and anabolic phosphorylation of 2',3'-dideoxynucleoside analogs in resting and activated human cells. *J Biol Chem* 1994;269:12633–8.

135. NIH AIDS Clinical Trials Group. AIDS Clinical Trials Group Protocol 175 Executive Summary. September 14, 1995.

136. Caliendo A, Savara A, An D, DeVore K, Kaplan J, D'Aquila R. Effects of zidovudine-selected human immunodeficiency virus type I reverse transcriptase amino acid substitutions on processive DNA synthesis and viral replication. *J Virol* 1996;70:2146–53.

137. Cavert W, Coombs RW, Grimes J *et al*. for the ACT6 Protocol 194 Clinics and Virology Laboratories. The therapeutic significance of switching to ddI or adding ddI in subjects with ZDV resistant HIV-1. Fourth International HIV Drug Resistance Workshop. Sardinia, Italy, 1995:41 and *J AIDS* (in press).

11

Non-Nucleoside Reverse Transcriptase Inhibitors — Mechanisms

EMILIO A. EMINI

STRUCTURE AND DESCRIPTION OF ACTIVITY

The non-nucleoside inhibitors of the human immunodeficiency virus type 1 (HIV-1) reverse transcriptase (RT) comprise a series of structurally diverse compounds that share a common mechanism of action and bind to a common site on the enzyme. Many of the non-nucleosides were originally identified by random screening of defined compounds and natural products for RT inhibitory activity. Subsequent chemical modifications resulted in the development of inhibitors that exhibited reasonable antiviral effects in cell culture. A number of the non-nucleosides have been evaluated in clinical trials for *in vivo* antiviral potential.

The first of the inhibitors to be described was the thiobenzimidazolone (TIBO) derivative R82150[1]. This was followed by description of an additional TIBO derivative R82913[2], as well as by accounts of the unrelated dipyridodiazepinone BI-RG-587 (nevirapine)[3,4] and the pyridinone L-697,661[5]. Numerous other non-nucleosides have been defined since. A list of the more extensively studied compounds is given in Table 11.1. However, additional members of this inhibitor class continue to be discovered and evaluated. Representative compound structures are presented in Figure 11.1.

As a group, the non-nucleoside inhibitors encompass notable structural diversity. Nonetheless, the compounds exhibit characteristic functional properties. All are specific for inhibition of the HIV-1 RT; none inhibit the HIV type 2 enzyme. Also, none inhibit other viral or mammalian cell nucleic acid polymerases. Unlike the nucleoside analog

Antiviral Drug Resistance. Edited by Douglas D. Richman © 1996 John Wiley & Sons Ltd

Table 11.1 *Non-nucleoside HIV-1 RT inhibitors*

Compound	References
Thiobenzimidazolone (TIBO) derivatives (R82150, R82913)	1,2
Dipyridodiazepinone BI-RG-587 (nevirapine)	3
Pyridinone derivatives (L-697,661, L-696,229)	5,46
Bisheteroarylpiperazine (BHAP) derivatives U-90152 (delavirdine) and U-87201 (atevirdine)	47–49
α-anilinophenyl acetamide (α-APA) derivatives (loviride)	50
TSAO analogs	51
1-[(2-hydroxy-ethoxy)methyl]-6-phenylthiothymine and derivatives (HEPT, E-EPU, I-EBU, MKC-442)	52–54
Quinoxaline derivatives (S-2720)	55
Calanolides	56
Quinoline derivatives (U-78036)	57
Thiazolo-iso-indolinones	58
Diarylsulfone derivatives	59
Inophyllums	60
Substituted naphthalenones	61
Pyrroles	62
Benzothiadiazine derivatives	63
Nitrophenyl phenyl sulfone (NPPS)	64
Oxathiin carboxanilide (UC-38)	64
[N-(2-phenly ethyl)-N'-(2-thiazolyl) thiourea (PETT) derivatives (trovirdine)	65,66
1, 4-dihydro-2H-3, 1-benzoxazin-2-ones (L-743, 726, DMP-266)	78

RT inhibitors, the non-nucleosides do not require metabolic activation to manifest their antiviral effects. As a result, there is typically a direct correlation between the compounds' *in vitro* anti-RT and cell-culture antiviral activities[5]. The non-nucleosides generally manifest additive to synergistic antiviral effects when used in combination with various nucleoside analog inhibitors or with anti-HIV-1 protease inhibitors[5-8].

MECHANISM OF ACTION

It was evident from early studies that the non-nucleoside inhibitors bind to a site on the RT enzyme that is distinct from the active site. Kinetic experiments showed that the compounds are non-competitive with respect to template-primer for inhibition of purified RT[9-13]. This suggested that the inhibitors bind directly to the free enzyme molecule, although the template-primer does appear to have some influence on the nature of the interaction[5,14-17]. It was eventually shown that the non-nucleosides bind to the enzyme–template-primer complex and adversely influence the enzyme's polymerizing activity[18].

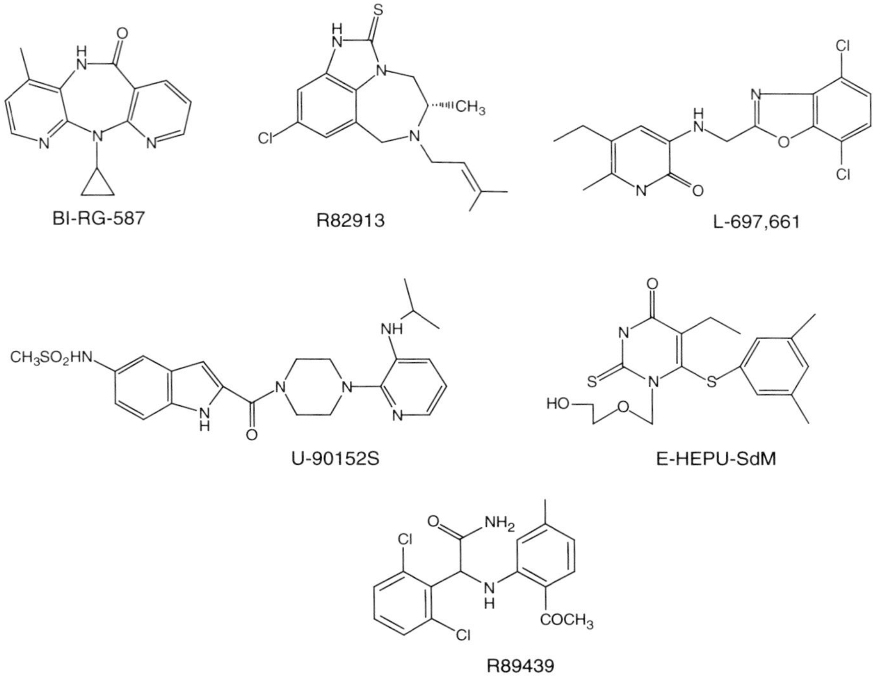

Figure 11.1 *The molecular structures of representative non-nucleoside HIV-1 RT inhibitors. BI-RG-587 (dipyridodiazepinone); R82913 (TIBO derivative); L-697,661 (pyridinone); U-90152S (BHAP derivative); E-HEPU-SdM (HEPT derivative); R89439 (α-APA derivative). Reproduced from reference 24 with permission*

Competition experiments with structurally different non-nucleosides demonstrated that the compounds occupy the identical binding site on the RT molecule[19,20]. The structural identification of the site was initially accomplished by Kohlstaedt *et al.*[21], who succeeded in determining a low-resolution crystal structure of the RT complexed with BI-RG-587 (nevirapine). The compound was bound in a hydrophobic 'pocket' located adjacent to the enzyme's active site. Assignment of RT amino acid alterations that engender loss of viral susceptibility to various non-nucleosides confirmed the site's location[22] (see Plate 2).

The RT enzyme is a heterodimer composed of p66 and p51 subunits. Activity resides with the larger subunit, whose structure has been described as being composed of three subdomains designated the thumb, palm and fingers. The thumb and fingers participate in the molecule's interaction with the template and primer, while the palm contains the enzyme's active site[21,23]. The non-nucleoside binding pocket lies below the base of the palm and appears to interact directly with the RT's active site. Binding of a non-nucleoside compound to the pocket apparently slows the rate of the RT-catalyzed chemical reaction[18]. This significantly interferes with the enzyme's ability to complete its task of converting the viral RNA genome into proviral DNA.

Various portions of the RT molecule contribute to the structure of the non-nucleoside binding pocket. These include the p66 subunit regions from amino acid residue 97 to residue 108, from 179 to 192, from 224 to 236 and from 317 to 321[24]. A fragment of the p51 subunit, delineated by residues 135–139, is also located proximal to the pocket. The side chains of many of the contributing residues point into the internal pocket cavity and, depending on the specific non-nucleoside, interact directly with the inhibitor[24]. Two of the more significant side chains are those of residues 181 and 188. Cross-linking experiments with BI-RG-587 resulted in the specific labeling of these residues[25]. Both are tyr residues in HIV-1 RT, whereas both are either leu or ile in the non-susceptible HIV-2 RT. Shih et al.[26] demonstrated that conversion of both residues to tyr in the type 2 enzyme results in a partial sensitization of the altered RT to inhibition by BI-RG-587. Similar results were obtained by Condra et al.[27] using type 1 and type 2 RT chimeras. The requirement for aromatic side chains at 181 and 188 for non-nucleoside activity was confirmed by Sardana et al.[28], who showed that inhibition of the purified type 1 enzyme by several non-nucleosides was not affected by substitution of phe residues for tyr at these positions. Non-aromatic substitutions resulted in varying degrees of susceptibility loss. Finally, amino acids that contribute to the binding pocket's structure, but whose side chains are oriented away from the pocket, can also affect non-nucleoside binding. For instance, alterations at residues 101 mediate susceptibility loss to some of the non-nucleosides (see below), suggesting the importance of local structural effects through the α-carbon backbone.

The exact means by which non-nucleoside binding adversely influences RT activity is not entirely clear. The enzyme's three active site asp residues are located at positions 110, 185 and 186. All three positions are reasonably proximal to the non-nucleoside binding pocket, so that inhibitor binding can be envisaged to alter the structure of the active site. Spence et al.[18] have direct evidence that the non-nucleoside pocket and the active site functionally interact. Binding of magnesium ions to the active site apparently lessens the binding of certain non-nucleoside inhibitors. Active site changes mediated by the non-nucleosides are presumably the result of structural shifts in the amino acid side chains that contribute to the pocket, particularly the tyr residues at 181 and 188. These shifts may occur subsequent to the RT's accommodation of the non-nucleoside compound. The crystal structure of unliganded RT suggests that notable structural rearrangements must take place for the RT to accept binding of a non-nucleoside[29].

This latter observation has implications for the universal application of so-called 'rational drug design'. The non-nucleoside inhibitors could not have been designed using the unliganded RT structure as the compound binding site is not obvious. The site is apparently manifest only following the protein rearrangements that occur to accommodate inhibitor binding.

LOSS OF HIV-1 SUSCEPTIBILITY TO NON-NUCLEOSIDE-MEDIATED INHIBITION

It has become abundantly evident that the primary limitation to the continued clinical antiviral effectiveness of HIV-1 therapeutic agents is the selection of resistant viral mutants and the rapid replacement of the wild-type virus population with such variants. Attempts to isolate variants expressing reduced susceptibility to the non-nucleosides in cell culture were almost immediately successful. The initial mutants were derived by passing wild-type virus in the presence of increasing concentrations of either BI-RG-587[30], a pyridinone derivative[31] or a TIBO compound[32]. The resulting viral mutants exhibited significantly reduced susceptibilities of 10- to 1000-fold. Genetic analyses of some of these variants mapped the susceptibility changes to amino acid substitutions at residue 181 and/or residues located in the 97–108 region. Varying degrees of cross-resistance were noted using different non-nucleoside structural classes[31]. This implied that each inhibitor interacted with the same binding site, but probably in a unique way. It also suggested that resistant virus selected with one inhibitor would express at least partial cross-resistance to other non-nucleosides, and that combinations of different non-nucleosides were likely to select for variants expressing a common loss of susceptibility.

At the time when these studies were performed, the structural identification of the non-nucleoside binding site had not yet been accomplished. Subsequent mapping of these susceptibility-altering substitutions, as well as others that were eventually defined, showed that all contributed to the inhibitor-binding site. This intimated that the functional basis for loss of susceptibility was modified interaction of the inhibitor with the RT molecule.

Table 11.2 summarizes the single amino acid substitutions that negatively influence virus susceptibility to individual inhibitors. The substitutions were identified either by selection of virus with reduced susceptibility in cell culture, by genetic analysis of resistant viral

Table 11.2 *RT amino acid substitutions that engender resistance to the non-nucleoside inhibitors*

Inhibitor	RT substitution	Reference
Thiobenzimidazolone (TIBO) derivatives	100 (leu → ile)	32–34,39
	103 (lys → asn)	34,67
	106 (val → ala)	39
	108 (val → ile)	33,68
	181 (tyr → cys)	33,69,70
	188 (tyr → leu/his)	28,70
BI-RG-587 (nevirapine)	103 (lys → asn)	31
	106 (val → ala)	39,40,67
	108 (val → ile)	33
	181 (tyr → cys)	30,31,33,34,39,40
	188 (tyr → leu)	25,28
	190 (gly → ala)	37
Pyridinone derivatives	98 (ala → gly)	67
	101 (lys → glu)	67
	103 (lys → asn/gln)	31,67
	108 (val → ile)	67
	179 (val → asp/glu)	67
	181 (tyr → cys)	31,34,67
	188 (tyr → leu/his)	28
Bisheteroarylpiperazine (BHAP) derivatives (delavirdine, atevirdine)	100 (leu → ile)	34,67
	181 (tyr → cys)	67
	236 (pro → leu)	38
α-APA (loviride)	181 (tyr → cys)	50
TSAO	138 (glu → lys)	34,69,71,72
	181 (tyr → cys)	69
HEPT, E-EPU, I-EBU, MKC-442	100 (leu → ile)	33
	103 (lys → arg/asn)	73,74
	106 (val → ala)	75
	108 (val → ile)	33,73
	181 (tyr → cys/ile)	33,73–76
	188 (tyr → cys/his)	75,76
	236 (pro → leu)	33
Quinoxaline derivatives (S-2720)	181 (tyr → cys)	36
	190 (gly → glu)	35,36
Calanolides	100 (leu → ile)	33
	103 (lys → asn)	74
	108 (val → ile)	33
	181 (tyr → ile)	74

(Continued)

Table 11.2 *Continued*

Inhibitor	RT substitution	Reference
Thiazolo-iso-indolines	181 (tyr → cys)	58
Inophyllums	188 (tyr → leu)	74
Pyrroles	181 (tyr → cys)	62
Benzothiadiazine derivatives	108 (val → ile)	33
	181 (tyr → cys)	33,63
Diphenylsulfone	100 (leu → ile)	33
	108 (val → ile)	33
	181 (tyr → cys)	33
Oxathiin carboxanilide	100 (leu → ile)	33
	108 (val → ile)	33
	181 (tyr → cys)	33
PETT derivatives (trovirdine)	100 (leu → ile)	65,66
	181 (tyr → cys)	65,66
	188 (tyr → his)	65
1,4-dihydro-2H-3,1-benzoxazin-2-ones	100 (leu → ile)	78
	103 (lys → asn)	78
(L-743, 726, DMP-266)	188 (tyr → leu)	78

populations from inhibitor-treated patients, by phenotypic analysis of specifically constructed HIV-1 mutants, or by *in vitro* analysis of constructed RT enzyme variants.

DIFFERENCES AMONG THE NON-NUCLEOSIDE INHIBITORS IN RT BINDING

The information given in Table 11.2 provides a perspective on both the common and the unique characteristics of the interaction between the RT enzyme and each structural class of non-nucleoside inhibitor. All of the non-nucleoside compounds are influenced by the amino acid residues at positions 181 and 188. As noted previously, the structural and enzymatic data demonstrate that both residues are primary contributors to the non-nucleoside binding pocket, and that the residues' respective aromatic side chains are essential for inhibitor activity. However, the degree of susceptibility loss engendered by substitution at either of these residues is not uniform among the non-nucleosides. For instance, the cys for tyr substitution at residue 181 mediates a 10-fold susceptibility loss to oxathiin carboxanilide, but it engenders a more than 100-fold resistance to BI-RG-587 (nevirapine)[33].

Similarly, certain non-nucleosides are uniquely affected by specific amino acid substitutions. TSAO analog activity is particularly influenced by substitutions at residue 138[34], whereas alterations at residue 190 have a noted effect on virus susceptibility to BI-RG-587 (nevirapine) and the quinoxaline derivatives[34-37]. The pro to leu substitution at RT residue 236 mediates specific negative effects for the BHAP derivatives and the HEPT compounds, yet it hypersensitizes the virus to inhibition by other non-nucleosides[33,38].

These observations reinforce the notion that, although the RT binding pocket for the non-nucleoside inhibitors represents a single structural entity, the binding specificities of individual compounds may be quite distinctive. Accordingly, it has been suggested that combination therapy with non-nucleosides representing different functionally interactive classes may be reasonable[33]. Multiple resistance would then require the selection of multiple, independent RT amino acid substitutions. It remains to be clinically established whether such a requirement would pose a significant hindrance to resistant virus selection. However, given the common RT binding site for the non-nucleosides, it is likely that single amino acid substitutions may be selected that would simultaneously adversely affect virus susceptibility to any combination non-nucleoside inhibitor therapy.

PHENOTYPIC INTERACTIONS AMONG RT SUSCEPTIBILITY-ALTERING AMINO ACID SUBSTITUTIONS

The viral susceptibility characteristics mediated by certain RT amino acid substitutions have been found to influence the phenotypes engendered by other amino acid alterations within the enzyme. Understanding the nature of these interactions is also important when considering the choice of agents for possible combination therapy.

Table 11.3 summarizes the effects of the residue 236 (pro→leu) substitution selected by the non-nucleoside BHAP compounds (e.g. U90152S)[38]. This alteration was shown to hypersensitize HIV-1 to unrelated non-nucleosides, such as BI-RG-587 (nevirapine), the pyridinone L-697,661 and the TIBO derivative R82913. In addition, co-expression of the residue 236 substitution with the 181 (tyr→cys) change significantly attenuates the loss of viral non-nucleoside susceptibility mediated by the latter mutation. The appropriate combination of non-nucleoside inhibitors could exploit this interaction to hinder

Table 11.3 *Effect of the 236 (pro → leu) RT amino acid substitution on HIV-1 susceptibility to various non-nucleoside inhibitors*[a]

Mutant virus	Inhibitor			
	U-90152S	BI-RG-587	L-697,661	R82913
Wild type	1×	1×	1×	1×
181 (tyr → cys)	32×	>20×	>75×	10×
236 (pro → leu)	70×	0.1×	0.1×	0.1×
181 (tyr → cys) +				
236 (pro → leu)	>230×	2×	12×	2×

[a] Values represent approximate fold-differences in virus susceptibility. Values were calculated from data in [38]

selection of HIV-1 variants expressing cross-resistance. This possibility awaits clinical testing.

An additional possibility for combination RT inhibitor therapy is presented by the interactions between certain non-nucleoside resistance-associated RT substitutions and RT mutations that mediate resistance to the nucleoside analog 3′-azido-3′,-deoxythymidine (AZT)[39–41]. Table 11.4 partially summarizes these observations. The expression of the 181 (tyr → cys) substitution, selected by many of the non-nucleoside compounds, resensitizes AZT-resistant HIV-1 to AZT. This is noted using AZT-resistant virus bearing AZT-specific mutations at residues 41 and 215, as well as with virus expressing alterations at residues 67, 70, 215 and 219. However, the degree of resensitization does appear to be influenced by the nature of the AZT-associated alterations. In addition to the 181 substitution, the 100 (leu → ile) change was also shown to mediate a profound resensitization to AZT[41]. Neither the 100 or 181 mutations affects the loss of virus susceptibility to the nucleoside analog ddI as mediated by the ddI-specific residue 74 (leu → val) substitution[39,41].

The selection of resistant viral variants during clinical studies of combined therapy with non-nucleoside inhibitors and AZT is apparently affected by these described phenotypic interactions. For instance, whereas monotherapy with the pyridinone L-697,661 results predominantly in the selection of variants that express the 181 (tyr → cys) alteration[42], co-treatment of therapy-naive patients with L-697,661 and AZT leads to the selection of virus exclusively expressing the non-nucleoside resistance substitution at residue 103[43]. Similar alternative substitution pathways were noted in clinical studies involving the combination of AZT and BI-RG-587 (nevirapine)[44].

The eventual clinical significance of these interactive phenotypic effects is not known. Given the numerous substitution patterns available for engendering resistance to the non-nucleoside inhibitors, it would

Table 11.4 *Interactive effects of RT amino acid substitutions on HIV-1 susceptibility to non-nucleoside inhibitors and to the nucleoside analog AZT*[a]

Mutant virus	AZT IC_{50}	AZT IC_{95}	BI-RG-587 IC_{50}	BI-RG-587 IC_{95}	L-697,661 IC_{95}	R82913 IC_{50}	R82913 IC_{95}
Wild type	1×	1×	1×	1×	1×	1×	1×
100 (leu→ile)	—[b]	1×	—	1×	2×	—	>4×
181 (tyr→cys)	1×	1×	200×	>8×	>30×	40×	>4×
41 (met→leu) + 215 (thr→tyr)	70×	1000×	1×	1×	1×	1×	1×
67 (asp→asn) + 70 (lys→arg) + 215 (thr→tyr) + 219 (lys→gln)	150×	8000×	1×	1×	1×	1×	1×
41 (met→leu) + 100 (leu→ile) + 215 (thr→tyr)	—	1×	—	1×	2×	—	—
67 (asp→asn) + 70 (lys→arg) + 100 (leu→ile) + 215 (thr→tyr) + 219 (lys→gln)	—	2×	—	1×	2×	—	>4×
41 (met→leu) + 181 (tyr→cys) + 215 (thr→tyr)	1×	60×	170×	>8×	>30×	25×	>4×
67 (asp→asn) + 70 (lys→arg) + 181 (tyr→cys) + 215 (thr→tyr) + 219 (lys→gln)	5×	8×	100×	>8×	>30×	25×	>4×

[a] Values represent approximate fold-differences in virus susceptibility. Differences were calculated using IC_{50}[39] or IC_{95}[41] assay determinations (see text)

[b] not done

seem that combinations of RT amino acid alterations are possible that will mediate co-resistance to the non-nucleosides and to the nucleoside analogs. In fact, HIV-1 variants with reduced susceptibility to AZT, ddI and BI-RG-587 (nevirapine) have been selected in cell culture[40]. Similar multiply resistant variants were also constructed by mutagenesis[45]. In both cases, either the 103 (lys → asn) or the 106 (val → ala) substitution was used to mediate loss of non-nucleoside susceptibility in the context of both AZT and ddI resistance.

THE FUTURE OF NON-NUCLEOSIDE RT INHIBITORS

The ease with which the HIV-1 RT can express loss of susceptibility to the non-nucleoside inhibitors would suggest that the clinical utility of these compounds as monotherapeutic agents is limited. This notion is supported further by the RT's ability to accommodate numerous substitutions within the inhibitor binding pocket and the enzyme molecule as a whole, thereby permitting multiple resistance to the various non-nucleosides as well as to the nucleoside analogs. However, the theoretical initial antiviral potency of some of the described non-nucleosides is substantial. This may allow for the use of such compounds in combined antiviral treatment with other potent anti-HIV-1 inhibitors. Such combination therapy could result in significant delay in the selection of HIV-1 variants resistant to each member of the combination. Also, additional drug discovery and inhibitor design efforts may allow for the development of compounds whose interaction with the non-nucleoside binding pocket is unique, and for which resistance selection pathways may be limited. It is also possible to conceive of inhibitors that can extend from the non-nucleoside pocket to the enzyme's active site, thereby mediating a possibly novel mechanism of RT inhibition[16]. The continued acquisition and analysis of structural, genetic, mechanistic and resistance data will provide the necessary basis for these efforts.

Acknowledgments

The author wishes to thank Dolores Wilson and Agnes Hendricks for their assistance in the preparation of the manuscript.

REFERENCES

1. Pauwels R, Andries K, Desmyter D *et al.* Potent and selective inhibition of HIV-1 replication *in vivo* by a novel series of TIBO derivatives. *Nature* 1990;243:470–4.

2. White EL, Buckheit RW, Ross LJ *et al*. A TIBO derivative, R82913, is a potent inhibitor of HIV-1 reverse transcriptase with heteropolymer templates. *Antiviral Res* 1991;16:257–66.

3. Merluzzi VJ, Hargrave KD, Labadia M *et al*. Inhibition of HIV-1 replication by a nonnucleoside reverse transcriptase inhibitor. *Science* 1990;250:1411–13.

4. Koup RA, Merluzzi VJ, Hargrave KD *et al*. Inhibition of human immuno-deficiency virus type 1 (HIV-1) replication by the dipyridodiazepinone BI-RG-587. *J Infect Dis* 1991;163:966–70.

5. Goldman ME, Nunberg JH, O'Brien JA *et al*. Pyridinone derivatives: specific human immunodeficiency virus type 1 reverse transcriptase inhibitors with antiviral activity. *Proc Natl Acad Sci USA* 1991;88:6863–7.

6. Vacca JP, Dorsey BD, Schleif WA *et al*. L-735,524, an orally bioavailable HIV-1 protease inhibitor. *Proc Natl Acad Sci USA* 1994;91:4096–100.

7. Richman DD, Rosenthal AS, Skoog M *et al*. BI-RG-587 is active against zidovudine-resistant human immunodeficiency virus type 1 and synergistic with zidovudine. *Antimicrob Agents Chemother* 191;35:305–8.

8. Pagano PJ, Chong KT. *In vitro* inhibition of human immunodeficiency virus type 1 by a combination of delavirdine (U-90152) with protease inhibitor U-75875 or interferon-alpha. *J Infect Dis* 1995;171:61–7.

9. Frank KB, Noll GJ, Connell EV, Sim IS. Kinetic interaction of human immunodeficiency virus type 1 reverse transcriptase with the antiviral tetrahydroimidazo [4,5,1,jk]-[1,4]-benzodiazepine-2-(1H)-thione compound R82150. *J Biol Chem* 1991;266:14232-6.

10. Kopp EB, Miglietta JJ, Shrutkowski AG *et al*. Steady state kinetics and inhibition of HIV-1 reverse transcriptase by a non-nucleoside dipyridodiazepinone BI-RG-587 using a heteropolymeric template. *Nucleic Acids Res* 1991;19:3035–9.

11. Althaus IW, Chou JJ, Gonzalez AJ *et al*. Steady-state kinetic studies with the non-nucleoside HIV-1 reverse transcriptase inhibitor U-87201E. *J Biol Chem* 1993;268:6119–24.

12. Carroll SS, Olsen DB, Bennett CD *et al*. Inhibition of HIV-1 reverse transcriptase by pyridinone derivatives. *J Biol Chem* 1993;268:276–81.

13. Zhang H, Vrang L, Unge T, Oberg B. Characterization of HIV-1 reverse transcriptases with tyr 181 → cys and leu 100 → ile mutations. *Antiviral Chem Chemother* 1993;4:301–8.

14. Taylor PB, Culp JS, Debouck C *et al*. Kinetic and mutational analysis of human immunodeficiency virus type 1 reverse transcriptase inhibition by inophyllums, a novel class of non-nucleoside inhibitors. *J Biol Chem* 1994:269:6325–31.

15. Debyser Z, Pauwels R, Andries K *et al*. An antiviral target on reverse transcriptase of human immunodeficiency virus type 1 revealed by tetrahydroimidazo-[4,5,1-jk] [1,4] benzodiazepine-2(1H)-one and -thione derivatives. *Proc Natl Acad Sci USA* 1991;88:1451–5.

16. Olsen DB, Carroll SS, Culberson JC, Shafer JA, Kuo LC. Effect of template secondary structure on the inhibition of HIV-1 reverse transcriptase by a pyridinone non-nucleoside inhibitor. *Nucleic Acids Res* 1994;22:1437–43.

17. Kopp EB, Miglietta JJ, Shrutkowski AG *et al*. Steady state kinetics and inhibition of HIV-1 reverse transcriptase by a non-nucleoside dipyridodiazepinone, BI-RG-587, using a heteropolymeric template. *Nucleic Acids Res* 1991;19:3035–9.

18. Spence RA, Kati WM, Anderson KS, Johnson KA. Mechanism of inhibition of HIV-1 reverse transcriptase by nonnucleoside inhibitors. *Science* 1995;267:988–93.

19. Wu JC, Warren TC, Adams J *et al*. A novel dipyridodiazepinone inhibitor of

HIV-1 reverse transcriptase acts through a nonsubstrate binding site. *Biochemistry* 1991;30:2022–6.

20. Dueweke TJ, Kezdy FJ, Waszak GA, Deibel MR, Tarpley WG. The binding of a novel bisheteroarylpiperazine mediates inhibition of human immunodeficiency virus type 1 reverse transcriptase. *J Biol Chem* 1992;267:27–30.

21. Kohlstaedt LA, Wang J, Friedman JM, Rice PA, Steitz TA. Crystal structure at 3.5Å resolution of HIV-1 reverse transcriptase complexed with an inhibitor. *Science* 1992;256:1783–90.

22. Smerdon SJ, Jager J, Wang J *et al.* Structure of the binding site for nonnucleoside inhibitors of the reverse transcriptase of human immunodeficiency virus type 1. *Proc Natl Acad Sci USA* 1994;91:3911–5.

23. Jacobo-Molina A, Ding J, Nanni RG *et al.* Crystal structure of human immunodeficiency virus type 1 reverse transcriptase complexed with double-stranded DNA at 3.0 Å resolution shows bent DNA. *Proc Natl Acad Sci USA* 1993;90:6320–4.

24. Tantillo C, Ding J, Jacobo-Molina A *et al.* Location of anti-AIDS drug binding sites and resistance mutations in the three-dimensional structure of HIV-1 reverse transcriptase. *J Mol Biol* 1994;243:369–87.

25. Cohen KA, Hopkins J, Ingraham RJ *et al.* Characterization of the binding site for nevirapine (BI-RG-587), a nonnucleoside inhibitor of human immunodeficiency virus type 1 reverse transcriptase. *J Biol Chem* 1991;266:14670–4.

26. Shih C-K, Rose JM, Hansen GL *et al.* Chimeric human immunodeficiency virus type 1/type 2 reverse transcriptases display reversed sensitivity to nonnucleoside analog inhibitors. *Proc Natl Acad Sci USA* 1991;88:9878–82.

27. Condra JH, Emini EA, Gotlib L *et al.* Identification of the human immunodeficiency virus reverse transcriptase residues that contribute to the activity of diverse nonnucleoside inhibitors. *Antimicrob Agents Chemother* 1992;36:1441–6.

28. Sardana VV, Emini EA, Gotlib L *et al.* Functional analysis of HIV-1 reverse transcriptase amino acids involved in resistance to multiple nonnucleoside inhibitors. *J Biol Chem* 1992;267:17526–30.

29. Rodgers DW, Gamblin SJ, Harris BA *et al.* The structure of unliganded reverse transcriptase from the human immunodeficiency virus type 1. *Proc Natl Acad Sci USA* 1995;92:1222–6.

30. Richman D, Shih C-K, Lowy I *et al.* Human immunodeficiency virus type 1 mutants resistant to nonnucleoside inhibitors of reverse transcriptase arise in cell culture. *Proc Natl Acad Sci USA* 1991;88:11241–5.

31. Nunberg JH, Schleif WA, Boots EJ *et al.* Viral resistance to human immunodeficiency virus type 1-specific pyridinone reverse transcriptase inhibitors. *J Virol* 1991;65:4887–92.

32. Mellors JW, Im G-J, Tramontano E *et al.* A single conservative amino acid substitution in the reverse transcriptase of human immunodeficiency virus-1 confers resistance to (+)-(59)-4,5,6,7-tetrahydro-5-methyl-6-(3-methyl-2-butenyl)imidazo[4,5,1-jk] [1,4] benzodiazepine-2(1H)-thione (TIBO R82150). *Mol Pharmacol* 1993;43:11–6.

33. Buckheit RW, Fliakas-Boltz V, Decker WD *et al.* Comparative anti-HIV evaluation of diverse HIV-1-specific reverse transcriptase inhibitor-resistant virus isolates demonstrates the existence of distinct phenotypic subgroups. *Antiviral Res* 1995;26:117–32.

34. Balzarini J, Karlsson A, Perez-Perez M-J, Camarasa MJ, DeClerq E. Knocking-out concentrations of HIV-1 specific inhibitors completely

suppress HIV-1 infection and prevent the emergence of drug-resistant virus. *Virology* 1993;196:576–85.

35. Kleim JP, Bender R, Kirsch R *et al*. Mutational analysis of residue 190 of human immunodeficiency virus type 1 reverse transcriptase. *Virology* 1994;200:696–701.

36. Balzarini J, Karlsson A, Meichsner C *et al*. Resistance pattern of human immunodeficiency virus type 1 reverse transcriptase to quinoxaline S-2720. *J Virol* 1994;68:7986–92.

37. Bacolla A, Shih C-K, Rose JM *et al*. Amino acid substitutions in HIV-1 reverse transcriptase with corresponding residues from HIV-1. *J Biol Chem* 1992;22:16571–7.

38. Dueweke TJ, Pushkarskaya T, Poppe SM *et al*. A mutation in reverse transcriptase of bis(heteraryl)piperazine-resistant human immunodeficiency virus type 1 confers increased sensitivity to other nonnucleoside inhibitors. *Proc Natl Acad Sci USA* 1993;90:4713–7.

39. Larder BA. 3'-azido-3'-deoxythymidine resistance suppressed by a mutation conferring human immunodeficiency virus type 1 resistance to nonnucleoside reverse transcriptase inhibitors. *Antimicrob Agents Chemother* 1992;36:2664–9.

40. Larder BA, Kellam PK, Kemp SD. Convergent combination therapy can select viable multi-drug resistant HIV-1 *in vitro*. *Nature* 1993;365:451–3.

41. Byrnes VW, Emini EA, Schleif WA *et al*. Susceptibilities of human immunodeficiency virus type 1 enzyme and viral variants expressing multiple resistance-engendering amino acid substitutions to reverse transcriptase inhibitors. *Antimicrob Agents Chemother* 1994;38:1404–7.

42. Saag MS, Emini EA, Laskin OL *et al*. A short clinical trial of L-697,661, a non-nucleoside inhibitor of HIV-1 reverse transcriptase. *New Engl J Med* 1993;329:1065–72.

43. Staszewski S, Massari FE, Kober A *et al*. Combination therapy with zidovudine prevents selection of HIV-1 variants expressing high-level resistance to L-697,661, a nonnucleoside reverse transcriptase inhibitor. *J Infect Dis* (in press).

44. Richman DD, Havlir D, Corbeil J *et al*. Nevirapine resistance mutations of human immunodeficiency virus type 1 selected during therapy. *J Virol* 1994;68:1660–6.

45. Emini EA, Graham DJ, Gotlib L *et al*. HIV and multidrug resistance. *Nature* 1993;364:679.

46. Goldman ME, O'Brien JA, Ruffing TL *et al*. L-696,229 specifically inhibits human immunodeficiency virus type 1 reverse transcriptase and possesses antiviral activity *in vitro*. *Antimicrob Agents Chemother* 1992;36:1019–23.

47. Dueweke TJ, Poppe SM, Romero DL *et al*. U-90152, a potent inhibitor of human immunodeficiency virus type 1 replication. *Antimicrob Agents Chemother* 1993;37:1127–31.

48. Vasudevachari MB, Battista C, Lane HC *et al*. Prevention of the spread of HIV-1 infection with nonnucleoside reverse transcriptase inhibitors. *Virology* 1992;190:269–77.

49. Romero DL, Morge RA, Biles C *et al*. Discovery synthesis and bioactivity of bis(heteroaryl) piperazines. 1. A novel class of non-nucleoside HIV-1 reverse transcriptase inhibitors. *J Med Chem* 1994;37:999–1014.

50. Pauwels R, Andries K, Debyser Z *et al*. Potent and highly selective human immunodeficiency virus type 1 (HIV-1) inhibition by a series of α-anilinophenylacetamide derivatives targeted at HIV-1 reverse transcriptase. *Proc Natl Acad Sci USA* 1993;90:1711–5.

51. Balzarini J, Perez-Perez MJ, San-Felix A et al. 2',5'-Bis -O-(tertbutyldimethylsilyl-3'-spiro-5"-(4"-amino-1",2"-oxathiol-2",2"-dioxide) pyrimidine (TSAO) nucleoside analogues: highly selective inhibitors of human immunodeficiency virus type 1 that are targeted at the viral reverse transcriptase. Proc Natl Acad Sci USA 1992;89:4392–6.

52. Baba M, Tanaka M, De Clercq E et al. Highly specific inhibition of human immunodeficiency virus type 1 by a novel 6-substituted acyclouridine derivative. Biochem Biophys Res Commun 1989;165:1375–81.

53. Baba M, DeClercq E, Tanaka H et al. Potent and selective inhibition of human immunodeficiency virus type 1 (HIV-1) by 5-ethyl-6-phenylthiou-racil derivatives through their interaction with the HIV-1 reverse transcriptase. Proc Natl Acad Sci USA 1991;88:2356–60.

54. Tanaka H, Baba M, Hayakawa H et al. A new class of HIV-1-specific 6-substituted acyclouridine derivatives: synthesis and anti-HIV-1 activity of 5- or 6-substituted analogues of 1-[(2-hydroxyethoxy)methyl]-6-(phenylthio)thymine (HEPT). J Med Chem 1991;34:349–57.

55. Kelim JP, Bender R, Billhardt UM et al. Activity of a novel quinoxaline derivative against human immunodeficiency virus type 1 reverse transcrip-tase and viral replication. Antimicrob Agents Chemother 1993;37:1659–64.

56. Kashman Y, Gustafson KR, Fuller RW et al. The calanolides, a novel HIV-inhibitory class of coumarin derivatives from the tropical rainforest tree, Calophyllum lanigerium. J Med Chem 1992;35:2735–43.

57. Althaus IW, Gonzales AJ, Chou JJ et al. The quinoline U-78036 is a potent inhibitor of HIV-1 reverse transcriptase. J Biol Chem 1993;268:14875–80.

58. Maass G, Immendoerfer U, Koenig B et al. Viral resistance to the thiazolo-iso-indolinones, a new class of nonnucleoside inhibitors of the human immunodeficiency virus type 1 reverse transcriptase. Antimicrob Agents Chemother 1993;37:2612–7.

59. McHamon JB, Gulakowski RJ, Weislow OW et al. Diarylsulfones, a new chemical class of nonnucleoside antiviral inhibitors of human immunodeficiency virus type 1 reverse transcriptase. Antimicrob Agents Chemother 1993;37:754–60.

60. Patil AD, Freyer AJ, Eggleston DS et al. The inophyllums, novel inhibitors of HIV-1 reverse transcriptase isolated from the Malaysian tree, Calophyllum inophyllum Linn. J Med Chem 1993;36:4131–8.

61. Alam M, Bechtold CM, Patick AK et al. Substituted naphthalenones as a new structural class of HIV-1 reverse transcriptase inhibitors. Antiviral Res 1993;22:131–41.

62. Antonucci T, Warmus JS, Hodges JC, Nickell DG. Characterization of the antiviral activity of highly substituted pyrroles: a novel class of non-nucleoside HIV-1 transcriptase inhibitors. Antiviral Chem Chemother 1995;6:98–108.

63. Buckheit RW, Fliakis-Boltz V, Decker WD et al. Biological and biochemical anti-HIV activity of the benzothiadiazine class of nonnucleoside reverse transcriptase inhibitors. Antiviral Res 1994;25:43–56.

64. Rubinek T, McMahon JB, Hizi A. Inhibition of reverse transcriptase of human immunodeficiency virus type 1 and chimeric enzymes of human immunodeficiency viruses type 1 and 2 by two novel non-nucleoside inhibitors. FEBS Lett 1994;350:299–303.

65. Ahgren C, Backro K, Bell FW et al. The PETT series, a new class of potent nonnucleoside inhibitors of human immunodeficiency virus type 1 reverse transcriptase. Antimicrob Agents Chemother 1995;39:1329–35.

66. Johansson N-G, Classon B, Engelhardt P et al. Optimization of antiviral and kinetic properties of PETT compounds, a class of potent non-nucleoside HIV-RT inhibitors. Antiviral Res 1995;26:A257.

67. Byrnes VW, Sardana VV, Schleif WA et al. Comprehensive mutant enzyme and viral variant assessment of human immunodeficiency virus type 1 reverse transcriptase resistance to nonnucleoside inhibitors. Antimicrob Agents Chemother 1993;37:1576–9.

68. Samanta H, Rose R, Patick AK et al. Characterization of a mutant HIV-1 reverse transcriptase resistant to (+)-(5S)-4,5,6,7-tetrahydro-5-methyl-6-(3-methyl-2-butenyl)-imidazo[4,5,1-jk] [1,4]benzodiazepin-2(1H)-thione (TIBO R82150). Antiviral Chem Chemother 1994;5:278–81.

69. Balzarini J, Karlsson A, Perez-Perez M-J et al. Treatment of human immunodeficiency virus type 1 (HIV-1)-infected cells with combinations of HIV-1-specific inhibitors results in a different resistance pattern than does treatment with a single-drug therapy. J Virol 1993;67:5353–9.

70. DeVreese K, Debyser Z, Vandamme A-M et al. Resistance of human immunodeficiency virus type 1 reverse transcriptase to TIBO derivatives induced by site-directed mutagenesis. Virology 1992;188:900–4.

71. Balzarini J, Karlsson A, Vandamme AM et al. Human immunodeficiency virus type-1-specific [2',5'-bis-O-(tert-butyldimethylsilyl)-β-D-ribofuranosyl]-3'-spiro-5'-(4'-amino-1',2"-oxathiole-2',2'-dioxide)-purine analogues show a resistance spectrum that is different from that of human immunodeficiency virus type 1-specific non-nucleoside analogues. Mol Pharmacol 1993;43:109–14.

72. Balzarini J, Karlsson A, Vandamme A-M et al. Human immunodeficiency virus type 1 (HIV-1) strains selected for resistance against the HIV-1-specific [2',5'-bis-O-(tert-butyldimethylsilyl)-3'-spiro-5"-(4"-amino-1",2"-oxathiole-2", 2"-dioxide)]-β-D-pentafuranosyl (TSAO) nucleoside analogues retain sensitivity to HIV-1-specific nonnucleoside inhibitors. Proc Natl Acad Sci USA 1993;90:6952–6.

73. Seki M, Sadakata Y, Yuasa S, Baba M. Isolation and characterization of human immunodeficiency virus type 1 mutants resistant to the non-nucleotide reverse transcriptase inhibitor MKC-442. Antiviral Chem Chemother 1995;6:73–9.

74. Boyer PL, Currens MJ, McMahon JB, Boyd MR, Hughes SH. Analysis of nonnucleoside drug-resistant variants of human immunodeficiency virus type 1 reverse transcriptase. J Virol 1993;67:2412–20.

75. Balzarini J, Karlsson A, DeClercq E. Human immunodeficiency virus type 1 drug resistance patterns with different 1[(2-hydroxyethoxy)methyl]-6-(phenylthio)thymine derivatives. Mol Pharmacol 1993;44:694–701.

76. Nguyen MH, Schinazi RF, Shi C et al. Resistance of human immuno-deficiency virus type 1 to acyclic 6-phenylselenyl- and 6-phenyl-thiopyrimidines. Antimicrob Agents Chemother 1994;38:2409–14.

77. Taylor PB, Culp JS, Debouck C et al. Kinetic and mutational analysis of human immunodeficiency virus type 1 reverse transcriptase inhibition by inophyllums, a novel class of non-nucleoside inhibitors. J Biol Chem 1994;269:6325–31.

78. Young SD, Britcher SF, Tran LO et al. L-743,726 (DMP-266): a novel, highly potent nonnucleoside inhibitor of human immunodeficiency virus type 1 reverse transcriptase. Antimicrob Agents Chemother 1995;39:2602–5.

12

Non-Nucleoside Reverse Transcriptase Inhibitors — Clinical Aspects

DIANE HAVLIR AND DOUGLAS D. RICHMAN

INTRODUCTION

The easy selection of HIV mutants resistant to non-nucleoside reverse transcriptase inhibitors (NNRTI) *in vitro*[1,2] predicted that such mutants would readily emerge in the clinic. The speed at which mutants emerged in the clinical setting permitted the compelling association of the loss of antiretroviral drug activity with the emergence of drug resistance much more easily than could be done with the nucleoside analogs. It also provided a tool to analyze the population dynamics of HIV *in vivo*, and insights with regard to interactions of drug-resistance mutations. The analysis of the relationships between resistance and therapeutic response may provide strategies for the development and use of this class of antiviral drugs.

RAPID SELECTION OF RESISTANCE WITH MONOTHERAPY

NNRTI-resistant virus readily and rapidly emerges in all patients receiving monotherapy with this class of compounds (Table 12.1)[3,4]. In contrast to zidovudine, where the cumulative acquisition of multiple mutations is required to generate large changes in susceptibility, point mutations in the reverse transcriptase (RT) genome are sufficient to confer a 100-fold increase in resistance to NNRTI. Mutations in the RT genome occur in codons which comprise the binding site of the NNRTI

Antiviral Drug Resistance. Edited by Douglas D. Richman © 1996 John Wiley & Sons Ltd

Table 12.1 Mutations to non-nucleoside reverse transcriptase inhibitors identified from clinical isolates*. Reproduced from reference 21 with permission

Compound	Amino acid substitution	Reference
TIBO derivatives (R 82913)	Y188L	5
TIBO derivatives (R 091767)	K101E	33
	K103N	33
	Y181C	33
	K238T	33
Nevirapine	L100I	3
	K103N	3
	V106A	3
	V108I	3
	Y181C/S	3,16,28
	Y188L/H/D	3,28
	G190A/S/L	3,28
Pyridinones (L-697,661)	A98G	13
	K101E/Q	13
	K103Q/N/E	4,13
	V108I	13
	V179D	13
	Y181C	4,13
	Y188C/H/L	13
U-87201 (atevirdine)	K101E	34
	L103A	35
	Y181C	35
	Y188H	34
	E233V	34
	K238T	34
	Y181C	35
U-90152 (delavirdine)	Y181C	36
	K103N/T	36–38
	P236L	36,38
α-APA (loviride)	Y181C/L	39
	K103N	39
	K101E	39
	118	39
	K238T	39
	Y188L/H/C	39
	A98G	39
	L100I	39
	V106A	39
	G190A	39

*Mutations selected *in vitro* are referenced in the previous chapter

in the enzyme. Substitutions at the 181 and 188 positions are common in isolates obtained from patients on the tetrahydroimidazobenzo-diaze-pinone (TIBO) inhibitor, L-697,661 and nevirapine.

Resistance develops quickly in the setting of monotherapy with the NNRTI. A tyrosine to leucine mutation at the 188 position (Y188L) was identified from a clinical isolate three weeks after administration of TIBO R82913 was initiated[5]. In the studies with L-697,661, a greater than eightfold reduction in susceptibility was detected in 11 of 16 subjects within six weeks of the initiation of treatment[4]. In the phase I/II studies of nevirapine, virus isolates obtained from all 24 patients (CD4 cell count <400/mm[3]) displayed at least 100-fold reductions in susceptibility to nevirapine by the eighth week of treatment[3]. Resistant virus was detected as early as one week in some subjects participating in this study, illustrating the dynamic turnover of circulating virus.

Rapid selection of resistant virus with the NNRTI is not limited to HIV-infected patients with advanced disease. Resistant virus was detected in all isolates by 12 weeks in a cohort of 19 patients with over 500 CD4 cells mm[3] administered 400 mg of nevirapine[6]. These observations imply that viral turnover is occurring at a sufficiently rapid rate in these subjects for the imposition of selective pressure with nevirapine to select for resistance rapidly.

The rapid selection of drug-resistant mutants with the initiation of NNRTI monotherapy is dependent on at least two factors. First, the drug-resistant mutant must be present prior to treatment. There are two reports where mutations in the 181 position were identified in subjects with no prior treatment with an NNRTI. In one study a 181 mutant population was selected in culture in the absence of drug in a subject with no prior exposure to NNRTI[7]. In the other study plasma RNA with the Y181C mutation comprised a significant subpopulation in the plasma of a patient before treatment[8]. After one week of nevirapine treatment no antiviral response was detected in this patient and his plasma RNA was predominantly mutant. The Y181C mutation appears to occur at a calculated frequency of 0.7–13 copies per 1000 HIV RNA copies based on mathematical models of virus kinetics[9].

The second factor which must be present for resistant virus to emerge is antiretroviral activity. In the phase I/II studies with L-697,661, resistance was not seen uniformly in patients receiving the lowest doses, in whom evidence of virologic activity was absent. Similarly, resistance to TIBO was not observed at inactive doses. In contrast, in the clinical evaluation of nevirapine, where even the lowest doses demonstrated antiviral activity, resistance was detected consistently in all isolates evaluated.

RESISTANCE WITH COMBINATION THERAPY

The simplest and earliest clinical strategy to delay or prevent resistance to NNRTI was to administer zidovudine in combination. Such combination studies were encouraged by preclinical data demonstrating that HIV resistant to either zidovudine or NNRTI was not cross-resistant to the other class of drugs, and that combination therapy was in fact synergistic[10]. Moreover, studies in animals suggested that NNRTI would not produce overlapping toxicity with zidovudine.

Combination zidovudine–nevirapine therapy neither delayed nor prevented the emergence of resistant virus[3]. Viral isolates obtained from all patients on combination therapy exhibited high-level resistance to nevirapine by 12 weeks of therapy. Although there was no difference in the *in vitro* inhibitory concentrations of the resistant strains between the nevirapine monotherapy and zidovudine–nevirapine combination therapy-treated patients, the point mutations conferring resistance differed between the two groups (Table 12.2). In the nevirapine mono-therapy group the predominant mutation was at the 181 position. In contrast, patients receiving nevirapine combined with zidovudine were more likely to have mutations at the 188 or 190 positions. There were no Y181C mutations identified in any of 44 isolates from the 14 patients on combination therapy.

The presence of zidovudine thus appears to exert a selective pressure upon the virus to utilize an alternative evolutionary pathway to evade inhibition by nevirapine. This effect of zidovudine on nevirapine-resistance mutations may be explained by *in vitro* studies by Larder[11].

Table 12.2 *Emergence of isolates of HIV with reduced susceptibility and resistance mutations with nevirapine therapy. From reference 3, with permission*

Weeks of therapy	1	2	4	8	≥12
Cumulative proportion with reduced susceptibility	3/3	12/14	23/26	32/32	38/38
Cumulative proportion with a known resistance mutation*		6/8	18/21	30/30	38/38
Either	3/3	12/15	24/26	33/33	38/38

* Mutations identified: K103N, V106A, V108I, Y181C, Y181S, Y188L, Y188H, Y188D, G190A, G190S, G190L. The effects of some allelic variations, i.e. 188D, 190S, 190L, on susceptibility to nevirapine have not been fully characterized by site-directed mutagenesis.
The table combines results of 24 patients receiving nevirapine monotherapy and 14 patients receiving combination therapy with AZT

The Y181C mutation that confers nevirapine resistance reverses the phenotypic effects of mutations at residue 215 which diminish susceptibility to zidovudine. This *in vitro* observation was confirmed by observations in patients with zidovudine-resistant virus treated with nevirapine[3,12]. In patients on nevirapine monotherapy, the reversal of zidovudine susceptibility has no immediate negative impact on virus replication; however, the combination of the 215 and 181 mutations is of some benefit to the virus. Under selective pressure of combination therapy with nevirapine and zidovudine alternative mutations conferring nevirapine resistance emerge, allowing the phenotypic expression of resistance to both drugs.

The combination of the pyridinone derivative L-697,661 with zidovudine similarly did not prevent the emergence of resistance, but did change the pattern of resistance mutations that quickly emerged with therapy[13]. As with nevirapine, the Y181C mutations emerge most readily with L-697,661 monotherapy to confer high-level resistance[3,4,13]; concomitant therapy with zidovudine prevented the emergence of this mutation[13]. In contrast to nevirapine, however, the alternative mutations that emerged with L-697,661 did not confer the greater than 100-fold reductions in susceptibility seen with the Y181C mutation. These data are not directly comparable to those of nevirapine because antiviral activity was not well documented and the susceptibility of virus isolates was not presented[13]. Nevertheless, these data provide support for the proposal of convergent combination therapy whereby combinations directed to the same viral target might constrain the flexibility of evolutionary options for successful drug resistance to one of the components of the combination[14].

NNRTI-resistant virus was also readily selected in combination studies with atevirdine (U-87201E) and zidovudine[15]. In a phase I trial, 15 HIV-infected patients with CD4 cell counts below 500 μl and no previous zidovudine experience were administered 600 mg of atevirdine and 200 mg of zidovudine every eight hours. Owing to the complex pharmacokinetics and high degree of interindividual variability, the daily doses of atevirdine were adjusted in order to maintain plasma levels in the 5–10 μmol range. Susceptibility to atevirdine gradually diminished over time; at 24 weeks the median IC_{50} increased from 1.83 to 37 μmol. Although five of 13 subjects exhibited significantly decreased susceptibility (defined as a 100-fold reduction in IC_{50} compared to baseline, or a single IC_{50} greater than 30 μmol to atevirdine at 24 weeks), an increasingly resistant atevirdine viral population was being selected over time. A failure to achieve therapeutic drug levels capable of producing an antiviral effect in all the patients may explain the absence of high-level resistance in this study.

As with combination therapy, an alternating regimen of nevirapine and zidovudine did not prevent the selection of drug-resistant virus[16]. The investigators had hypothesized that a treatment strategy of cycles of one week nevirapine followed by three weeks of zidovudine might be able to delay the emergence of drug-resistant virus by either limiting the exposure to nevirapine and thereby reducing the selective pressure, or by producing competitive selective pressures that might favor virus susceptible to nevirapine. Serum p24 antigen values declined after the first, but not subsequent cycles, of nevirapine. After two courses of therapy (eight weeks), the susceptibilities of viral isolates to nevirapine from two patients had diminished by 40- and 1000-fold. The absence of continuous selective pressure did not appear to prevent resistance or to favor reversion to nevirapine-susceptible virus.

The finding that combination or alternating NNRTI–zidovudine therapy could not prevent the emergence of resistant mutants was discouraging but not unexpected. Multidrug therapy has successfully prevented the development of resistance in settings such as tuberculosis, where at least one of the drugs effectively reduces the organism burden to a level where the remaining population is not large enough to contain mutants resistant to the second drug. The available nucleoside analogs and the NNRTI are capable of reducing the circulating HIV RNA by less than 100-fold. Circulating plasma HIV RNA levels range from 10^2 to 10^7 copies/ml. Higher virus levels are seen in lymphoid tissue. Thus, even a combination regimen of zidovudine and NNRTI permits the survival of a large virus population in the plasma and lymphoid tissues that can serve as a reservoir for the selection of resistant virus. At the present time, then, the rationale for combination therapy with nucleosides and NNRTI is to identify combinations of drugs that might improve the suppression of the viral burden by additive or synergistic antiviral activity, rather than by preventing resistance.

COMPLEXITY OF VIRAL MIXTURES *IN VIVO* AND VIRAL FITNESS

Although rapid selection *in vitro* for virus resistant to NNRTI predicted the rapid emergence of resistance during clinical trials, the virus population that emerged in patients administered NNRTI were much more genetically complex. Genetic heterogeneity of HIV within and between individuals is well documented, especially when examining *env* sequences; however, genetic variation is more limited in the gene for reverse transcriptase[17]. Mixtures of wild-type and mutant virus and mixtures of different mutants were frequently observed after the initiation of nevirapine therapy[3]. Table 12.3 depicts the complex combinations of virus identified in a patient with a one-year history of prior zidovudine therapy.

Prior to the addition of 12.5 mg of nevirapine daily, this patient carried an RT sequence that already included two zidovudine (AZT)-resistance mutations, M41L and T215Y. After a single passage in peripheral blood mononuclear cells of virus isolated from this patient, the RT gene was sequenced both by asymmetric RT PCR and from four clones from independent PCRs of DNA from the cells in which the virus propagated. A number of observations could be made. First, with only a few exceptions the population sequence for the supernatant RNA reflected the sequences of clones in the cell pellet DNA. Secondly, even with the baseline specimen, a swarm or genetic mixture of virus was isolated from the patient, as indicated by amino acid residue 43. Thirdly, a nevirapine-resistance mutation (K103N) emerged within only four weeks of nevirapine therapy. Fourthly, at 16 weeks two different populations of nevirapine-resistant virus were co-circulating (K103N and V106A). Fifthly, at 32 weeks nevirapine-resistant virus with a third mutation had emerged (G190A) in the K103N background sequence but not in the V106A subpopulation of this genetic mixture. The G190A mutation also appeared in the earlier circulating virus that contained neither the K103N nor the V106A mutation. The population containing both the K103N and G190A mutations was observed on a background of signature amino acids at residues 44, 67 and 75 distinct from any viruses previously sequenced. Of note, D67N represents an additional zidovudine resistance mutation to M41L and T215Y. Sixthly, drug susceptibility values for both nevirapine and zidovudine generated with independent isolates at each time point showed a much greater variability than usually found. These genetic sequence data would explain this great phenotypic variability.

Data from this patient indicated that populations or genetic variants were in constant flux, with the frequent appearance of additional and different mutations. Examination of the sequences from various patients has suggested that the greatest number of mixtures and the highest frequency of new mutations occurred within the first 12 weeks of therapy, after which time a more stable population appeared to establish itself. This observation is consistent with the general principles of RNA virus population genetics, in which a master sequence (the most fit member of a mutant spectrum) emerges under selective pressures to generate a new consensus sequence (see Chapter 14).

The fitness of this genotypically altered virus selected by drug pressure is indicated by the observation that six patients who were withdrawn from nevirapine therapy retained their drug-resistant virus

Table 12.3 Amino acid sequences deduced from nucleotide sequencing of portions of the RT gene of sequential isolates of HIV-1 from patient 453 treated with AZT and nevirapine. From reference 3, with permission

Amino acid residue number		41	43	44	67	70	75	103	106	135	181	188	190	210	215	219	254
Consensus amino acid		M	K	E	D	K	V	K	V	I	Y	Y	G	L	T	K	V
Week 0	clone 1	L	.	.	.	.	.	.	.	T	.	.	.	W	Y	.	.
	clone 2	L	.	.	.	.	.	.	.	T	.	.	.	W	Y	.	.
	clone 3	L	Q	.	.	.	.	.	.	T	.	.	.	W	Y	.	.
	clone 4	L	Q	.	.	.	.	.	.	T	.	.	.	W	Y	.	.
	population sequence	L	Q/K$_{mix}$	.	.	.	.	.	.	T	.	.	.	W	Y	.	.
Week 4	population sequence	L	Q	.	.	.	.	N	.	T	.	.	.	W	Y	.	.
Week 16	clone 1	L	Q	.	.	.	.	.	A	T	.	.	.	W	Y	.	.
	clone 2	L	Q	.	.	.	.	N	.	T	.	.	.	W	Y	.	.
	clone 3	L	Q	.	.	.	.	.	A	T	.	.	.	W	Y	T	.
	clone 4	L	Q	.	.	.	.	.	A	T	.	.	.	W	Y	.	.
	population sequence	L	Q	.	.	.	.	.	V/A$_{mix}$	T	.	.	.	W	Y	.	.
Week 32	clone 1	L	Q	.	.	.	.	.	.	T	.	.	A	W	Y	.	G
	clone 2	L	.	D	N	.	M	N	.	T	.	.	A	W	Y	.	.
	clone 3	L	.	D	N	.	M	N	.	T	.	.	A	W	Y	.	.
	clone 4	L	.	D	N	.	M	.	.	T	.	.	A	W	Y	.	.
	population sequence	L	Q	.	.	.	.	.	.	T	.	.	A	W	Y	.	.

A, alanine; D, aspartic acid; E, glutamic acid; G, glycine; I, isoleucine; K, lysine; L, leucine; M, methionine; N, asparagine; Q, glutamine; T, threonine; V, valine; W, tryptophane; Y, tyrosine

for at least 20 months (unpublished data). Thus, the wild-type pheno-type and genotype did not quickly re-emerge after the withdrawal of the selective pressure of nevirapine therapy, similar to *in vitro* observations. In addition, the pathogenicity of the altered virus was evident by the immunologic and clinical deterioration that occurred in patients with resistant virus[18].

RELATIONSHIP BETWEEN RESISTANCE AND ANTIVIRAL ACTIVITY

Although L-697,661 and nevirapine rapidly selected for drug resistance *in vivo*, the critical question in terms of the ultimate utility of these drugs as therapeutic agents for HIV infection was whether this selection resulted in the complete loss of antiviral activity. The answer to this question initially appeared to be quite straightforward, based on the observations made during the initial studies with L-697,661 and nevirapine[3,4,16,18,19]. The selection of resistant virus was associated with the loss of antiviral activity.

The majority of patients treated with L-697,661 experienced a reduction of p24 antigen and an increase in CD4 cell counts a week after drug therapy initiation. Six weeks later these signs of antiviral activity were lost, coincident with the emergence of resistant virus[4]. Similar results were reported by Cheeseman *et al.* in the phase I/II dose escalation studies with nevirapine[18]. Patients were treated with doses of nevirapine ranging from 12.5 to 200 mg daily. Based on previous single-dose pharmacokinetic studies, it was predicted that drug levels that exceeded the inhibitory concentration of the wild-type virus by at least 100-fold would be achieved[20]. Although hepatic enzyme induction resulted in plasma concentrations of nevirapine slightly lower than predicted at the highest dose, these levels still far exceeded *in vitro* inhibitory concentrations. In all patients studied, p24 antigen rapidly diminished and CD4 cell count increased within the first few weeks of drug initiation (Figure 12.1). Within weeks the antiviral effect was lost and was associated with the selection of nevirapine-resistant virus. In more detailed studies of viral burden utilizing PCR-based assays, the transient changes in antiviral effect have been confirmed. Thus, in contrast to zidovudine, where the relationship between *in vitro* resistance and antiviral activity is complex and variable between individuals (see Chapter 10), data generated during the early clinical studies with L-697,661 and nevirapine suggested a very straightforward relationship between the selection of resistance *in vivo* and antiviral activity.

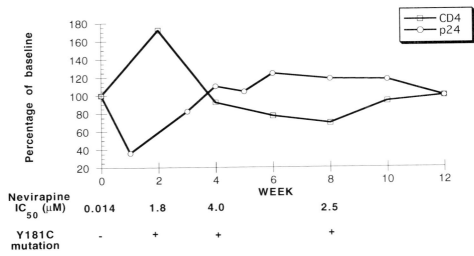

Figure 12.1 *Effect of nevirapine therapy on viral markers, CD4 cell counts, and drug resistance. Patient 154 was administered 12.5 mg of nevirapine daily. The responses at the indicated weeks with regard to CD4 lymphocyte count, HIV p24 antigen level in serum, nevirapine susceptibility and the Y181C-resistance mutation of the patient's virus isolate are depicted. From reference 3, with permission*

ACTIVITY DESPITE RESISTANCE

For a number of reasons the clinical development of the NNRTI proceeded despite the observations that resistance was associated with a loss of activity. In general, this class of compounds was relatively easy to synthesize, had very favorable pharmacokinetics in terms of oral bioavailability and half-life, and appeared relatively non-toxic. Further dose escalation studies of nevirapine were conducted to test the hypothesis that by obtaining drug levels that exceeded the inhibitory concentrations of resistant virus, sustained antiviral activity could be attained.

The initial results of dose-escalation studies with nevirapine produced some very promising data[21]. Twenty-one patients were administered 400 mg of nevirapine daily and in eight of these a sustained reduction of p24 antigen was achieved (Figure 12.2). There was no delay in the selection of nevirapine-resistant virus, and the genotypic changes conferring resistance resembled those seen at lower doses. Not all subjects studied demonstrated sustained antiviral effect with the 400 mg dose of nevirapine. The 'responders' (those with sustained suppression of p24 antigen) and the 'non-responders' could be different-iated in this small study by the presence of higher plasma nevirapine

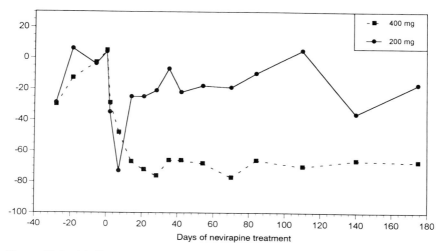

Figure 12.2 *Median percentage change from baseline of immune complex-dissociated (ICD) serum HIV p24 antigen levels over time in patients receiving 200 or 400 mg/day nevirapine. From reference 21, with permission*

levels[22] (Figure 12.3). Plasma nevirapine levels exceeded the IC_{50} of the patients' isolates by three- to fourfold. A multivariate analysis of three nevirapine clinical studies has confirmed that drug levels are an independent predictor of response. The risk of being a non-responder is seven times higher in patients with nevirapine trough levels less than 4 μg/ml[12]. Similar observations demonstrating drug exposure–activity relationships with delavirdine have been made.

Achieving even higher plasma levels could potentially produce more durable and consistent suppression of NNRTI-resistant virus. Unfortunately, dose escalation beyond 600 mg of nevirapine daily has not been possible owing to drug toxicity. Almost 50% of patients developed a rash at the 400 mg daily dose. Although the incidence of rash was reduced using a dose escalation strategy (200 mg for two weeks, followed by 400 mg), at 600 mg daily dosing the incidence and severity of rash was felt to be intolerable[23]. Rash is also a dose-limiting toxicity for delavirdine.

The level of resistance is a second parameter that distinguishes responders from non-responders[12]. Although all patients who are treated with nevirapine have isolates that are more than 100 times less susceptible to drug than their pretherapy isolates, the isolates from treated patients who sustain suppression of p24 antigen or HIV RNA tend to have susceptibilities below 10 μM. In contrast, patients with only transient responses develop isolates with IC_{50}s above 20 μM. The isolates

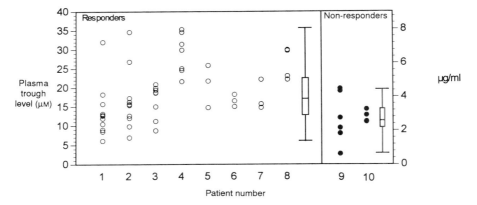

Figure 12.3   *Steady-state plasma trough levels of nevirapine in responders (patients with sustained reduction in p24 antigen at eight weeks) and non-responders (no sustained antiviral response). Horizontal lines in bars, median plasma trough levels for groups: upper and lower ends of bars are 25th and 75th percentiles, respectively: vertical lines represent to 1.5 times range of boxes. From reference 21, with permission*

with the highest IC_{50} values tended to contain both drug-resistance mutations V108I and Y181C if they were on nevirapine monotherapy, and Y188L or G190A mutations if they were on AZT combination therapy. The question arises why highly resistant viruses with these mutations emerge only in some patients. Perhaps the backbone sequence of reverse transcriptase may affect the phenotypic consequences and evolutionary options of any given resistance mutation. Other factors that do not determine whether a patient becomes a sustained or transient responder to nevirapine include such pretreatment characteristics as stage of disease, CD4 cell count, HIV RNA, and the presence of isolate with syncytium-inducing phenotype.

NNRTI COMBINED WITH MULTIPLE NUCLEOSIDE ANALOGS

Although the same rationale that exists for two-drug combination therapy applies for triple-drug therapy, i.e. to achieve additive or synergistic effects, the clinical testing of triple-drug therapy with the NNRTI was launched at an unprecedented pace in the hope of achieving the same results *in vivo* as were reported by Chow *et al. in vitro*[14]. Combining multiple drugs active against a single viral target, reverse transcriptase for example, was proposed as a strategy to exploit the different resistance mutations that emerge with each drug. This strategy, termed convergent combination therapy, would succeed if the combinations of mutations forced by these multiple drugs impaired the replicative capacity of the virus. Viral evolution would then have to choose between an attenuated virus resistant to the drug combination, or a more virulent virus susceptible to a component of the chemotherapy. Unfortunately, some of the data in the original paper were flawed; resistance to NNRTI and multiple nucleoside were constructed *in vitro*[24,25] and identified in clinical isolates[3].

Nevertheless, the benefit of adding an NNRTI to a two-drug regimen of zidovudine and ddI was tested directly in the AIDS Clinical Trials Group (ACTG) study 241[26]. In this double-blinded randomized study the combination of zidovudine and ddI was compared to zidovudine, ddI and nevirapine. All patients had more than six months' prior zidovudine experience and CD4 cell counts below 350/mm[3]. Four hundred patients were randomized and followed for 48 weeks. CD4 cell counts were 25% higher in patients on triple-drug therapy at the end of the study. Reductions in HIV RNA and quantitative HIV cultures favored triple-drug therapy at eight weeks, but not at the end of the study. Additional analyses of RNA and virus susceptibility are under way, but it is likely that resistant virus was selected in both treatment arms. As with the phase I/II studies with nevirapine, some subjects exhibited a sustained suppression of HIV RNA whereas others appeared to lose the antiviral response. Investigations are in progress to confirm whether characteristics (nevirapine plasma levels and susceptibilities) that correlated with sustained responses in the phase I/II studies predict responses in ACTG 241.

Similarly, the addition of delavirdine to zidovudine plus ddI has been reported to be superior to the two-drug therapy in all of the virologic and immunologic parameters evaluated[27]. Sixty percent of 47 subjects in the three-drug versus none of the subjects in the two-drug regimen had a 50% reduction in p24 antigen. Plasma RNA decreased by 44% in the three-drug regimen, versus 12.5% in the two-drug regimen. A tenfold decrease in plasma viremia was seen in 77% of the patients on three drugs compared to 25% of patients on the two-drug regimen. Resistance assays and genotypic analysis of viral isolates from study participants have not been published, although in another unpublished study of delavirdine and zidovudine 70% of subjects had at least 100-fold reduction in susceptibility in the first 24 weeks. Despite the selection of resistant virus, sustained suppression of p24 antigen was still observed in some patients and was more likely to occur in subjects with higher delavirdine levels.

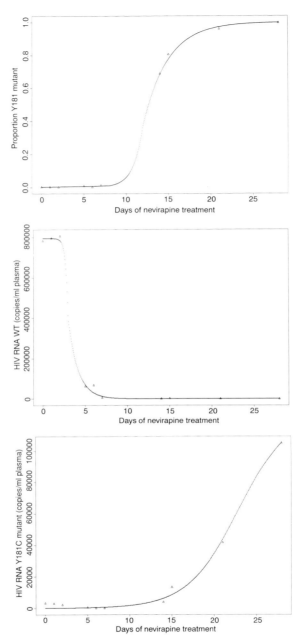

Figure 12.4 Dynamics or populations of HIV RNA in plasma of a patient treated with nevirapine. Proportion of Y181C mutant (top panel), logistic curve fitted to 181 wild-type virus population (middle panel) and 181 mutant (lower panel). The half-life of wild-type virus was 0.81 days and the doubling time of the Y181C mutant was 2.1 days. The estimated frequency of the Y181C mutant prior to treatment is $6.8/10^5$ HIV RNA copies. From reference 9 with permission

KINETICS OF RESISTANCE

The rapid selection of resistant virus which had been detected in isolates from patients on the phase I/II studies of L-697,661 and nevirapine suggested that the virus must be rapidly turning over in order to produce such dynamic changes in viral genotype[3,4]. Wei *et al.*[28] used mathematical models to estimate rates of viral clearance and production in patients who added nevirapine to a stable regimen of nucleoside antiviral therapy.

The rate of decline of HIV RNA followed an exponential decay curve, and estimates of viral half-life ranged from 1.5 to 2 days depending on the mathematical model used. These estimates of viral half-life did not appear to vary among the patients within the range of CD4 cell counts ($18-355$ cells/mm^3) or baseline HIV RNA (10^4-10^7) copies per ml. Direct viral population sequencing was used to evaluate the viral populations of four subjects in detail. Virus with nevirapine mutations replaced the wild-type virus completely within two to four weeks of initiation of drug therapy. The ratios of mutant to wild-type virus over time were utilized to calculate viral doubling time, which was estimated to be two days.

The turnover of wild-type to resistant virus was much slower and not as complete in the PBMC as in the plasma. By 20 weeks only $50-80\%$ of the PBMC pool harbored nevirapine-resistant virus. Thus it is the plasma viral pool which rapidly responds to drug pressure and selects for a more viable population with a distinct survival advantage. Although drug pressures eventually result in the turnover of a proportion of the reverse transcripts in the PBMC, the majority of these cells do appear not to be the reservoir for the rapidly replicating plasma viral pool. It is not clear whether this DNA in PBMC represents HIV genome that is latent or replication defective.

Similar findings were observed in a small study of viral dynamics in patients starting nevirapine monotherapy[9]. More frequent measurements of HIV RNA than those performed by Wei *et al.* during the first 72 hours of treatment led to estimates of slightly faster viral production and clearance ($0.61-1.45$ days). Utilizing differential PCR to quantify viral wild-type and mutant populations during the course of therapy it was estimated that the frequency of nevirapine-resistant mutations in an untreated population ranges from 0.7 to 13.3 per 1000 plasma HIV RNA copies (Figure 12.4). This estimate is in close agreement with purely theoretical estimates made on viral population dynamics[29]. The doubling time ($3.3-5.7$ days) of nevirapine-resistant virus appears longer than that of wild type in treated individuals. This may represent either a decrease in fitness of the mutant compared to wild-type virus, which would be consistent with the low frequency of mutants in untreated patients, or partial suppression by continuing nevirapine treatment of the more resistant viral population.

USE OF SUSCEPTIBILITY MEASUREMENTS IN PATIENT MANAGEMENT

Would susceptibility testing or the determination of drug-resistance mutations permit more effective use of NNRTIs? At present there is not sufficient information to justify these costly procedures for individual patient management. We know that for doses of NNRTI that exhibit antiviral activity, whether as monotherapy or in combination, the rapid emergence of drug-resistant virus occurs in all patients within several months. As mentioned earlier, sustained responses correlate with higher plasma nevirapine levels and lower IC_{50} values for resistant virus. It is likely that measuring plasma drug levels may prove more useful for drug administration than drug susceptibility measurements.

The detailed analysis of resistance which has been performed on this class of compounds has led to important advances and insights into drug activity. At present the assessment of a patient's response to therapy by evaluating changes in immunologic parameters (CD4 cell counts) or viral burden (HIV RNA), which assess the cumulative effects of drug activity, antiviral drug resistance and viral replicative capacity, will be more likely to contribute to patient management than will a determination of virus phenotype. The most effective ways to use NNRTI, should they in fact prove useful, clearly requires additional study.

TRANSMISSION OF NNRTI-RESISTANT VIRUS

Transmission of zidovudine-resistant virus is well documented (see Chapter 10). To date, there have been no reports of the transmission of NNRTI-resistant virus, although there is no theoretical reason to think that NNRTI virus is any less transmissible than wild-type virus. The primary existence of amino acids in codon 181 of the RT genome that confer resistance to NNRTI has been found in clinical isolates[7,30], as well as in HIV-2[31] and 'O' group HIV-1 isolates[32]. As mentioned earlier, such resistant variants occur naturally in HIV-1 at a frequency of about 1 in 1000, and rapidly emerge with NNRTI therapy. Even with the discontinuation of therapy, the continued presence of a nevirapine-resistant population has been documented for up to two years, thus providing ample opportunity for transmission of strains from individuals even with only brief exposure to nevirapine[3].

IMPLICATIONS FROM THE CLINICAL SIGNIFICANCE OF NNRTI RESISTANCE FOR THE DEVELOPMENT OF OTHER ANTIRETROVIRAL AGENTS

The systematic evaluation of NNRTI and the drug resistance associated with treatment with this class of compounds have provided important insights regarding HIV population dynamics and potential approaches to design effective chemotherapy despite the emergence of drug resistance. Time is required to determine whether these efforts will also result in more effective chemotherapy for HIV infection.

The lessons learned from these clinical studies of NNRTI may prove directly applicable to other drugs, especially protease inhibitors which, like NNRTI, are not subject to complex intracellular metabolism:

1. The emergence of drug resistance occurs with drugs and doses that exhibit antiretroviral activity.
2. The loss of antiretroviral drug activity is associated with the loss of drug susceptibility and the acquisition of drug-resistance mutations.
3. The mutations that emerge *in vivo* tend to be more varied and complex than those that emerge with selection *in vitro*.
4. The co-administration of other reverse transcriptase inhibitors confers selective pressures that may force the emergence of alternative drug-resistance mutations. It is possible that certain resistant mutants would have impaired replicative capacities, resulting in diminished virulence.
5. Genetic variants that include drug-resistant mutants circulate as minor subpopulations in the absence of treatment. Treatment selects for the emergence of these variants as the predominant population.
6. There may be constraints on the mutability of the reverse transcriptase of HIV, such that the cumulative acquisition of mutations does not usually occur. Thus effective treatment of virus resistant to NNRTI with sustained activity may be possible if high plasma drug levels can be attained that sufficiently exceed the susceptibility of the resistant virus. These conclusions would encourage the search for drugs with greater potency and superior pharmacologic properties that permit sustained high drug levels.

Clinical trials continue with this class of compounds. Studies of antiviral activity and drug resistance should provide additional insights into drug discovery and viral pathogenesis. The best lessons would be how to provide more effective chemotherapeutic management of HIV infection.

NOTE IN PROOF

Recent data demonstrate that resistance to nevirapine is prevented for up to a year when administered in combination with two other nucleoside analogues (AZT and ddI) as a triple drug regimen in previously untreated HIV-infected patients. This observation implies that a level of viral suppression sufficient to prevent the emergence of virus resistant to nevirapine is achievable, and indicates a very promising clinical utility of non-nucleoside reverse transcriptase inhibitors as part of combination regimens to completely suppress HIV replication.

REFERENCES

1. Nunberg JH, Schleif WA, Boots EJ et al. Viral resistance to human immunodeficiency virus type 1-specific pyridinone reverse transcriptase inhibitors. *J Virol* 1991;65:4887–92.
2. Richman DD, Shih C-K, Lowy I et al. HIV-1 mutants resistant to non-nucleoside inhibitors of reverse transcriptase arise in tissue culture. *Proc Natl Acad Sci USA* 1991;88:11241–5.
3. Richman DD, Havlir D, Corbeil J et al. Nevirapine resistance mutations of human immunodeficiency virus type 1 selected during therapy. *J Virol* 1994;68:1660–6.
4. Saag MS, Emini EA, Laskin OL et al. A short-term clinical evaluation of L-697,661, a non-nucleoside inhibitor of HIV-1 reverse transcriptase. *New Eng J Med* 1993;329:1065–72.
5. Vandamme A-M, Debyser Z, Pauwels R et al. Characterization of HIV-1 strains isolated from patients treated with TIBO R82913. *AIDS Res Hum Retroviruses* 1994;10:39–46.
6. Havlir D, McLaughlin MM, Richman DD. A pilot study to evaluate the development of resistance to nevirapine in asymptomatic human immuno-deficiency virus-infected patients with CD4 cell counts of >500/mm^3: AIDS Clinical Trials Group Protocol 208. *J Infect Dis* 1995;172:1379–83.
7. Nájera I, Richman DD, Olivares I et al. Natural occurrence of drug resistance mutations in the reverse transcriptase of human immunodeficiency virus type 1 isolates. *AIDS Res Hum Retroviruses* 1994;10:1479–88.
8. de Jong MD, Schuurman R, Lange JMA, Boucher CAB. Replication of a pre-existing resistant HIV-1 subpopulation *in vivo* after introduction of a strong selective drug pressure. *Antiviral Ther* 1996;1:33–41.
9. Havlir D, Eastman S, Gamst A, Richman DD. Nevirapine resistant virus: kinetics of replication and estimated prevalence in untreated patients. *J Viol* 1996 (in press).
10. Richman DD, Rosenthal AS, Skoog M et al. BI-RG-587 is active against zidovudine-resistant human immunodeficiency virus type 1 and synergistic with zidovudine. *Antimicrob Agents Chemother* 1991;35:305–8.
11. Larder BA. 3'-Azido-3'-deoxthymidine resistance suppressed by a mutation conferring human immunodeficiency virus type 1 resistance to nonnucleoside reverse transcriptase inhibitors. *Antimicrob Agents Chemother* 1992;36:2664–9.
12. Havlir DV, Johnson VA, Hall DB et al. Factors determining sustained antiviral response to nevirapine. *J AIDS* 1995;10(suppl. 3):S10–11.

13. Staszewski S, Massari FE, Kober A *et al.* Combination therapy with zidovudine prevents selection of human immunodeficiency virus type 1 variants expressing high-level resistance to L-697,661, a nonnucleoside reverse transcriptase inhibitor. *J Infect Dis* 1995;171:1159–65.

14. Chow Y-K, Hirsch MS, Merrill DP *et al.* Replication incompatible and replication compromising combinations of HIV-1 RT drug resistance mutations. *Nature* 1993;361:650–4.

15. Reichman RC, Morse GD, Demeter LM *et al.* Phase I study of atevirdine, a nonnucleoside reverse transcriptase inhibitor in combination with zidovudine for human immunodeficiency virus type 1 infection. *J Infect Dis* 1995;171:297–304.

16. de Jong MD, Loewenthal M, Boucher CAB *et al.* Alternating nevirapine and zidovudine treatment of human immunodeficiency virus type 1-infected persons does not prolong nevirapine activity. *J Infect Dis* 1994;169:1346–50.

17. Richman DD. Drug resistance in relation to pathogenesis. *AIDS* 1995; 9(Suppl A):S49–53.

18. Cheeseman SH, Havlir D, McLaughlin MM *et al.* Phase I/II evaluation of nevirapine alone and in combination with zidovudine for infection with human immunodeficiency virus. *J AIDS* 1995;8:141–51.

19. Davey RT, Dewar RL, Reed GF *et al.* Plasma viremia as a sensitive indicator of the antiretroviral activity of L-697,661. *Proc Natl Acad Sci USA* 1993;90:5608–12.

20. Cheeseman SH, Hattox SE, McLaughlin MM *et al.* Pharmacokinetics of nevirapine: initial single-rising-dose study in humans. *Antimicrob Agents Chemother* 1993;37:178–82.

21. Havlir D, Cheeseman SH, McLaughlin M *et al.* High dose nevirapine: safety, pharmacokinetics, and antiviral effect in patients with human immunodeficiency virus infection. *J Infect Dis* 1995;171:537–45.

22. Havlir D, The ACTG 164 and 168 Study Teams. Antiviral activity of nevirapine at 400 mg in p24 antigen positive adults. IXth International Conference on AIDS/IVth STD World Congress, Berlin, Germany. 6–11 June 1993; [Abstract].

23. Havlir D, Murphy R, Saag M *et al.* Nevirapine: further dose escalation of monotherapy (600 mg daily) and combination therapy with zidovudine. First National Conference on Human Retroviruses and Related Infections, Washington DC, December 1993;101 [Abstract].

24. Larder BA, Kellam P, Kemp SD. Convergent combination therapy can select viable multidrug-resistant HIV-1 *in vitro. Nature* 1993;365:451–3.

25. Emini EA, Graham DJ, Gotlib L *et al.* HIV and multidrug resistance. *Nature* 1993;364:679.

26. D'Aquila R, Hughes M, Liou S-H. A comparative study of a combination of zidovudine, didanosine, and double-blinded nevirapine versus a combination of zidovudine and didanosine. Second National Conference on Human Retroviruses and Related Infections. Washington DC, 29 January–2 February 1995; [Abstract].

27. Freimuth WW. Update on delavirdine mesylate non-nucleoside RTI: virology, PK, safety and clinical surrogate marker response. Fourth Triennial Symposium on New Directions in Antiviral Chemotherapy. San Francisco, CA: 10–12 Nov 1994; [Abstract].

28. Wei X, Ghosh SK, Taylor ME *et al.* Viral dynamics in human immunodeficiency virus type 1 infection. *Nature* 1995;373:117–22.

29. Coffin JM. HIV population dynamics *in vivo*: implications for genetic variation, pathogenesis and therapy. *Science* 1995;267:483–9.
30. Nájera I, Holguín A, Quiñones-Mateu ME *et al. pol* gene quasispecies of human immunodeficiency virus: mutations associated with drug resistance in virus from patients undergoing no drug therapy. *J Virol* 1995;69:23–31.
31. Shih C-K, Rose JM, Hansen GL *et al.* Chimeric human immunodeficiency virus type 1/type 2 reverse transcriptase display reversed sensitivity to nonnucleoside analog inhibitors. *Proc Natl Acad Sci USA* 1991;88:9878–82.
32. Descamps D, Collin G, Loussert-Ajaka I *et al.* HIV-1 group O sensitivity to antiretroviral drugs. *J AIDS* 1995;10(suppl. 3):S8 .
33. Moeremans M, De Raeymaeker M, Van den Broek R *et al.* Virological analysis of HIV-1 isolates in patients treated with the non-nucleoside reverse transcriptase inhibitor R091767, (-)-(S)-8-chloro-4,5,6,7-tetrahydro-5-methyl-6-(3-methyl-2-butenyl)imidazo[4,5,1-jk][1,4]benzodiazepine-2(1H)-tihone monohydrochloride (8-chloro-tibo). *J AIDS* 1995;10(Suppl. 3):S15.
34. Demeter LM, Resnick L, Tarpley WG *et al.* HIV-1 resistance to atevirdine (ATV), a bisheteroaryl piperazine (BHAP) non-nucleoside reverse transcriptase inhibitor (NNRTI), is associated with multiple reverse transcriptase (RT) mutations. Second International HIV Drug Resistance Workshop, Noordwijk, The Netherlands. 3–5 June 1993; [Abstract].
35. Demeter L, Resnick L, Nawaz T. Phenotypic and genotypic analysis of atevirdine (ATV) susceptibility of HIV-1 isolates obtained from patients receiving ATV monotherapy in a phase I clinical trial (ACTG 187): comparison to patients receiving combination therapy with AZT and zidovudine. Third Workshop on Viral Resistance. Gaithersburg, MD: 19–22 September 1993; [Abstract].
36. Demeter LM, Shafer RW, Para M *et al.* Delavirdine (DLV) susceptibility of HIV-1 isolates obtained from patients (PTS) receiving DLV monotherapy (ACTG 260). *J AIDS* 1995;10(Suppl. 3):S11.
37. Wathen LK, Freimuth WW, Batts DH, Cox SR. Phenotypic and genotypic characterization of HIV-1 viral isolates from patients treated with combined AZT and delavirdine mesylate (DLV) therapy. Third International HIV Drug Resistance Workshop, Kauai, Hawaii, 2–5 August 1994; [Abstract].
38. Been-Tiktak AMM, Joly V, Sitbon G *et al.* Combination therapy with delavirdine mesylate (DLV) and AZT: virology data from a European phase II trial. *J AIDS* 1995;10(Suppl. 3):S23–4.
39. Moeremans M, De Raeymaeker M, Van den Broek R, Stoffels P, Andries K. Genotypic analysis of HIV-1 isolates from patients receiving loviride alone, or in combination with nucleoside reverse transcriptase inhibitors. *J AIDS* 1995;10(Suppl. 3):S15–16.

13

Protease Inhibitors—Mechanisms and Clinical Aspects

MARTIN MARKOWITZ AND DAVID D. HO

INTRODUCTION

The development of clinically relevant inhibitors of HIV-1 protease represents the successful combined efforts of the medicinal chemist, the virologist and the structural biochemist. These agents have been rationally designed based on the knowledge of the enzyme's structure and function and modified to exhibit favorable pharmacologic properties which have allowed for their clinical development. In this chapter we will describe the basic structural and functional features of the HIV-1 protease. Emphasis will be placed on the design of inhibitors based on protease–substrate interactions. Finally we will describe the current experience concerning both *in vitro* and *in vivo* viral resistance, emphasizing the mechanisms by which the virus becomes less susceptible to the effects of these novel antiretroviral compounds.

HIV-1 PROTEASE: FUNCTION

The lifecycle of HIV-1 can be divided into three main stages: entry and reverse transcription, integration, and finally expression and release of mature infectious particles that are capable of initiating another round of infection[1]. HIV-1 protease is required for the production of infectious virus particles[2]. Translation of the gag open reading frame results in a 55 kD polyprotein, referred to as p55 gag.

Antiviral Drug Resistance. Edited by Douglas D. Richman © 1996 John Wiley & Sons Ltd

Similarly, the gag–pol message is expressed by a ribosomal frame shift as a 160 kD polyprotein, referred to as p160 gag–pol. These polyproteins are directed to the plasma membrane in a ratio of approximately 10 : 1 (gag:gag–pol), where they are cleaved and packaged into virions[3,4]. The HIV-1 protease cleaves these polyproteins via hydrolysis of a peptide bond at one of the scissile sites, as shown in Figure 13.1[5]. The result of this process is the generation of the structural proteins (matrix, capsid, nucleocapsid and p6) as well as the virally encoded enzymes reverse transcriptase, integrase and protease. The actual mechanism by which proteolytic processing is initiated is yet unknown.

HIV-1 protease function is required for the production of infectious viral particles. Using site-directed mutagenesis, Kohl *et al.*[6] demonstrated that an asparagine for aspartic acid replacement at residue 25, the enzyme's active site, eliminated the proteolytic activity of the enzyme. By constructing a mutant provirus containing Asn-25, they produced a viral particle which contained p55 gag but no p24. These mutant particles were incapable of infecting a cell line, unlike the wild-type virus. Subsequently, pharmacologic inhibition of the enzyme has

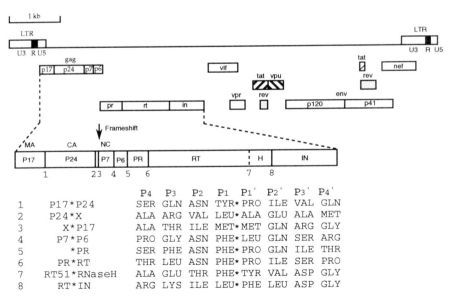

Figure 13.1 *Genomic organization of HIV-1, structure of the p55 gag and p160 gag–pol polyproteins and the cleavage sites for HIV-1 protease. The (*) symbol marks the position of the scissile bond. The P1, P2 etc. subsite terminology is according to Schecter and Berger[14]. Reproduced and modified from reference 5 with permission*

resulted in similar inhibition of infectivity, in both acutely infected and chronically infected cell lines[7,8]. Loss of protease activity thus results in the interruption of the last stages of the viral lifecycle, thereby blocking the next round of infection.

The effect of protease inhibition on the structure of HIV-1 has been visualized with electron microscopy[9]. As shown in Figure 13.2b, H9 cells

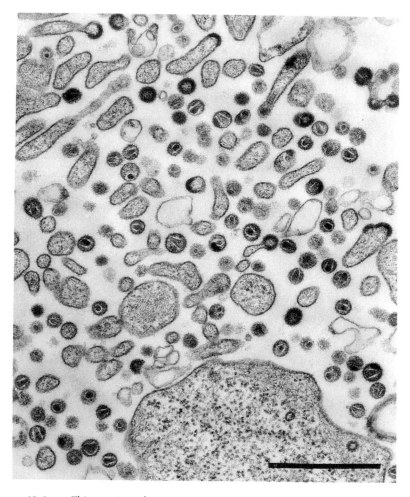

a

Figure 13.2 **a** *Thin-section electron microscopy of part of an H9 cell productively infected with HIV-1 IIIB.* **b** *Thin-section electron microscopy of H9 cells chronically infected with HIV-1 IIIB after treatment for three days with Ro 31-8959. HIV-1 particles released from the cells have and maintain immature morphology. Reproduced from reference 9 with permission*

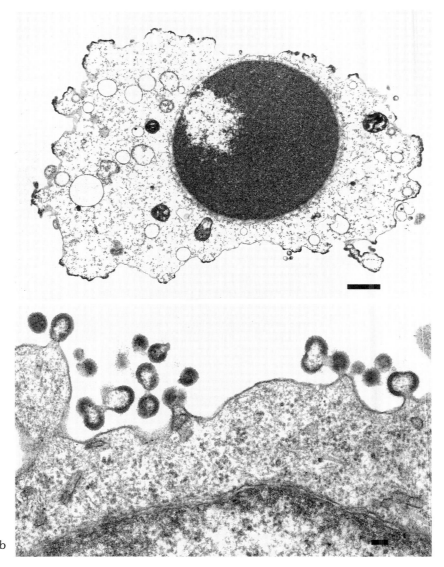

b

Figure 13.2   *Continued*

chronically infected with HIV-1 IIIB and treated with a protease inhibitor
release particles which lack the characteristic dense core (Figure 13.2a).
These budding particles are immature, devoid of processed gag and
gag–pol polyproteins, and are non-infectious.

HIV-1 PROTEASE: STRUCTURE

HIV-1 protease is an aspartyl protease composed of two identical 99-amino acid monomers, combining to form a C_2-symmetrical homodimer whose single active site contains the signature sequence Asp-Thr-Gly at residues 25–27 of each monomer[10]. The active site is stabilized by hydrogen bonds involving the threonine residue at position 26, which form a rigid network referred to as a 'fireman's grip'[11]. These features are common to catalytic sites in all aspartyl proteases, be they cellular or retroviral. In addition, the HIV-1 protease contains two folded β hairpins that form a flap which covers the enzyme active site[12,13]. Upon binding substrate or a competitive inhibitor, the protease undergoes structural changes, particularly in the area of the flaps[13]. These shift to form a tunnel-like structure which becomes the enzyme's active site (Plate 3). Starting from the central aspartates, and using the notation of Schecter and Berger[14], there are distinct subsites termed S1, S2, S3 ..., as well as the symmetry-related S1', S2', S3' ..., which form binding pockets capable of interacting with the side chain of inhibitors, referred to as P1/P1', P2/P2' etc. The borders of S1/S1' are formed by the side chains of Asp 25/125, Ile 23/123, Ile 50/150, Ile 84/184, Pro 81/181, the γ-carbon of Thr 80/180 and the carbonyl oxygens of Gly 27/127. In this notation amino acid residues are numbered 1–99 on one protease monomeric subunit and 101–199 on the symmetric second subunit. The S2/S2' subsites are bounded by Val 32/132, Ile 50/150, Ile 47/147, Leu 76/176, and the side chains of Ala 28/128 and Asp 30/130. The S3/S3' subsites are bordered by Leu 23/123, Val 82/182, Pro 81/181 and the guanidinium groups of Arg 8/108, which form a salt bridge with Asp 29/129[13]. These amino acid residues are clearly important in the interaction of the enzyme with both its substrates and its inhibitors. An appreciation of these interactions is essential for understanding the mechanisms by which the virus becomes less susceptible to the effects of inhibitors of HIV-1 protease.

PROTEASE–SUBSTRATE INTERACTION

The cleavage sites in gag and gag–pol are quite variable in their sequences (see Figure 13.1). However, there appear to be some favored motifs which aid in understanding how the enzyme maintains specificity. Poorman *et al.*[15] have analyzed over 40 cleavage sites and have concluded that amino acids preferentially occupying the same location on both sides of the hydrolyzable or scissile bond are not identical. The residues from P2 to P2' appear to be the most important in conferring enzyme specificity. The positional preference for a particular amino acid is greatest for P2' which is generally occupied by a glutamine or glutamic acid. In addition, a hydrophobic residue (Phe, Leu, Met, Asn, Tyr) is preferred at the P1 and P1' sites. Valine, asparagine and isoleucine are favored at the P2 site[16]. These observations are critical in appreciating the design of the protease inhibitors, which are essentially mimics of these amino acid motifs.

PROTEASE–INHIBITOR INTERACTION

The cornerstone of the design strategies used to create inhibitors of HIV-1 protease has been the introduction of a non-hydrolyzable bond in the place of the amide bond linking the P1–P1' sites. To date, three basic design strategies have been described: the peptidomimetic method by Roberts *et al.*[17], the C_2-symmetry-based concept advanced by Erickson *et al.*[18], and the non-peptide cyclic ureas described by Lam and co-workers[19].

As the amide bond of proline residues is not hydrolyzable by mammalian endopeptidases, Roberts *et al.* reasoned that this particular cleavage site, Phe-Pro or Tyr-Pro, would be an ideal starting point for the design of specific selective inhibitors of HIV-1 protease. They described compounds based on the pol fragment Leu 165-Ile 169 with inhibitory activity in the nanomolar range which were highly specific for HIV-1 protease. Indeed, the inhibitory properties of the compounds translated consistently into antiviral activity as measured by inhibition of p24 antigen production in C8166 cells infected with HIV-1 RF[17].

Shortly thereafter, Erickson and co-workers argued that peptide-based compounds exhibited adverse pharmacologic properties, such as poor solubility, poor oral absorption and rapid metabolism. They therefore set out to use the C_2-symmetric nature of the enzyme's active site to design novel compounds which would be less peptide-like in nature. The initial compound, A-74704, had phenylalanine groups occupying the P1/P1' sites, a preferred valine at P2/P2', and a carbobenzyl group at the P3/P3' site. This compound proved to be a potent competitive inhibitor of the HIV-1 protease, with a K_i of 4.5 nM. As observed with the peptide-based transition-state analogs, the inhibitory activity translated well into antiviral activity as assessed by inhibition of HIV-1 IIIB replication in H9 cells *in vitro*[18]. Modeling of the inhibitor–protease complex revealed that the initial hypothesis was indeed true: the inhibitor, a symmetric non-peptide, bound tightly and symmetrically to the enzyme[18].

Finally, Lam and co-workers developed a third structurally based approach to the design of inhibitors of the HIV-1 protease. As discussed above, the protease is a dimer, with paired aspartic residues at the floor of the active site. When bound to an inhibitor, a water molecule is juxtaposed between the inhibitor and the isoleucine residues at position 50/150 in the flap of the enzyme (Plate 4). Starting with a C_2-symmetric diol, Lam and co-workers modified the diol to form a ring structure, added a urea group to strengthen hydrogen binding to the flap, and optimized the side chains to facilitate a favorable drug–enzyme interaction at the first and second binding pockets. As achieved by the two previous groups, compounds with K_is in the nanomolar to sub-nanomolar range with potent *in vitro* antiviral activity were synthesized, among them XM323[19]. In addition to activity against laboratory and clinical isolates *in vitro*, this agent initially showed favorable pharmacokinetics in animal studies[19].

Clearly, knowledge of the structure of HIV-1 protease, along with an intimate understanding of its function, has allowed for the development of numerous new compounds with potent activity and promising pharmacologic profiles. Three compounds are well into clinical development and are approved in the USA: saquinavir or Ro 31-8959 (Roche)[21], indinavir or MK-639 (Merck)[22], and the C_2-symmetry-based ritonavir or ABT-538 (Abbott Laboratories)[23]. Additional peptidomimetic compounds, including those developed by Vertex[24] and Agouron[25], are in earlier phases of clinical development.

RESISTANCE TO INHIBITORS OF HIV-1 PROTEASE

Viral resistance to the nucleoside and non-nucleoside inhibitors of reverse transcriptase has been well characterized and discussed in previous chapters. With the development of the inhibitors of HIV-1 protease, investigators queried whether HIV-1 protease could escape from the inhibitory effects of these agents. Given the diversity of the cleavage site recognition needed for function, as well as the small size of the enzyme and the fact that, being a dimer, mutations would be 'felt' twice, it was hoped that an attempt by the virus to mutate would result in a non-viable or less viable mutant. Unfortunately, this proved not to be the case and numerous reports of viral resistance to protease inhibitors have been published.

P9941 (Dupont Merck)

The first report of protease resistance by Otto *et al.*[27] described the *in vitro* selection of HIV-1 variants with reduced susceptibility to P9941, a C_2-symmetric diol inhibitor, not now clinically relevant. By serially passaging HIV-1RF in H9 cells in the presence of increasing concentrations

of the inhibitor, HIV-1 variants with six- to eightfold reduced susceptibility to P9941 were isolated. Sequence analysis of the protease coding
region from proviral DNA of infected H9 cells revealed a single point
mutation, a valine to alanine at position 82. The residue at position 82
forms a van der Waals contact between the enzyme's S1/S1' subsite and
the P1/P1' phenyl groups of the inhibitor. Enzymatic analysis of the
mutant versus wild-type enzyme confirmed the relative resistance of the
V82A mutant protease in an *in vitro* protease activity assay performed in
the presence of inhibitor. Thus, a point mutation in a known contact site
between enzyme and inhibitor could result in relatively low-level
resistance to a protease inhibitor.

A-77003 (Abbott)

A-77003, a C_2-symmetric inhibitor of HIV-1 protease, was also used to
select for the stepwise reduction in susceptibility with serial passages of
the virus in the presence of the drug[28]. A virus with 30-fold reduced
susceptibility to the protease inhibitor was characterized. The deduced
amino acid sequences of the proteases from resistant viruses revealed
the predominance of a R8Q/M46I double mutation. Additional passages
resulted in the emergence of additional mutations, including R8K. These
mutations were introduced singly, and in selected combinations, into an
NL4-3 background using site-directed mutagenesis. The R8Q mutant
replicated poorly, but the addition of M46I, which itself confers no
change in susceptibility to A-77003, resulted in a mutant that replicated
with greater efficiency. The two-step mutation R8K also resulted in a
variant which grew as well as the parental virus. Mutant enzymes (R8Q,
M46I) as well as that of the wild type (NL4-3) were expressed and
purified for the determination of the K_i to A-77003. The K_is for the wild
type and the M46I enzymes were nearly identical, but the value for the
R8Q mutant was 32 times higher, suggesting that this mutation critically
reduced viral susceptibility to A-77003. As shown in Plate 5, modeling of
the inhibitor complexed to wild-type protease revealed a critical
interaction between the aromatic pyridine occupying the P3/P3' site on
the inhibitor with the arginine residue forming the S3/S3' binding
pocket. The mutant, R8Q, makes less extensive van der Waals contacts
with the pyridine groups. In addition, it was noted that the electrostatic
interaction between the inhibitor and the enzyme should be weakened
owing to the reduced positive charge of the side chain of the glutamine
residue. Finally, in testing the mutants for their sensitivities to two
peptidomimetic compounds, Ro 31-8959 and L-689,502, no cross-
resistance was found, as was predicted by the lack of significant contact
of both protease inhibitors with the S3/S3' binding pocket of the mutant

protease. These findings were shortly followed by a report from Kaplan *et al.*[29], who described similar findings using another *in vitro* selection strategy in the presence of the A-77003. In addition, double mutations involving residues 32 and 82 in combination were also reported. Mutations at these sites interrupt critical binding pockets in both the S2/S2' and S1/S1' subsites respectively, and result in a mutant protease with less avidity for binding inhibitor. These reports clearly document that resistance to protease inhibitors could be mediated by genetic changes in the protease coding region. In addition, strong selective pressure is also exerted for compensatory mutations, capable of restoring the full replicative capacity of a drug-resistant virus.

Ritonavir ABT-538 (Abbott)

ABT-538 (Ritonavir) is an orally absorbed C_2-symmetric inhibitor with potent *in vivo* activity and is currently FDA approved and available in the US for the treatment of HIV-1 infection[26,30]. Using a selection method identical to that described for A-77003, HIV-1 variants of the laboratory strain NL4-3 which were five times less susceptible to ABT-538 were generated after 19 passages[31]. In just three additional passages a variant with a 25-fold increase in IC_{50} was isolated. Genetic analysis of the proteases of these resistant viruses revealed that the fivefold resistance was associated with the appearance of the M46I/I84V mutations. The more resistant variant also contained the L63P, A71V and V82F mutations. These mutations were constructed into pNL4-3. The I84V and V82F mutants were found to confer eight- to 10-fold and four- to fivefold resistance to ABT-538, respectively. The double mutant V82F/I84V exhibited poor replication kinetics, and drug susceptibility data on this viral construct could not be obtained. Interestingly, the remaining three amino acid substitutions, L63P, A71V and M46I, did not appear to affect susceptibility to ABT-538 when introduced singly into pNL4-3. L63P and A71V mutations are remote from the active site, and may, along with M46I, be compensatory for the two mutations at residues 82 and 84. Plate 6 is a computer-generated model of ABT-538 complexed with the wild-type and mutant proteases. I184 and V182 contact the benzyl group of the inhibitor at the S1' subsite. The modeled mutations I84V and I82F have different effects. The I84V change decreases the interaction with the C_β group of the benzyl side chain of ABT-538, whereas the I82F mutation results in severe spatial overlap, requiring considerable conformational changes which are likely to result in further decreased interactions between inhibitor and enzyme. The effects on the S1 subsite are similar. As was shown in the case of A-77003 and the R8Q mutant, these changes at critical binding subsites in the protease result in decreased protease–inhibitor interactions which are translated into loss of drug activity.

A phase I/II clinical trial of ABT-538 has recently been completed. Using plasma viremia as an indicator of antiviral activity, a 98.5% reduction in viral load was obtained in patients treated with 600–1200 mg of ABT-538 daily[30,32]. This was followed by a rebound viremia in many of the patients, particularly in those treated with less than 1200 mg daily[26]. In testing sequential viral isolates from selected patients in a PBMC-based drug sensitivity assay, HIV-1 variants with reduced susceptibility to ABT-538 have been demonstrated. Sequence analysis of protease coding regions from patient proviral DNA has revealed the accumulation of mutations in the HIV-1 protease at sites including 10, 36, 54, 63, 77, 82, 84, 93 and 95[46]. Norbeck *et al.* have determined that there is a marked delay in the appearance and accumulation of these drug-resistance mutations in ritonavir-treated subjects, with prolonged reduction in plasma RNA values compared to those subjects experiencing a return of viral load to pretreatment baseline[47]. Resistance to ritonavir may therefore require numerous steps, and may be delayed or even prevented by the use of non-cross resistant protease inhibitors or other agents which may effectively suppress viral replication and prevent the emergence of highly resistant viral variants *in vivo*.

Saquinavir (Roche)

Jacobsen *et al.*[33] reported the *in vitro* selection of a variant with 40-fold reduced susceptibility to the inhibitor Ro 31-8959 (Saquinivir). Genetic analysis of the resistant virus revealed G48V and L90M amino acid substitutions in the HIV-1 protease. Sequence heterogeneity was also observed at other sites (12, 36, 37, 57 and 63), but these changes were not as dominant as the two previously mentioned mutations. The glycine at position 48 is found on the enzyme's flap, whereas residue 90 is distant from the enzyme's active site. The precise structural mechanism by which this combination of mutations accounts for reduced susceptibility to Ro 31-8959 remains unclear; however, it is clear that this combination of mutations is responsible for the observed resistance. Introduction of either G48V alone or the combination of G48V/L90M resulted in a significant increase in the inhibitory constant (K_i) of Ro 31-8959. In addition, resistance was virologically confirmed by constructing the specific mutations into HIV-1 HXB2. The single mutant virus G48V resulted in an eightfold increase in IC_{90}, whereas the combination resulted in a 20-fold increase in IC_{90}. Interestingly, despite its distance from the active site, the L90M mutant virus was three to four times less sensitive to Ro 31-8959 than the parental virus. Clearly, further evaluation of the structural features of the inhibitor–enzyme interaction, as well as of the structural consequences of the observed amino acid substitutions, is necessary to understand the precise mechanism by which the virus escapes the effect of the inhibitor.

Data on *in vivo* resistance to Ro 31-8959 have also been reported by Jacobsen *et al.*[34]. Genetic analysis of sequential isolates from patients treated with Ro 31-8959 has exhibited both G48V and L90M changes, with the latter single mutant predominating. The difference between the *in vitro* and *in vivo* patterns may in part be explained by the limited bioavailability of saquinavir. This may result in significantly lower drug levels than those obtained during the *in vitro* selection experiments. The reduced selection pressure may therefore account for the difference in the incidence of the G48V mutation when comparing the *in vitro* and *in vivo* data. Alternatively, the mutations at 48 or 90 may be unfavorable to the virus *in vivo*, thus diminishing the likelihood of emerging. Current high-dose studies using saquinavir suggest that at doses of 3600 and 7200 mg daily, the incidence of mutations at codons 48 and 90, using rapid selective hybridization assays, were less frequent[48]. It may be the case that by achieving higher drug levels and increasing selective pressures, alternative paths to drug resistance with different arrays of point mutations may well emerge.

Indinavir or MK-639 (formerly L-735,524) (Merck)

Indinavir (MK-639), formerly known as L-735,524, is a peptidomimetic compound with oral bioavailability and substantial *in vivo* activity[22]. It is currently FDA approved and available in the US for the treatment of HIV-1 infection. It has been difficult to generate virus resistant to MK-639 using the *in vitro* selection methods as detailed above. Significant cross-resistance (10-fold) to MK-639 for the mutant virus was generated after multiple passages in the presence of ABT-538[31]. In addition, when the I84V mutation is introduced into pNL4-3, the virus exhibits an eightfold reduction in susceptibility to MK-639. Finally, using a series of *in vitro* selection experiments, a highly resistant virus which is 80 times less susceptible to MK-639[35] was obtained.

The Merck group has recently reported the emergence of resistant variants of HIV-1 in patients receiving MK-639[36]. In addition to testing susceptibility to MK-639, they also tested the susceptibility of viral isolates to a panel of protease inhibitors (Table 13.1). Cross-resistance of MK-639 clearly developed in the isolates from these four patients to A-80897, a compound related to ABT-538[37], and XM-323, a cyclic urea developed by Dupont Merck[20]. In evaluating Ro 31-8959[21], VX-478, a sulfonamide-based transition state analog[24], and SC-52151, the Searle urea-based hydroxyethylene isostere[38], an interesting pattern emerged in Patient A. At week 24 the isolate was four- to sevenfold resistant to

Table 13.1   *Patterns of* in vivo *resistance to selected protease inhibitors*

Patient (time)	MK-639	XM323	A-80897	Ro-31-8959	VX-478	SC-52151
A week 0	100 nm	200 nm	800 nm	25 nm	100 nm	200 nm
A week 24	2×	7.5×	3.5×	2×	2×	1×
A week 40	15×	15×	3.5×	16×	4×	15×
A week 52	>30×	>15×	>3.5×	16×	8×	>15×
B week 52	15×	4×	>3.5×	8×	4×	4×
C week 44	15×	15×	>3.5×	4×	15×	4×
D week 44	8×	7.5×	>3.5×	4×	15×	7.5×

MK-639, A-80897 and XM-323, whereas it remained susceptible to Ro 31-8959, VX-478, and SC-52151. However, with prolonged exposure to MK-639 *in vivo*, a seven- to 30-fold reduction in susceptibility to all six inhibitors was documented. Genetic analysis revealed a fair degree of diversity in the HIV-1 protease coding region prior to therapy in all four patients. In addition, at week 20 protease sequences from Patient A revealed a further reduction in susceptibility, mediated via the appearance of a V82T change in addition to the previously seen I84V, M46I and L63P substitutions. With continued exposure to drug additional changes were seen at other sites, but the I84V mutation did not persist. The remaining three patients were similarly studied at only one time point after the initiation of therapy, and rather diverse protease genotypic patterns were observed, with an average of approximately 10 amino acid substitutions. Substitutions at residues 32, 82 and 84 were commonly substituted, and these sites are known to form binding pockets for the inhibitor. However, changes at residues distant from the active site, such as 71, 63 and 90, and sites of intermediate distance such as 10, 16, 24, 35, 36 and 37, were also commonly observed. Again, the precise effects of these amino acid substitutions on protease structure and function and how they affect the interactions with the panel of inhibitors require continued investigation. These data do, however, strongly suggest that the development of high-level resistance to one inhibitor may result in cross-resistance to certain structurally diverse inhibitors.

Additional compounds and cross-resistance

As shown in Table 13.2, many groups have reported the *in vitro* selection of resistant variants to nearly all protease inhibitors in preclinical and clinical development. A wide array of amino acid substitutions have been similarly reported, probably reflecting some degree of structural

Table 13.2   In vitro resistance to inhibitors of HIV-1 protease

Drug	Degree of resistance	Genotype	Reference
C₂-symmetric inhibitors			
P-9941	6–8-fold	V82A	Otto[27]
A-77003 (Abbott)	30-fold	R8Q or R8K/M46I	Ho[28]
A-77003 (Abbott)	20-fold	V32I/V82I	Kaplan[29]
	60-fold	R8Q	
	4-fold	M46F	
A-80897 (Abbott)	5–8-fold	V32I/M46L	Vasavanonda[40]
ABT-538 (Abbott)	10–20-fold	M46I/L63P/A71V/V82F/I84V	Markowitz[31]
Peptidomimetics			
R031-8959 (Roche)	40-fold	G48V/L90M	Jacobsen[33]
MK-639 (Merck)	10–30-fold	V32I/M46L/V82A	Tisdale[41]
	10-fold	I84V	Vacca[22]
SC-52151 (Searle)	10-fold	G48V/V82A	Potts[42]
VB-11,328 (Vertex)	10–100-fold	L10F/M46I/I50V/I84V	Partaledis[43]
RPI-312	not stated	I84V	El Farrash[44]
AG-1284 (Agouron)	10–30-fold	A71V/V77I/V82A/T91A	Tisdale[41]
Cyclic ureas			
XM-323 (Dupont-Merck)	50-fold	V82F/I84V	King[45]
DMF-450 (Dupont-Merck)	25-fold	I84V	Mo[35]

heterogeneity among the various inhibitors. Table 13.3 summarizes the resistance patterns of six structurally diverse and clinically relevant protease inhibitors to an array of resistant viruses generated in our laboratory[35]. We have included four patterns of resistance: the first to A-77003 basically mediated by a change at position 8; the second to Ro 31-8959 and SC-52151 involving residue 48; the third to ABT-538 involving residues 82 and 84; and the fourth and most significant, I84A, a mutation found *in vitro* after prolonged exposure to ABT-538[35]. Despite some early segregation into patterns, after prolonged exposure to ABT-538 a highly cross-resistant virus is generated. These *in vitro* findings echo the *in vivo* findings of Condra et al. summarized above[36].

To date, investigators have concentrated on changes within the protease as the path to viral resistance. Interestingly, Lamarre and co-workers[49] have discovered variants with mutations not only within the protease coding region, but also at gag cleavage sites. *In vitro* experiments have generated highly resistant viruses to compounds BILA 1906/2011 BS and BILA 2185 BS. Protease mutants with changes at codons 32, 46, 63, 71 or 84 were documented to the first two drugs, whereas changes at residues 10, 23, 46, 47, 54, 71 and 84 were obtained in experiments using the latter compound. In addition, a lysine to phenylalanine substitution was seen in the p1/p6 cleavage site and a QA

Table 13.3 *Patterns of in vitro resistance to selected inhibitors of HIV-1 protease*

HIV-1 variant	IC_{90}	ABT-538 80 nm	MK-639 80 nm	Ro 31-8959 30 nm	AG-1343 25 nm	SC-52151 40 nm	DMF-450 250 nm
R8Q/M46I		3×	3×	1×	5×	3×	3×
G48V		2×	2×	5×	3×	16×	3×
I84V		10×	8×	3×	5×	10×	25×
M46I/L63P/A71V/V82F/I84V		20×	10×	3×	20×	15×	25×
M46I/L63P/I84A		80×	80×	80×	125×	125×	125×

was replaced by an RV at the P2–P3 positions of the p7/p1 cleavage site. Decapeptides incorporating these changes were more readily cleaved *in vitro* by HIV proteases than similar-sized wild-type peptides studied under similar conditions. In addition, these cleavage site mutations appeared to be important in maintaining viral viability. In other words, not only is the protease flexible in accommodating resistance-inducing mutations, but compensatory changes in the enzyme's target also appear to be permissive and may contribute to the emergence of resistance.

CONCLUSIONS

The successful development of a new class of antiretroviral compounds, the protease inhibitors, represents an important application of modeling based on structure and function, as well as the efforts of the medicinal chemist to modify a compound to achieve a pharmacologically effective result. Three compounds, saquinavir, ritonavir and indinavir, are approved for use in the treatment of HIV-1 infection, and additional compounds have entered or will be entering phase I/II trials in the near future.

Based on the results of both *in vitro* selection and recently reported analysis of patient isolates, it is clear that the HIV-1 protease is capable of tolerating multiple amino acid substitutions which result in reduced susceptibility to all of the inhibitors we have discussed. The mechanism of resistance to the various compounds would appear to be mediated by these observed changes in the enzyme's structure. We have presented models of the mutant protease–inhibitor interactions which clearly demonstrate the altered interaction between the inhibitor and the enzyme at critical binding sites. It is clear, however, that there are more complex interactions between the wide array of amino acid substitutions observed and the structural and functional consequences for the viral protease. There are certain mutations at critical hot spots, such as 8, 32, 48, 82 and 84, which are adjacent to the active site and which in modeling clearly result in reduced enzyme–inhibitor interactions. However, there are additional mutations at sites such as 46, 63, 71 and 90 which, despite being distant from the active site, are clearly important in accommodating the changes observed at the active site residues.

Resistance to inhibitors of HIV-1 protease emerges as a consequence of genetic variation. Based on these findings, as well as recent insights into the highly kinetic nature of viral replication at all stages of HIV-1 infection[32,39], it follows that the immediate goal is to design potent non-cross resistant compounds with non-overlapping toxicities which may be used in combination. Such an approach may prevent the emergence of viral variants highly resistant to this family of compounds.

REFERENCES

1. Ratner L. HIV life cycle and genetic approaches. *Perspect Drug Disc Design* 1993;1:3–22.
2. Peng C, Ho B, Chang T, Chang N. Role of human immunodeficiency virus type 1 specific protease in core maturation and viral infectivity. *J Virol* 1989;63:2550–6.
3. Jacks T, Power MD, Masiarz FR *et al*. Characterization of ribosimal frameshifting in HIV-1 gag–pol expression. *Nature* 1988;331:280–3.
4. Kaplan AH, Zack JA, Knigge M *et al*. Partial inhibition of the HIV-type 1 protease results in aberrant virus assembly and the formation of non-infectious particles. *J Virol* 1993;67:4050–5.
5. DeBouck C. The HIV-1 protease as a therapeutic target for AIDS. *AIDS Res Hum Retroviruses* 1992;8:153–64.
6. Kohl NE, Emini EA, Schleif WA *et al*. Active human immunodeficiency virus protease is required for viral infectivity. *Proc Natl Acad Sci USA* 1988;85:4686–90.
7. Craig JC, Duncan IB, Hockley D *et al*. Antiviral properties of Ro 31-8959, an inhibitor of human immunodeficiency virus (HIV) proteinase. *Antiviral Res* 1991;16:295–305.
8. Craig JC, Grief C, Mills JS *et al*. Effects of a specific inhibitor of HIV proteinase (Ro 31-8959) on virus maturation in a chronically infected promonocytic cell line (U1). *Antiviral Chem Chemother* 1991;2:181–6.
9. Gelderblom H. Assembly and morphology of HIV: potential effects of structure on viral function. *AIDS* 1991;5:617–38.
10. Navia MA, Fitzgerald PM, McKeever BM *et al*. Three-dimensional structure of aspartyl protease from human immunodeficiency virus HIV-1. *Nature* 1989;337:615–20.
11. Wlodawer A, Miller M, Jaskolski M *et al*. Conserved folding in retroviral proteases: crystal structure of a synthetic HIV-1 protease. *Science* 1989;245:616–21.
12. Appelt K. Crystal structures of HIV-1 protease-inhibitor complexes. *Perspect Drug Disc Design* 1993;1:23–48.
13. Wlodawer A, Erickson JW. Structure based inhibitors of HIV-1 protease. *Annu Rev Biochem* 1993;62:543–80.
14. Schecter I, Berger B. On the size of the active site in proteases. *Biochem Biophys Res Commun* 1967;27:157–62.
15. Poorman RA, Tomaselli AG, Heirikson RL, Kezdy FJ. A cumulative specificity model for proteases from human immunodeficiency virus types 1 and 2, inferred from statistical analysis of an extended substrate data base. *J Biol Chem* 1991;266:14554–61.
16. Pettit SC, Simsic J, Loeb DD *et al*. Analysis of retroviral protease cleavage sites reveals two types of cleavage sites and the structural requirements of the P1 amino acid. *J Biol Chem* 1991;266:14539–47.
17. Roberts NA, Martin JA, Kinchington D *et al*. Rational design of peptide-based HIV proteinase inhibitors. *Science* 1990;248:358–61.
18. Erickson JW, Meidhart DJ, Van Drie J *et al*. Design, activity and a 2.8 Å crystal structure of a C_2 symmetric inhibitor complexed to HIV-1 protease. *Science* 1990;249:527–33.
19. Lam PYS, Jadhav PK, Eyermann CJ *et al*. Rational design of potent, bioavailable nonpeptide cyclic ureas as HIV-1 protease inhibitors. *Science* 1994;263:380–4.

20. Otto MJ, Reid CD, Garber S *et al. In vitro* anti-human immunodeficiency virus (HIV) activity of XM323, a novel HIV protease inhibitor. *Antimicrob Agents Chemother* 1993;37:2606–11.
21. Kitchen VS, Skinner C, Ariyoshi K *et al.* Safety and activity of saquinavir in HIV-1 infection. *Lancet* 1995;345:952–5.
22. Vacca JP, Dorsey BD, Schleif WA *et al.* L-735,524: an orally bioavailable human immunodeficiency virus type 1 protease inhibitor. *Proc Natl Acad Sci USA* 1994;91:4096–100.
23. Kempf DJ, Marsh KC, Denissen JF *et al.* ABT-538 is a potent inhibitor of human immunodeficiency virus protease and has high oral bioavailability in humans. *Proc Natl Acad Sci USA* 1995;92:2484–8.
24. Kim EE, Baker CT, Dwyer MD *et al.* Crystal structure of HIV-1 protease in complex with VX-478, a potent and orally bioavailable inhibitor of the enzyme. *J Am Chem Soc* 1995;117:1181–2.
25. Patick A, Mo H, Markowitz M, Ho D, Webber S. *In vitro* antiviral and resistance studies of AG1343, an orally bioavailable inhibitor of HIV-1 protease. Second National Conference on Human Retroviruses and Related Infections, Washington DC, 29 January–2 February 1995; [Abstract].
26. Danner SA, Carr A, Leonard JM *et al.* Safety, pharmacokinetics, and antiviral activity of ritonavir, an inhibitor of HIV-1 protease. Fourth International Workshop on HIV Drug Resistance, Sardinia, Italy, 6–9 July 1995.
27. Otto MJ, Garber S, Winslow DL *et al. In vitro* isolation and identification of HIV-1 variants with reduced sensitivity to C_2 symmetrical inhibitors of HIV type 1 protease. *Proc Natl Acad Sci USA* 1993;90:7543–7.
28. Ho DD, Toyoshima T, Mo H *et al.* Characterization of HIV-type 1 variants with increased resistance to a C_2 symmetric protease inhibitor. *J Virol* 1994;68:2016–20.
29. Kaplan AH, Michae SF, Wehbie RS *et al.* Selection of multiple human immunodeficiency virus type 1 variants that encode viral proteases with decreased sensitivity to an inhibitor of HIV-1 protease. *Proc Natl Acad Sci USA* 1994,91:5597–601.
30. Markowitz M, Jalil L, Hurley A *et al.* Evaluation of the antiviral activity of orally administered ABT-538, an inhibitor of HIV-1 protease. Second National Conference on Human Retroviruses and Related Infections, Washington DC, 29 January–2 February 1995; [Abstract].
31. Markowitz M, Mo H, Kempf DJ *et al.* Selection and analysis of human immunodeficiency virus type 1 variants with increased resistance to ABT-538, a novel protease inhibitor. *J Virol* 1995;69:701–6.
32. Ho DD, Neumann A, Perelson AS *et al.* Rapid turnover of plasma virions and CD4 lymphocytes in HIV-1 infection. *Nature* 1995;373:123–6.
33. Jacobsen H, Yasargil K, Winslow DL *et al.* Characterization of human immunodeficiency virus type 1 mutants with decreased sensitivity to proteinase inhibitor Ro 31-8959. *Virology* 1995;206:527–34.
34. Jacobsen H, Brun-Vezinet F, Duncan I *et al.* Genotypic characterization of HIV-1 from patients after prolonged treatment with proteinase inhibitor, saquinavir. Third International Workshop on HIV Drug Resistance, Kauai, Hawaii, 2–5 August 1994; [Abstract].
35. Mo H, Markowitz M, Ho DD. Patterns of specific mutations in HIV-1 protease that confer resistance to a panel of protease inhibitors. Second National Conference on Human Retroviruses and Related Infections, Washington DC, 29 January–2 February 1995; [Abstract].

36. Condra JH, Schleif WA, Blahy OM *et al. In vivo* emergence of HIV-1 variants resistant to multiple protease inhibitors. *Nature* 1995; 374:569–71.
37. Kempf DJ, Marsh KC, Paul DA *et al.* Antiviral and pharmacokinetic properties of C_2 symmetric inhibitors of the human immunodeficiency virus type 1 protease. *Antimicrob Agents Chemother* 1991;35:2209–14.
38. Getman D, De Crescenzo GA, Hientz RM *et al.* Discovery of a novel class of potent HIV-1 protease inhibitors containing the (R)-(hydroxyethyl)urea isostere. *J Med Chem* 1993;36:288–91.
39. Wei X, Ghosh SK, Taylor ME *et al.* Viral dynamics in human immunodeficiency virus type 1 infection. *Nature* 1995; 373:117–22.
40. Vasavanonda S, Clement J, Robins T. Selection and characterization of HIV-1 mutants that are resistant to HIV-1 protease inhibitors. Thirty-third Interscience Conference on Antimicrobial Agents and Chemotherapy. 1993; [Abstract 39:126].
41. Tisdale M, Myers R, Parry NR *et al.* Comprehensive analysis of HIV-1 variants individually selected for resistance to six HIV protease inhibitors. Third International Workshop on HIV Drug Resistance, Kauai, Hawaii, 2–4 August 1994; [Abstract].
42. Potts KE, Smidt M, Stallings WC *et al. In vitro* selection and characterization of human immunodeficiency virus type 1 (HIV-1) with decreased sensitivity to hydroxyethylurea isostere containing protease inhibitors. Third International Workshop on HIV Drug Resistance, Kauai, Hawaii, 2–4 August 1994; [Abstract].
43. Pataledis JA, Yamaguchi K, Byrn RA, Livingston DJ. *In vitro* selection and characterization of HIV-1 viral isolates with reduced sensitivity to inhibitors of HIV protease. Third International Workshop on HIV Drug Resistance, Kauai, Hawaii, 2–4 August 1994; [Abstract].
44. El-Farrash MA, Kuroda MJ, Kitzaki T *et al.* Generation and characterization of a human immunodeficiency virus type 1 (HIV-1) mutant resistant to an HIV-1 protease inhibitor. *J Virol* 1994;68:233–9.
45. King RW, Garber S, Reid CD, Otto MJ. An HIV-1 (RF) variant encoding a protease with V82F and I84V mutations exhibit resistance to cyclic urea and C_2 linear diol protease inhibitors. Third International Workshop on HIV Drug Resistance, Kauai, Hawaii, 2–4 August 1994; [Abstract].
46. Molla A, Boucher C, Korneyeva M *et al.* Evolution of resistance to the protease inhibitor ritonavir in HIV infected patients. Fourth International Workshop on HIV Drug Resistance, Sardinia, Italy, 6–9 July 1995.
47. Norbeck D, Hsu A, Granneman R *et al.* Virologic and immunologic response to ritonavir, an inhibitor of HIV protease. Fourth International Workshop on HIV Drug Resistance, Sardinia, Italy, 6–9 July 1995.
48. Schapiro JM, Winters M, Merigan T. Mutational analysis of the saquinavir high dose monotherapy study. Fourth International Workshop on HIV Drug Resistance, Sardinia, Italy, 6–9 July 1995.
49. Lamarre D, Doyon L, Croteau G *et al.* Molecular basis of HIV resistance to protease inhibitors. Structural flexibility of the protease and second-site compensatory mutations in cleavage sites. Fourth International Workshop on HIV Drug Resistance, Sardinia, Italy, 6–9 July 1995.

14
Population Dynamics of HIV Drug Resistance

JOHN M. COFFIN

INTRODUCTION

Despite more than 10 years of a research effort unparalleled in intensity and productivity, we are still unable to apply knowledge of the basic biology of AIDS to its effective prevention or treatment. HIV infection remains a death sentence whose duration has so far been improved only modestly by antiviral therapy. Attempts to develop effective vaccination strategies have been even less successful. Within the past year a number of studies have led to a re-examination of our thinking about the mechanisms of HIV infection and pathogenesis. Instead of viewing the 10-year clinical latency of the virus as a period of inactivity, we now picture this period as reflecting active replication and cell killing by the virus, very nearly balanced by replacement of the infected cells. As I will discuss in the following sections, this one simple revelation has significantly illuminated our view not only of HIV replication *in vivo*, but also of genetic variation, evolution, pathogenesis and potential strategies for treatment. In this brief review I will first present the current picture of HIV replication *in vivo*, and then extend that picture to attempt to answer important but unsolved basic questions and apply the answers to potential therapeutic avenues. Much of what I present will be speculative in that it represents extensions of current understanding that I find logical, but incisive experimentation is clearly needed to validate these thoughts and extend them further.

Antiviral Drug Resistance. Edited by Douglas D. Richman © 1996 John Wiley & Sons Ltd

DYNAMICS OF HIV INFECTION

The HIV steady state

The central concept for understanding AIDS dynamics is that of the HIV steady state, which is established shortly after the end of the acute infection phase[6] and lasts until the collapse of the immune system in terminal AIDS patients. This phase might more properly be called a 'quasi steady state', since there is a steady decline in the number of CD4+ T cells and an increase in the virus load, as measured by levels of viral RNA in plasma[17,53] during this time (Figure 14.1). However, these changes are glacially slow compared to the underlying replication activity, and over periods of days, weeks and even months, can be considered to be invariant. Although there can be some short-term fluctuation in virus load and CD4 T-cell number—perhaps reflecting the overall state of immune activation consequent on infection or some other external cause—there seems to be a well established 'set point' at defined levels of these parameters.

That the apparently quiescent state of the infection belies an extraordinarily active state of underlying virus replication was first suspected from analysis of the high level of variation in nucleotide

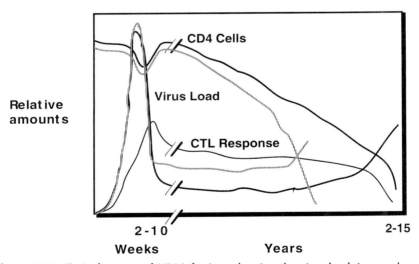

Figure 14.1 *Typical course of HIV infection, showing the virus load (as number of genomes in blood) and CD4 cell count in two infected individuals (one shown by solid lines; the other by dotted lines) as a function of time after infection. Note the correlation between high virus load, pace of CD4 + T-cell decline and progression to AIDS*

sequence occurring during the course of infection of a single individual[10,11,66]. Initial superficial analyses suggested that HIV variability simply reflected a very high mutation rate of HIV RT (reverse transcriptase). A closer look at the pattern of variability, particularly in monkeys infected with cloned simian immunodeficiency virus (SIV)[4,48], strongly implied that selective forces acting on the virus population were far more important in generating variability. Our experience with other retroviruses[5-7] led to the conclusion that the underlying mutation rate is quite unimportant in generating this kind of variability; what is important is the rate of replication in number of cycles per unit time. Under conditions where thousands of replication cycles separate cloning (transmission) events, selective advantages of substantially less than 1% are sufficient to turn over the entire population to mutant type.

The combination of high cycle numbers with the apparent stasis in cell and virus during years of infection implied the presence of a steady state, shown in its simplest form in Figure 14.2, top. This figure shows a single, kinetically uniform population of virus and cells, in which virus produced by infected cells infects susceptible cells at a constant rate. Infected cells proceed through an eclipse phase, followed by a period of virus production and then death, caused either directly by the virus or as a consequence of the immune response. At any given time the number of cells in each of these phases is proportional to its relative duration. The rate of cell replacement, by division of pre-existing CD4 cells or by *de novo* differentiation, is equal to the rate of death of infected (plus uninfected) cells. Under these conditions the total numbers of uninfected and infected cells remain constant, as does the rate of free virus released, which is simply proportional to the number of virus-producing cells. Some fraction of this virus escapes the site of replication (solid lymphoreticular tissue[49,50]) into the bloodstream. This virus itself establishes a steady state between its constant rate of release and a constant rate of clearance, due either to specific or non-specific mechanisms.

Although the productively infected cells just described are by far the most kinetically and pathogenically important class, there are three other outcomes of infection that should be mentioned. Latently infected and chronically producing cells (Figure 14.2) do not die rapidly, but instead have a much more extended lifetime, either producing virus only after encountering some external stimulus (such as an activation signal[27,42]) or producing virus constantly. Combined, these cells do not contribute more than 1% of the virus present at any one time[22,67], but they could be an important reservoir of genomes capable of rekindling an apparently cured infection.

The final cell type to be considered is pathogenically unimportant, but capable of confounding analyses. This comprises cells which have

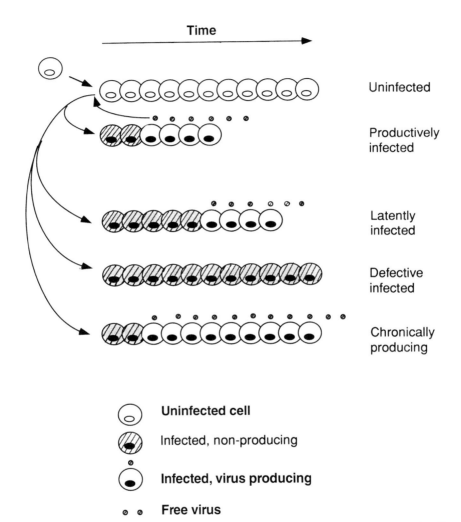

Figure 14.2   *The HIV steady state. Virus is shown as the small clots, infected cells have filled nuclei and uninfected cells are shown with open nuclei. The different rows show different kinetic classes of infected cells. The number of cells in each row reflects the relative time spent in each state. At the top are shown uninfected cells; below these the productive cycle, followed by latent infection (note the increased time spent in a non-producing state), chronic infection (a class which may not exist), and infection with defective proviruses*

received defective genomes, as a consequence of mutations incurred during reverse transcription, so that they do not yield infectious virus and are not killed by the infection. Although the accumulation of such cells may be quite slow, if they survive for much longer periods of time than productively infected cells, defective proviruses will become the majority after years of infection. Indeed, there is strong evidence for the occurrence of this process, in that genomes with inactivating mutations (in *env* and *tat*, for example) are frequently found in DNA amplified from PBMCs of HIV or SIV-infected individuals[26,32,66]. More recent analysis also indicates that the majority of slowly turning over proviral DNA in PBMCs is incapable of expression as infectious virus (G. Shaw, personal communication). The stability of cells containing defective proviruses most likely accounts for the relatively poor quality of PBMC as a prognostic indicator, compared to virion RNA (see below), and for the earlier misconceptions regarding the rate of appearance of resistant virus after anti-HIV drug therapy.

Use of antiviral drugs to probe the steady state

Considering only the productively infected class of cells, at steady state the proportion of cells in any one phase of the virus lifecycle is a measure of the relative time that an average infected cell spends in that phase. The underlying dynamics cannot be revealed by static measurements. For example, a finding that a small fraction of the viral DNA-containing cells express unspliced RNA[15] does not imply extensive latency, but could mean only that an infected cell on average produces virus for the last small fraction of its lifetime. (It could also mean that a large fraction of the infected cells contain defective proviruses.) The only way to uncover the kinetic parameters underlying the steady state is to perturb it. In HIV-infected individuals this has been accomplished by treatment with inhibitors of viral replication and measurement of the decline in virus in blood, as measured most sensitively and reliably by the amount of virus RNA in plasma[28,53].

Experiments reported by several groups using a variety of different inhibitors (Figure 14.3, for example) have given remarkably consistent results[21,44,60,67]. Within one to two weeks following initiation of therapy, the plasma virus declines to about 1% of its initial value, inevitably and rapidly rising again as resistant mutants take over the population. Simple modeling implies that both the average lifetime of an infected cell and the half-life of virus in circulation must each be less than about two days. A more sophisticated recent analysis using an inhibitor of HIV protease permitted separation of the parameters to give a value of about six hours for the half-life of circulating virus, and about one and a half

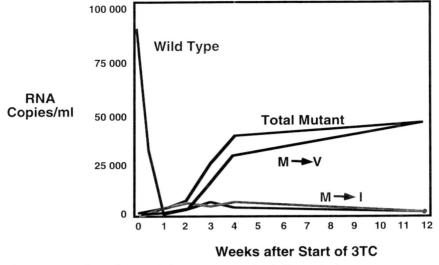

Figure 14.3 *Effect of antiviral therapy on virus load. Shown is the average response of wild-type and resistant mutant virus in HIV-infected subjects to treatment with 3TC[60]. Solid line, wild-type virus; dashed line, M184I mutant; dotted line, M184V mutant virus*

days for the lifetime of the average infected cell (A. Perelson and D. Ho, personal communication). These values mean that the average virion is produced by cells infected within the last day and a half, and the vast majority (>99%) of all virus in circulation is made by cells infected within the previous two weeks. Thus, the contribution of latently infected cells to the bulk of the infection process must be quite small; indeed, less than 1% of all infected cells enter this pathway. The number of cells containing latent proviruses must be larger: like cells containing defective proviruses, they will tend to accumulate with time.

The studies that support these conclusions appear to be quite robust: virtually identical results have been obtained in at least four different studies using at least six different inhibitors[6]. It is important to keep in mind, however, that their conclusions require two major assumptions. First, the inhibitors must be acting as they are expected to. That is, they must block infection of cells without side effects that affect the lifetime of infected cells, their ability to produce virions, or the stability of virus in circulation. Secondly, the virus in circulation must be an accurate sample (although it could be quite a small one) of the virus at the major sites of replication in solid lymphoid tissue. The former assumption is supported by the consistency of results with multiple inhibitors; the latter is still more difficult to assess. Although events in lymphoid tissue following inhibitor treatment are grossly similar to those in blood[8], studies comparing detailed kinetics of virus in tissue to that in circulation are still required to assess this issue. These would be difficult in humans, but could probably be carried out effectively in SIV models.

The studies presented above have generally been interpreted to mean that the inferred dynamics extend over the entire period of clinical latency; however, to date they have only been done in individuals with fewer than 500 CD4 cells per microliter, which is relatively advanced disease. However, the lack of correlation of variation in kinetic parameters with disease state from over a very wide range—two to 500 cells—strongly implies that the process is constant throughout the latent phase. Direct experimentation is still required to conform this point.

Another issue still requiring deeper experimental analysis is the actual number of infected cells. From the rate of increase of CD4 cells in blood shortly after drug treatment, it was estimated that some 10^9-10^{10} cells are infected and die every day[22]. Calculation of this number requires an assumption of the total number of CD4 cells in lymphoid tissue, as well as their normal turnover rate—both values that are not accurately known. It also requires the assumption (which has been challenged[41,62]) that the distribution of cells between solid tissue and blood remains constant throughout the experiment. Again, more direct experimentation in animals will help to clear up this important point.

The significance of viral load

As noted above, the concentration of free virus in blood, when accurately measured, is remarkably constant, especially in light of the rapid pace of the underlying events. Furthermore, a number of studies have indicated that the virus load, as established in the early stages of infection following the primary infection phase, is a good prognostic indicator. Individuals with relatively low levels of virus will progress to AIDS more slowly than those with higher levels[24,40,51,57] (P. Skolnik and J. Ioannidis, personal communication). In addition, several recent studies imply that reduction in virus load is well correlated with relatively successful clinical outcome in trials of antiviral therapy[28,58]. Thus, it is very likely that this measurement will assume increasing importance in routine clinical practice, both to identify patients more likely to benefit from aggressive therapy and to monitor therapy. It is therefore important that the underlying meaning of this measurement be well understood, and the steady-state model provides an approach to such an understanding.

Assuming that most virus replication takes place in cells in solid tissue, then the amount of virus in blood at steady state can be simply related to the number of productively infected cells (Figure 14.4) using simple differential equations as follows. The rate of change in virus concentration (V_L) at the site of replication is given by the rate of production, itself proportional to the number of infected cells (I), and the sum of decay at this site and the rate of release into blood. At steady state this value will be 0.

$$dV_L/dT = pI - c_L V_L - rV_L = 0$$
$$V_L = pI/(c_L - r)$$

where the parameters are defined in Figure 14.4. The rate of change of the virus concentration in blood (V_B) is the difference between its rate of release into the bloodstream from the site of replication and its rate of clearance.

$$dV_B/dT = rV_L - c_B V_B = 0$$
$$V_B = rV_L/c_B$$

Combining, we get

$$V_B = (rp/(c_B(c_L - r)))I$$

i.e., the concentration of virus in circulation is equal to the number of productively infected cells times a combination of parameters. Thus, the virus load is a direct measure of the number of infected cells, so long as

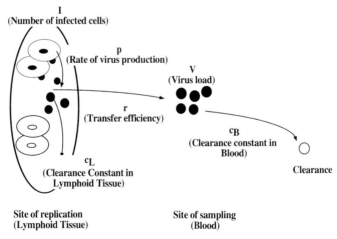

Figure 14.4 *Virus load at steady state. The cartoon shows the steady state of HIV replication on the left, with virus produced by infected cells at the site of replication at an average rate of p virions per cell per day; decaying at that site with a rate constant of c_L then released into the blood at an efficiency of r; and cleared from blood with a rate constant c_B*

the parameters remain constant. Furthermore, at steady state, the number of infected cells is a direct measure of the rate of infection of new cells, itself equal to the rate of death due to infection. To illustrate the latter point, if there are 10^9 infected cells at steady state, and their mean lifetime is 1.5 days, then $10^9/1.5$ or about 6.7×10^8 new cells are infected every day, and an equal number die.

It is important to remember that the virus load is not important for its own sake (and, despite rather foolish assertions to the contrary[13], the proportion of infectious virus is irrelevant). It has been estimated that an infected individual releases about 10^9–10^{10} virions into the blood each day[21], but this only corresponds to 1–10 μg of virions. Except for consideration of blood borne transmission, the virus in blood is itself probably unimportant to pathogenesis, since the infection is most likely maintained by cell–cell transmission of virus in lymphoid tissue. Its value as a marker, then, should reflect its relationship to the rate of infection and death of cells in the productive replication cycle.

Complete understanding of virus load measurements will also require understanding of the nature of the underlying constants, and whether they remain constant between infected individuals or within an individual at different times. For example, factors (such as a humoral immune response) could increase the clearance of free virus from blood without greatly affecting the number of infected cells. This would correspond to an increase in the value of k in the equation, causing an apparent decrease in V without any change in C. Similarly, if changes in lymphoid architecture late in infection[50] lead to increases in the release of virus from sites of its production, then the increase in r leads to an increase in V without a corresponding change in C. Finally, the comparison of virus load values among infected individuals could be compromised by genetic differences in both host and virus, so that different viruses produce differing numbers of virions per infected cell in different hosts, corresponding to different values of p, and again uncoupling the relationship between V and C. In the latter case, the correlation between low virus load and longer disease-free survival suggests either that differences in replication efficiency are relatively small, or that such differences are directly associated with effects on the steady-state numbers of infected cells. Experimentation to dissect out the various constants is required to resolve these important issues.

What maintains the steady state?

Given the short lifetime of the virus in circulation, the constancy over time of the virus load is remarkable, since it implies that there is little variation in the number of cells that are producing virus from one time to the next. It is not absolutely constant, however, exhibiting some

288 J. M. Coffin

day-to-day fluctuation as well as more significant increases in response to immunostimulatory treatments such as vaccination[24,47] or administration of IL-2 (interleukin 2). It is also remarkable that the apparent 'set point' of virus load in an infected individual treated with an antiviral is re-established by mutant virus at nearly the initial value, even after a 100-fold decline owing to the treatment.

Given all of these observations, we can speculate on the forces that maintain the steady state. There are two general mechanisms that can be imagined: a balance between virus replication and the immune response, and a limitation on the number of available target cells for infection. Arguing in favor of the former hypothesis is the observation that the immune response (particularly the cellular response) seems to play a significant role in the establishment of the steady state following primary infection, and the appearance of apparent immune escape mutations in somewhat cyclic patterns during infection[45]. Arguing against it is the stability of the virus load. One would expect a steady-state base on the immune response to be inherently unstable, and that at least some of the time the immune system would prevail and clear the infection, particularly after perturbation such as treatment with antiviral drugs. Furthermore, one would not expect immunostimulatory agents to cause an increase in virus load, as observed.

It is more probable that the viral steady state is maintained by limitation of target cells. Although at any one time the fraction of CD4 cells that are productively infected with HIV is small, it could easily represent all cells available for infection. As with other retroviruses, HIV replication requires that the cell be competent for DNA synthesis. In resting T cells only fragmentary viral DNA is made, and the infection is aborted[64,68]. This requirement would limit infection to those cells which had been stimulated into an activated state. These would include two types of cells, those specifically stimulated by the immune response and those generated *de novo* to maintain the correct CD4 cell number. This would have two important effects, both observed. First, the virus load would be sensitive to immune stimulation. Secondly, as the CD4 cell number declines the rate of replacement, and thus the number of available target cells, would be expected to increase, also leading to an increase in virus load. This provides an explanation for the seemingly paradoxical observation of increasing levels of virus replication in the face of declining CD4 cell numbers.

If all activated CD4 cells are available as targets for HIV infection, then HIV would effectively block their replacement. This effect could be the basis for AIDS. If so then there would also be a requirement for some other effect leading to loss of pre-existing cells. The CD4 cell decline could reflect simple attrition for natural reasons, or another specific effect of the infection process. For example, infection of cells activated in response to an antigen could specifically block replacement of this set of cells, leading eventually to its total loss. Alternatively, some other side effect of virus replication (of which a great many have been proposed, from induction of apoptosis by envelope protein to inappropriate cytokine induction[17,34]) might be important. Sorting out these effects is obviously an important goal.

Genetic variation

The mode of replication of HIV, and probably all lentiviruses, *in vivo* can be seen as a new paradigm of virus infection. It stands in sharp contrast to the relatively small numbers of replication cycles per infected host of 'traditional' viruses, such as influenza and polio, which replicate in one host for only a short time (probably less than 10 cycles) before transmission, or DNA viruses such as herpesviruses, which have a protracted phase of true latency, existing as a non-replicating molecule of DNA for many years.

This mode of replication carries with it an important consequence. Given the relatively high error rate of RNA replicating enzymes, an RNA virus replicating repetitively as a large population becomes exquisitely sensitive to the molding effects of subtle selective forces. This effect is illustrated in Figure 14.5, which shows the predicted frequency of point mutations in a virus population as a function of the forward and reverse mutation rates, the contribution to selective advantage or disadvantage conferred by the mutation on the virus, and the number of replication cycles as a population. As can be seen, the accumulation of mutations that confer a selective advantage becomes sensitive to very small selective forces when the number of replication cycles becomes large enough. At numbers of replication cycles now known to be characteristic of HIV infection, selective advantages (or disadvantages) of less than 1% lead to significant deviation of the pattern of change in mutant frequency from that expected for a 'neutral' mutation. This sort of deterministic accumulation of mutation in a virus population must be the rule whenever it undergoes sufficient numbers of sequential replication cycles as a sufficiently large population. A feeling for the number of replication cycles that is necessary for this effect can be obtained from Figure 14.6, where the number of replication cycles necessary for the frequency of a mutation to become 50% of its eventual equilibrium value (A) or to deviate by a factor of 2 from that expected from neutrality (B) is plotted as a function of its selective advantage, assuming a mutation rate of 3×10^{-5}. This replotting makes apparent the role of large numbers of replication cycles in allowing very small selective forces to mold the virus population. It also highlights the fundamental difference between HIV

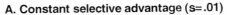

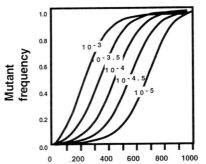

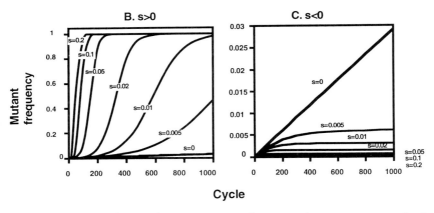

Cycle

Figure 14.5 *Accumulation of mutations as a function of mutation rate, selective forces and numbers of replication cycles. The values shown were obtained by iteratively 'replicating' a virus in a simple computer program, incrementing the proportion of a given mutant by new mutation (at a rate μ) and by the selective advantage (s) and decrementing it by reverse mutation (μ_r) and selective disadvantage. In all panels the frequency of a mutation is plotted against replication cycles. A The selective advantage is held constant at 0.01 and a family of curves for different mutation rates is shown. B The mutation rate is fixed at 3×10^{-5}, the present best estimate for the mutation rate of HIV[36] and a variety of curves at various positive values of s is shown. C The same as B, but at negative values of s (selectively disadvantageous mutations). Note the 30-fold greater scale on the ordinate. For simplicity, the value of μ_r has been set equal to μ. In practice it has very little effect*

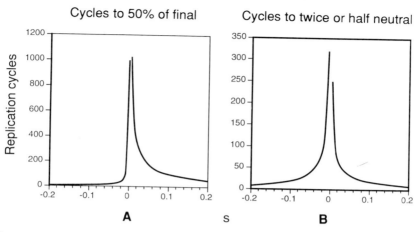

Figure 14.6 *Impact of replication cycles on generation of diversity. Results of the calculations shown in Figure 14.5 have been replotted to show, as a function of s, the number of cycles needed for mutation frequencies to (A) reach one half their final values or (B) differ by a factor of two from the value for s = 0. The forward and mutation rates have been set at 3×10^{-5}. The value for s = 0 in A is about 100 000, and in B is infinite. Note the different scales on the ordinate*

and viruses which have relatively few replication cycles per infection. The curves show a fairly sharp break at 50 cycles, where the influence of selection becomes noticeably greater.

It is important to keep in mind that this formulation is the simplest possible model for the generation of diversity. So called 'simple' models that assume neutrality[19,52] or linearity (i.e. calculate a 'rate' of accumulation of mutations[12,19,61]) in fact require additional complicating assumptions that the selective forces or number of replication cycles over the time being measured are significantly less than indicated in Figure 14.6. It is also important to note that the effect of higher mutation rates is not to reduce the force of selection, but simply to make the clock run faster (see Figure 14.5A). Thus, at very high mutation rates the effects of selection are even more pronounced. It is also important to be aware that the size of the population has no effect on this process so long as it is greater than the minimum necessary to have all mutations represented at predictable frequencies. What is important is how fast the virus is replicating, not how much. Thus, no correlation between virus load and genetic diversity is expected, in agreement with at least some observations (S. Wolinsky, personal communication).

Although the situation *in vivo* cannot be any simpler than described by this model, it is likely to be more complex. Replication of the virus is not, unfortunately, taking place in the 'well stirred pot' of the blood, but rather in solid lymphoid tissue. Virus and infected cells observed in circulation are those that, by whatever mechanism, are released from the sites of replication. The consistency of this release from time to time and from site to site remains to be investigated, as does the extent to which the virus populations are in genetic contact. Thus the *in vivo* viral quasispecies is likely to consist of a set of subpopulations, seeded with different founding viruses, replicating independently of one another and assayed together in the blood. Related to this is the problem of temporal variation. Although the consistency of the virus load throughout the clinically latent phase argues against significant fluctuations in population size, it still remains possible that the replicating virus population passes through significant bottlenecks, and genetic analyses of virus populations as a function of time imply the sort of dramatic population shifts consistent with such bottlenecks[11]. Such shifts could also result from differential seeding of the bloodstream from different replication sites at different times. Further study of the structure of virus populations at the sites of replication will be required to resolve this point. It is important to remember, however, that the existence of population shifts and bottlenecks does not permit one to ignore or simplify the underlying laws of mutation and selection.

DRUG RESISTANCE

The most important practical consequence of the genetic variation that accompanies the replication dynamics of HIV is the problem of rapid acquisition of resistance to chemotherapeutic agents exhibited by HIV *in vivo*. The studies discussed above make it quite clear that antiviral agents can be very effective at blocking virus replication *in vivo* and restoring CD4 cell numbers. They strongly imply that the pathogenically important virus population is that which turns over most rapidly, and which leads to extensive death of infected cells. Were it not for the occurrence of resistant mutants, this population would be readily controlled by existing therapies, HIV infection would almost certainly be manageable, if not curable, and AIDS would have ceased to be a significant problem, at least in countries wealthy enough to afford the treatment.

Despite the initial effect of antiviral treatment, however, the virus population replicating in infected individuals has so far demonstrated a remarkable ability to become resistant to all antivirals so far tested. In the case of the study with 3TC presented above[60] (Figure 14.3), resistant virus is detectable in as little as a week after the onset of treatment, and rapidly becomes the majority of the virus population, restoring the virus load to nearly pretreatment levels within a month or so. As the mutant virus increases, the initial gain in CD4 cells is lost and the pre-existing steady state seems to be restored. To a greater or lesser extent this pattern has been observed with all antivirals tested so far. Many, including most non-nucleoside RT inhibitors, give rise to the same rapid reversion to the original steady state as does 3TC[1,2,14,46,54,55], with single point mutations associated with the appearance of resistance[59,65]. Others, like AZT (zidovudine), seem to have a more prolonged rebound of virus load, with complex patterns of mutations in the RT of the resistant virus[29,31,39]. Others, especially the protease inhibitors, typically also have a much more prolonged course, which is quite variable from patient to patient[63], and also show complex patterns of mutation in the target gene[23,37,38]. Even combinations of treatments, such as AZT and ddI, are incapable of preventing the appearance of resistant mutants[16,20,56]. Obviously, understanding the mechanism of resistance to chemotherapeutic agents and the evolutionary events which give rise to them is essential for the development of truly effective antiviral treatment.

As with all other mutations, those that give rise to drug resistance will accumulate according to the rules discussed above. Most importantly, any such mutation will be expected to have a negative effect on fitness in the absence of drug. As can be seen in Figure 14.5, any mutation that was advantageous or even neutral would already be represented at such a high level in natural virus populations that the drug would have been discarded as ineffective in the first place. For the purpose of discussion, I will refer to the selective disadvantage (i.e. $-s$) conferred by a drug-resistant mutation in the absence of drug as the 'cost' of that mutation. Figure 14.5C shows the accumulation of negatively selected mutations at a variety of costs. As with positively selected mutations, costs of significantly less than 0.01 cause significant deviation from neutrality at high numbers of replication cycles. Unlike the sigmoidal curves seen with positive selection, however, negative mutations accumulate with a continuously decreasing slope, initially equal to the mutation rate, and approaching a steady-state value at high cycle number. This value is equal to

$$\mu/(-s + \mu + \mu_r)$$

For $-s \gg \mu \approx \mu_r$ this becomes $\sim\mu/-s$
For $s = 0$ (a neutral mutation) the steady-state frequency is $\mu/(\mu + \mu_r)$ ($\sim 1/2$ if $\mu \approx \mu_r$)
For $s = -1$ (a lethal mutation) the steady-state frequency is $\sim\mu$ (as one would expect).

At steady state the increase in frequency due to new mutations becomes exactly equal to its loss by reverse mutation and counterselection. Note that, unlike the accumulation of selected mutations, which is only weakly dependent on μ, the steady-state frequency of a negative mutation is equally dependent on μ and s. For example, a mutation with s = 10^{-2} and $\mu = 3 \times 10^{-5}$ will have a steady-state frequency in the virus population of slightly less than 3×10^{-3}. Thus, it is not the rate with which mutations arise that is important for drug resistance, but rather their frequency in the virus population at the time of treatment. For virus mutants resistant to multiple agents, the frequency of resistance is given not by the product of the mutation rates, but rather by the product of the steady-state frequencies (assuming the mutations do not antagonize or synergize). In a replicating virus population with a steady-state value of 10^{10} infected cells, all possible combinations of independent double mutations with the properties given in the example will be present about 10^5 times, and all triple combinations about 300 times.

It is a common misconception that drug-resistant mutations arise only after the onset of treatment, and can therefore be prevented by more effective therapy. No matter how effectively a drug treatment suppresses replication of wild-type virus, its real effectiveness will be limited by the frequency of resistant mutant present at the start of treatment, and the ability of these to replicate in the presence of drug.

Several lines of experimental evidence support the theoretical argument just presented. First, analysis of large numbers of *pol* genes from HIV-infected drug-naive individuals has revealed the presence of mutations potentially encoding resistance to a number of antivirals at frequencies around 1%[43]. Secondly, the cost of mutations to resistance to many antivirals currently in use or under test is clearly quite low. For example, the principal mutation conferring resistance to AZT, T215Y/F[30], can be maintained during repeated passage of the virus in cell culture for long periods of time without obvious reversion[18], and AZT-resistant virus can be transmitted from one individual to another. These observations imply that the selective advantage of wild-type virus is relatively small. A recent observation shows that such AZT-resistant mutant virus is slowly replaced by wild-type virus in infected individuals with kinetics implying a cost of about 0.01 (J. Goudsmit and A. Perelson, personal communication).

Another observation supporting the theory presented here comes from the study with 3TC treatment presented above[60]. As shown in Figure 14.7, two different mutations to 3TC resistance were observed, with different kinetics. The first to appear was M184I, detectable about two weeks after treatment. This mutant was rapidly replaced by M184V, which became the dominant virus after a few more weeks. The rapid appearance of both mutations implies that neither has a very high cost, consistent with *in vitro* studies[18,65]. The nucleotide

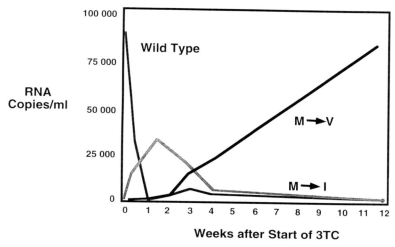

Figure 14.7 *Kinetics of appearance of drug-resistant mutations after treatment. The concentration of wild type (M, codon ATG) and mutant (I, codon ATA; and V, codon GTG) shown in Figure 14.3 are replotted as a fraction of total virus*[60]

sequences of the mutations selected by 3TC *in vivo* are revealing. The pattern observed is

$$\text{ATG (M)} \rightarrow \text{ATA (I)} \rightarrow \text{GTG (V)}.$$

Since both GTG and GTA encode valine, the sequence of changes implies that the V mutation arose directly by a single change from the wild-type ATG, rather than sequentially from the first mutant ATA. The simplest explanation for this pattern is that both mutations were present in the virus population prior to treatment, but that the ATA sequence was present at a higher level than GTG, either because it had a lower cost or because the mutation rate of the initial A to G was higher than G to A, or both. *In vitro* observations support the difference in mutation rate as being the stronger determinant in this case, since reverse transcriptase seems to have a higher rate of A to G than G to A mutations[3], but this point should be checked directly.

IMPLICATIONS FOR THERAPY

Despite the apparent inevitability of drug-resistant virus, the prospects for developing more effective therapy for HIV infection are quite good, assuming that adequate effort continues to be applied to the problem. However, development of new therapeutic strategies needs to take into account some important general principles that derive directly from the arguments I have presented here.

First, it should not be necessary to achieve complete elimination of the infection to have a significant clinical effect. The relationship between virus load and time of conversion to AIDS among infected individuals implies that permanent reduction of the number of infected cells at steady state by a relatively small factor might greatly prolong survival. Although direct tests remain to be done to elucidate the precise relationship, in the simplest case the time to disease is in simple inverse proportion to the integral of virus load since the end of the primary infection (J. Ioannidis and P. Skolnik, personal communication). In such a case, reducing the load by a factor of two would double the time remaining. Obviously, this strategy would require early intervention. Initiating treatment at the threshold of conversion to AIDS, as has been standard practice, would provide little benefit and require much greater levels of prolonged suppression to achieve any benefit at all. Starting treatment near the time of AIDS onset also raises the issue of the time at which the damage done to the immune system becomes irreversible. For example, it may do relatively little good to treat the underlying infection when the lymphoid architecture is so badly damaged that recovery of normal immune response is impossible.

Secondly, consideration of the inevitability of the appearance of drug-resistant mutants must be at the center of strategies for treatment of HIV infection. In comparison to this problem, the discovery of effective and pharmacologically acceptable inhibitors of HIV infection seems relatively easy. Although difficult, the problem does not seem impossible and some headway has already been made. There are several possible strategic approaches that are being, or should be, considered.

1. *Early treatment.* The mutant frequency arguments presented above assume a virus population of an age approaching mutational steady state. With a very few exceptions (such as suspected occupational exposure), this is probably an accurate description of the present situation. In general, treatment is not begun until many years after infection. At 200 or so replication cycles a year, the virus being treated is often more than 1000 generations old, substantially more than needed for all but the most neutral mutations to be near equilibrium frequency (see Figure 14.5C). If treatment could be initiated at or near the time of infection, then all mutations would be present at levels close to the mutation frequency, and there is a reasonable probability that rapid combined therapy with drugs that would be quite ineffective later (such as non-nucleoside RT inhibitors) could be quite effective. At very early times there would be the additional advantage of relatively small populations of infected cells. By the time of obvious primary infection (a

few weeks) the advantage of small population size is lost, but the population is only 10 or so generations old and even neutral mutations will be present at frequencies of a few times 10^{-4} or so. There is thus some reason to believe that it might be possible to eradicate the infection by sufficiently early treatment. At early times it is also reasonable to expect that there will be many fewer latently infected cells than at later times, since such cells must accumulate much more slowly than productively infected cells. Thus, unlike the situation late in infection, the possibility exists that aggressive treatment might be curative and could perhaps even be discontinued after a limited time.

The obvious difficulty with this strategy is the practical one of identifying newly infected individuals. The infection event itself usually passes completely unnoticed, and even the full-blown primary infection is symptomatic in only a minority of cases[17].

2. *High cost of resistance.* Clearly, the only compounds truly effective against established infection will be those for which mutations to resistance have a high cost to virus replication. The use of such compounds has two potential benefits. First, the steady-state level of resistant mutants in the pretreatment virus population will be low, and it will thus take longer for the population to recover after treatment. Secondly, the mutant viruses will replicate more slowly, affecting both the rate at which they recover and the steady-state population level after recovery. Of these, the first effect is the stronger: a mutation with a cost of 0.1 will be present at about 10-fold lower concentration prior to treatment than one with a cost of 0.01, whereas the former mutant will have a steady state level about 90% that of the latter (assuming essentially complete resistance). Also, such mutations will rapidly revert to wild type on transmission and when treatment is discontinued, allowing—at least in theory—the possibility of cycling on and off a given treatment.

In practice, analysis of resistance mutations should be built into the drug discovery process at a very early stage. Because cross-resistance is common, screening against panels of viruses containing known resistance mutations is an obvious first step. Compounds that survive this screen should then be used to select resistant mutants in cell culture. Resistant mutants that arise can then be tested (by competitive growth with wild-type virus) for the cost of the resistance mutation. Although this strategy will not guarantee that the virus cannot evolve *in vivo* to lower cost resistance than is seen *in vitro*, it will allow one to rapidly screen out compounds which have no hope of being any more effective than those presently in use.

3. *Combined therapy.* The same considerations apply to combination therapy as to monotherapy. If mutations resistant to the set of compounds used do

not interact (as will usually be the case for different molecular targets), then the equilibrium frequency of multiply resistant mutants will be the product of the individual frequencies. If the mutations synergize for virus replication (i.e. the cost of the multiple mutant is less than the cost of each mutation alone), then multiple mutations will be present at greater frequency than predicted for each alone; if they antagonize (i.e. the cost of a mutation in the presence of another is greater than in its absence), then less than predicted. A similar effect will also be seen on the virus load after the multiply mutant virus grows out. The latter is obviously the desirable situation. At present there would seem to be little future in combinations of drug therapies for which the individual mutations to resistance are of low cost and independent of one another.

An interesting application of antagonistic mutation seems to be the combination of AZT and 3TC. Although mutations conferring resistance to either compound alone seem to be of quite low cost, in combination treatment a significantly prolonged reduction in virus load can be maintained for a year or more[9]. When the virus in treated patients is examined it is found to have the RT mutation at amino acid 184 characteristic of 3TC resistance, but AZT-resistant mutations are not seen[33]. Apparently the change at position 184 creates AZT sensitivity in virus containing mutations that would otherwise make it AZT resistant. It is likely that other mutations to AZT resistance will eventually appear, but these must have much higher cost to the virus. Thus, the role of 3TC in the combination is to force the virus to remain in the mutant genotype that is AZT sensitive. An alternative explanation for the effect of 3TC on AZT resistance—that RT containing the 184 mutations has a lower error rate (M. Wainberg, personal communication)—seems unlikely, since this would not affect mutations present at the time treatment was initiated.

4. *Other therapies.* Although the preceding discussion has been focused on treatment with 'classical' chemical agents, virtually identical considerations apply to a number of other potential therapeutic treatments, such as stimulation of the antiviral immune response in already infected individuals, and the use of gene therapy techniques to introduce antiviral genes (antisense or ribozymes) into target cells. A number of therapeutic strategies against HIV infection that do not depend on direct interaction with virus replication have been proposed. These include generalized stimulation of the immune response (by IL-2, for example) and treatment with agents, such as hydroxyurea, that reduce nucleotide pools in target cells[25,35]. It is unlikely (but not impossible) that the mutant virus resistant to such treatments can arise. However, they are unlikely to be suitable for long-term control of infection, but might be usefully applied in combination with antivirals to reduce the burden of infected

cells at the time of initiation of treatment. As noted above, immuno-stimulation is probably counterproductive, since it seems only to increase the number of available target cells. The converse strategy might be worth considering: temporary ablation of all (or at least all activated) CD4 cells. This treatment would 'starve' the replicating virus population and eliminate latently infected cells as well. As the survival of the virus is dependent on constant replication, removal of suitable host cells should cause its rapid decline. Since the half-life of free virus is about six hours, even a few days without target cells should lead to significant reductions in load.

CONCLUSION

The rapid and inevitable appearance of drug-resistant variants of HIV may make the possibility of ever developing effective antiviral therapies seem remote. The real situation is far from desperate, but, as should be clear from the preceding discussion, understanding the full conse-quences of the replication dynamics of HIV in infected individuals is crucial if effective therapeutic strategies are to be developed. Indeed, it was experiments involving some relatively ineffective agents that provided some of the key insights into HIV replication dynamics. At the time of writing we are still far short of a complete understanding of this important subject, and many key issues remain to be addressed experimentally, including:

- the relationship between virus replication in solid tissue and virus detected in blood
- the forces responsible for maintaining the steady state
- the reasons behind its eventual decay and progression to AIDS
- the uniformity of viral diversity from site to site in the body
- the constancy of the steady state parameters over time within an infected individual and between individuals
- the numbers of total and infected target cells
- the mechanism driving T-cell replacement
- the point in disease progression at which immune damage becomes irreversible
- testing some of the predictions of the steady-state model, including the pre-existing levels of drug-resistant mutants
- the value of viral load testing in managing HIV therapy.

Addressing these issues should provide a firm base of understanding valuable for both the development and eventual application of the next generations of antiviral agents.

REFERENCES

1. Balzarini J, Karlsson A, Sardana VV *et al.* Human immunodeficiency virus 1 (HIV-1)-specific reverse transcriptase (RT) inhibitors may suppress the replication of specific drug-resistant (E138K)RT HIV-1 mutants or select for highly resistant (Y181C → C181I)RT HIV-1 mutants. *Proc Natl Acad Sci USA* 1994;91:6599–603.
2. Balzarini J, Karlsson A, Perez-Perez M-J *et al.* Treatment of human immunodeficiency virus type 1 (HIV-1)-infected cells with combinations of HIV-1 specific inhibitors results in a different resistance pattern than does treatment with single-drug therapy. *J Virol* 1993;67:5353–9.
3. Bebenek K, Kunkel TA. The fidelity of retroviral reverse transcriptases. In: Skalka AM, Goff SP, eds. *Reverse Transcriptase.* Cold Spring Harbor, NY: Cold Spring Harbor Laboratory Press, 1993:85–102.
4. Burns DPW, Desrosier RC. Selection of genetic variants of simian immunodeficiency virus in persistently infected rhesus monkeys. *J Virol* 1991;65:1843–54.
5. Coffin JM. Genetic variation in retroviruses. In: Kurstak E, Marusyk RG, Murphy FA, Regenmortel MHVV, eds. *Applied Virology Research: Volume 2. Virus Variability, Epidemiology, and Control.* New York: Plenum Press, 1990:11–33.
6. Coffin JM. HIV replication dynamics *in vivo*: implications for genetic variation, pathogenesis, and therapy. *Science* 1995;267:483–8.
7. Coffin JM, Tsichlis PN, Barker CS, Voynow S. Variation in avian retrovirus genomes. *Ann N Y Acad Sci* 1980;354:410–25.
8. Cohen OJ, Pantaleo G, Holodniy M *et al.* Decreased human immunodeficiency virus type 1 plasma viremia during antiretroviral therapy reflects downregulation of viral replication in lymphoid tissue. *Proc Natl Acad Sci USA* 1995;92:6017–21.
9. Condra JH, Schleif WA, Blahy OM *et al. In vivo* emergence of HIV-1 variants resistant to multiple protease inhibitors. *Nature* 1995;374:569–71.
10. Delassus S, Cheynier R, Wain-Hobson S. Evolution of human immunodeficiency virus type 1 nef and long terminal repeat sequences over 4 years *in vivo* and *in vitro. J Virol* 1991;65:225–31.
11. Delwart EL, Sheppard HW, Walker BD, Goudsmit J, Mullins JI. Human immunodeficiency virus type 1 evolution in vivo tracked by DNA hetero-duplex mobility assays. *J Virol* 1994;68:6672–83.
12. Doolittle RF, Feng DF, McClure MA, Johnson MS. Retrovirus phylogeny and evolution. In: Swanstrom R, Vogt PK, eds. *Retroviruses. Strategies of Replication.* New York: Springer-Verlag, 1990:1–18.
13. Duesberg P, Bialy H. HIV results in the frame. HIV an illusion. *Nature* 1995;375:197.
14. Dueweke TJ, Pushkarskaya T, Poppe SM *et al.* A mutation in reverse transcriptase of bis(heteroaryl)-peperazine-resistant human immuno-deficiency virus type 1 that confers increased sensitivity to other nonnucleoside inhibitors. *Proc Natl Acad Sci USA* 1993;90:4713–17.
15. Embretson J, Supancic M, Ribas JL *et al.* Massive covert infection of helper T lymphocytes and macrophages by HIV during the incubation period of AIDS. *Nature* 1993;362:359–62.
16. Emini EA, Graham DJ, Gotlib L *et al.* HIV and multidrug resistance. *Nature* 1993;364:679.

17. Fauci AS. Immunopathogenesis of HIV infection. *JAIDS* 1993;6:655–62.
18. Gao Q, Gu Z, Parniak MA, Li X, Wainberg MA. *In vitro* selection of variants of human immunodeficiency virus type 1 resistant to 3'-azido-3'-deoxythymidine and 2',3'-dideoxyinosine. *J Virol* 1992;66:12–19.
19. Gojobori T, Moriyama EN, Kimura M. Molecular clock of viral evolution, and the neutral theory. *Proc Natl Acad Sci USA* 1990;87:10015–18.
20. Hammer SM, Kessler HA, Saag MS. Issues in combination antiretroviral therapy: a review. *JAIDS* 1994;7:S24–S27.
21. Ho DD, Neumann AU, Perelson AS *et al.* Rapid turnover of plasma virions and CD4 lymphocytes in HIV infection. *Nature* 1995;373:123–6.
22. Ho DD, Sarngadharan MG, Hirsch MS *et al.* Human immunodeficiency virus neutralizing antibodies recognize several conserved domains on the envelope glycoprotein. *J Virol* 1987;61:2024–8.
23. Ho DD, Toyoshima T, Mo H *et al.* Characterization of human immunodeficiency virus type 1 variants with increased resistance to a C_2-symmetric protease inhibitor. *J Virol* 1994;68:2016–20.
24. Hogervorst E, Jurrians S, de Wolfe F *et al.* Predictors for non and slow progression in human immunodeficiency virus (HIV) type 1 infection: low viral RNA copy numbers in serum and maintenance of high HIV-1 p24-specific but not V3-specific antibody levels. *J Infect Dis* 1995;171:811–21.
25. Ichimura H, Levy JA. Polymerase substrate depletion: a novel strategy for inhibiting the replication of the human immunodeficiency virus. *Virology* 1995;211:554–60.
26. Johnson PJ, Hamm TE, Goldstein S, Kitov S, Hirsch VM. The genetic fate of molecular cloned simian immunodeficiency virus in experimentally infected macaques. *Virology* 1991;185:217–28.
27. Jones KA, Kadonaga JT, Luciw PA, Tjian R. Activation of the AIDS retrovirus promoter by the cellular transcription factor. *Science* 1986;232:755–9.
28. Kappes JC, Saag MS, Shaw GM *et al.* Assessment of antiretroviral therapy by plasma viral load testing: standard and ICD HIV-1 p24 antigen and viral RNA (QC-PCR) assays compared. *JAIDS* 1995;10:139–49.
29. Kellam P, Boucher CAB, Larder BA. Fifth mutation in human immunodeficiency virus type 1 reverse transcriptase contributes to the development of high-level resistance to zidovudine. *Proc Natl Acad Sci USA* 1992;89:1934–8.
30. Kovacs J, Baseler M, Dewar R *et al.* Increases in CD4 T lymphocytes with intermittent courses of interleukin-2 in patients with human immunodeficiency virus infection. A preliminary study. *New Engl J Med* 1995;332:567–75.
31. Kozal MJ, Shafer RW, Winters MA, Katzenstein DA, Merigan TC. A mutation in human immunodeficiency virus reverse transcriptase and decline in CD4 lymphocyte numbers in long-term zidovudine recipients. *J Infect Dis* 1993;167:526–32.
32. Kusumi K, Conway B, Cunningham S *et al.* Human immunodeficiency virus type 1 envelope gene structure and diversity *in vivo* and after cocultivation *in vitro. J Virol* 1992;66:875–85.
33. Larder BA, Kemp SD, Harrigan PR. Potential mechanism for sustained antiretroviral efficacy of AZT-3TC combination therapy. *Science* 1995;269:696–9.
34. Levy JA. Pathogenesis of human immunodeficiency virus infection. *Microbiol Rev* 1993;57:183–289.

35. Lori F, Malykh A, Cara A *et al.* Hydroxyurea as an inhibitor of human immunodeficiency virus-type 1 replication. *Science* 1994;266:801–5.
36. Mansky LM, Temin HM. Lower *in vivo* mutation rate of human immunodeficiency virus type 1 than that predicted from the fidelity of purified reverse transcriptase. *J Virol* 1995;69:5087–94.
37. Markowitz M, Mo H, Kempf DJ *et al.* Selection and analysis of human immunodeficiency virus type 1 variants with increased resistance to ABT-538, a novel protease inhibitor. *J Virol* 1995;69:701–6.
38. Maschera B, Furfine E, Blair ED. Analysis of resistance to human immunodeficiency virus 1 protease inhibitors by using matched bacterial expression and proviral infection vectors. *J Virol* 1995;69:5431–6.
39. Mayers DL, McCutchan FE, Sandersbuell EE *et al.* Characterization of HIV isolates arising after prolonged zidovudine therapy. *J AIDS* 1992;5:749–59.
40. Michael NL, Mo T, Merzouki A *et al.* Human immunodeficiency virus type 1 cellular RNA load and splicing patterns predict disease progression in a longitudinally studied cohort. *J Virol* 1995;69:1868–77.
41. Mosier DE. CD4+ cell turnover. *Nature* 1995;375:193–4.
42. Nabel G, Baltimore D. An inducible transcription factor activates human immunodeficiency virus expression in T cells. *Nature* 1987;326:711–13.
43. Najera I, Holguin A, Quinones-Mateu ME *et al. pol* gene quasispecies of human immunodeficiency virus: mutations associated with drug resistance in virus from patients undergoing no drug therapy. *J Virol* 1995;69:23–31.
44. Nowak MA, Bonhoeffer S, Loveday C *et al.* Results confirmed. *Nature* 1995;375:193–203.
45. Nowak MA, May RM, Phillips RE *et al.* Antigenic oscillation and shifting immunodominance in HIV-1 infections. *Nature* 1995;375:605–11.
46. Nunberg JH, Schleif WA, Boots EJ *et al.* Viral resistance to human immunodeficiency virus type 1-specific pyridinone reverse transcriptase inhibitors. *J Virol* 1991;65:4887–92.
47. O'Brien W, Grovit-Ferbas K, Namaz IA *et al.* Human immunodeficiency virus-type 1 replication can be increased in peripheral blood of seropositive patients after influenza vaccination. *Blood* 1995;86:1082–9.
48. Overbaugh J, Rudensey LM. Alterations in potential sites for glycosylation predominate during evolution of the simian immunodeficiency virus envelope gene in macaques. *J Virol* 1992;66:5937–48.
49. Pantaleo G, Graziosi C, Butini L *et al.* Lymphoid organs function as major reservoirs for human immunodeficiency virus. *Proc Natl Acad Sci USA* 1991;88:9839–42.
50. Pantaleo G, Graziosi C, Demarest JF *et al.* HIV infection is active and progressive in lymphoid tissue during the clinically latent stage of disease. *Nature* 1993;362:355–9.
51. Pantaleo G, Menzo S, Vaccarezza M *et al.* Studies in subjects with long-term nonprogressive human immunodeficiency virus infection. *New Engl J Med* 1995;332:209–16.
52. Pelletier E, Saurin W, Cheynier R, Letvin NL, Wain-Hobson S. The tempo and mode of SIV quasispecies development *in vivo* calls for massive viral replication and clearance. *Virology* 1995;208:644–52.
53. Piatak MJ, Saag MS, Yang LC *et al.* High levels of HIV-1 in plasma during all stages of infection determined by competitive PCR. *Science* 1993;259:1749–54.
54. Richman D, Shih C-K, Lowy I *et al.* Human immunodeficiency virus type 1

mutants resistant to nonnucleoside inhibitors of reverse transcriptase arise in tissue culture. *Proc Natl Acad Sci USA* 1991;88:11241–5.

55. Richman DD, Havlir D, Corbeil J *et al.* Nevirapine resistance mutations of human immunodeficiency virus type 1 selected during therapy. *J Virol* 1994;68:1660–6.
56. Richman DD, Meng TC, Spector SA *et al.* Resistance to AZT and DDC during long-term combination therapy in patients with advanced infection with human immunodeficiency virus. *J AIDS* 1994;7:135–8.
57. Rinaldo C, Huang X-L, Fan Z *et al.* High levels of anti-human immunodeficiency virus type 1 (HIV-1) memory cytotoxic T-lymphocyte activity and low viral load are associated with lack of disease in HIV-1-infected long-term nonprogressors. *J Virol* 1995;69:5838–42.
58. Ruffault A, Michelet C, Jacquelinet C *et al.* The prognostic value of plasma viremia in HIV-infected patients under AZT treatment: a two-year follow-up study. *J AIDS* 1995;9:243–8.
59. Schinazi R, Larder B, Mellors J. Mutations in HIV-1 reverse transcriptase and protease associated with drug resistance. *Int Antiviral News* 1994;2:72–5.
60. Schuurman R, Nijhuis M, van Leeuwen R *et al.* Rapid changes in human immunodeficiency virus type 1 RNA load and appearance of drug-resistant virus populations in persons treated with lamiudine. *J Infect Dis* 1995;171:1411–19.
61. Smith TF, Srinivasan A, Schochetman G, Marcus M, Myers G. The phylogenetic history of immunodeficiency viruses. *Nature* 1988;333:573–5.
62. Sprent J, Tough D. CD4+ cell turnover. *Nature* 1995;375:194.
63. Staprans SI, Hamilton BL, Follansbee SE *et al.* Activation of virus replication following vaccination of HIV-1-infected individuals. *J Exp Med* 1995; (in press).
64. Stevenson M, Stanwick TL, Dempsey MO, Lamonica CA. HIV-1 replication is controlled at the level of T cell activation and proviral integration. *EMBO J* 1990;9:1551–60.
65. Tisdale M, Kemp SD, Parry NR, Larder BA. Rapid *in vitro* selection of human immunodeficiency virus type 1 resistant to 3'-thiacytidine inhibitors due to a mutation in the YMDD region of reverse transcriptase. *Proc Natl Acad Sci USA* 1993;90:5653–6.
66. Vartanian J-P, Meyerhans A, Asjo B, Wain-Hobson S. Selection, recombination, and G–A hypermutation of human immunodeficiency virus type 1 genomes. *J Virol* 1991;65:1779–88.
67. Wei X, Ghosh S, Taylor ME *et al.* Viral dynamics in human immunodeficiency virus type 1 infection. *Nature* 1995;373:117–22.
68. Zack JA, Haislip AM, Krogstad P, Chen ISY. Incompletely reverse-transcribed human immunodeficiency virus type 1 genomes in quiescent cells can function as intermediates in the retroviral life cycle. *J Virol* 1992;66:1717–25.

Index

Index compiled by A. Campbell Purton